GENETIC
HEARING LOSS

GENETIC
HEARING LOSS

EDITED BY
PATRICK J. WILLEMS
GENDIA
Antwerp, Belgium

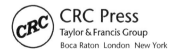

CRC Press
Taylor & Francis Group
Boca Raton London New York

CRC Press is an imprint of the
Taylor & Francis Group, an **informa** business

CRC Press
Taylor & Francis Group
6000 Broken Sound Parkway NW, Suite 300
Boca Raton, FL 33487-2742

First issued in paperback 2019

© 2003 by Taylor & Francis Group, LLC
CRC Press is an imprint of Taylor & Francis Group, an Informa business

No claim to original U.S. Government works

ISBN-13: 978-0-8247-4032-0 (hbk)
ISBN-13: 978-0-367-39534-6 (pbk)

Library of Congress Cataloging-in-Publication Data
A catalog record for this book is available from the Library of Congress.

Visit the Taylor & Francis Web site at
http://www.taylorandfrancis.com

and the CRC Press Web site at
http://www.crcpress.com

Preface

Lend me your ears

Shakespeare, *Julius Caesar*

Hearing loss, affecting millions of people, is the most common form of sensory impairment. In most cases it is due to an unfavorable interaction between genetic and environmental factors. Whereas environmental factors such as exposure to noise, infection, trauma and ototoxic drugs have been recognized for years, the genetic factors contributing to hearing loss have long remained unknown. Although molecular biology formed the cutting edge in most medical disciplines, until recently the ear remained a black box filled only with sounds of silence. It was not until 1995 that the first nuclear gene responsible for nonsyndromic hearing loss was isolated. Since then, however, the pace of research has been unprecedented, and more than 60 loci and 25 genes have been implicated in hearing loss over the last decade.

This book is one of the first to describe the molecular genetics of hearing loss. It presents the first crop of genes, which is the harvest of an international effort to identify all the key players in hearing loss using the tremendous power of positional cloning.

As only a limited number of an estimated total of 100 genes implicated in hearing loss had been identified at the time this book was written, we are looking at only the tip of the iceberg. Consequently, the real understanding of the biology and pathology of the auditory system will require the identification of many more genes, with the elucidation of their function being the major challenge.

For the time being, lend me your ears to listen to those who are cracking the auditory genetic code.

Patrick J. Willems

Contents

Genes Responsible for Nonsyndromic Hearing Loss

Miscellaneous Factors

Contributors

Nadav Ahituv, Ph.D. Department of Human Genetics and Molecular Medicine, Sackler School of Medicine, Tel Aviv University, Tel Aviv, Israel

Stylianos E. Antonarakis, M.D., D.Sc. Division of Medical Genetics, University of Geneva Medical School and University Hospitals, Geneva, Switzerland

Karen B. Avraham, Ph.D. Department of Human Genetics and Molecular Medicine, Sackler School of Medicine, Tel Aviv University, Tel Aviv, Israel

Orit Ben-David, M.Sc. Department of Human Genetics and Molecular Medicine, Sackler School of Medicine, Tel Aviv University, Tel Aviv, Israel

Tamar Ben-Yosef, Ph.D. Section on Human Genetics, Laboratory of Molecular Genetics, National Institute on Deafness and Other Communication Disorders, National Institutes of Health, Rockville, Maryland, U.S.A.

Ingrid Breuskin Center for Cellular and Molecular Neuroscience, University of Liège, Liège, Belgium

John A. Butman, M.D., Ph.D. Department of Diagnostic Radiology, Warren G. Magnuson Clinical Center, National Institutes of Health, Bethesda, Maryland, U.S.A.

Paul Coucke, Ph.D.   Connective Tissue Laboratory, Department of Medical Genetics, University Hospital Ghent, Ghent, Belgium

Cor W. R. Cremers, M.D.   Department of Otorhinolaryngology, University Hospital Nijmegen, Nijmegen, The Netherlands

Else de Leenheer   Department of Otorhinolaryngology, University Hospital Nijmegen, Nijmegen, The Netherlands

Koenraad Devriendt, M.D., Ph.D.   Centre for Human Genetics, University of Leuven, Leuven, Belgium

Jill Dixon, Ph.D.   School of Biological Sciences and Department of Dental Medicine and Surgery, University of Manchester, Manchester, England

Michael J. Dixon, B.D.S., Ph.D.   Department of Dental Medicine and Surgery, School of Biological Sciences, University of Manchester, Manchester, England

Nathan Fischel-Ghodsian, M.D.   Department of Pediatrics, Cedars-Sinai Medical Center and David Geffen School of Medicine at UCLA, Los Angeles, California, U.S.A.

Thomas B. Friedman, Ph.D.   Laboratory of Molecular Genetics, Section on Human Genetics, National Institute on Deafness and Other Communication Disorders, National Institutes of Health, Rockville, Maryland, U.S.A.

Paolo Gasparini, M.D.   Division of Medical Genetics, Department of General Pathology, Second University of Naples and Telethon Institute of Genetics and Medicine, Naples, Italy

Richard J. Goodyear, D.Phil.   School of Biological Sciences, University of Sussex, Brighton, England

Paul J. Govaerts, M.D., Ph.D.   The Eargroup, Antwerp, Belgium

Andrew J. Griffith, M.D., Ph.D.   Hearing Section and Section on Gene Structure and Function, National Institute on Deafness and Other Communication Disorders, National Institutes of Health, Rockville, Maryland, U.S.A.

Ronna Hertzano, B.Sc. Department of Human Genetics and Molecular Medicine, Sackler School of Medicine, Tel Aviv University, Tel Aviv, Israel

Egbert H. Huizing, M.D. Department of Otorhinolaryngology, University Hospital of Utrecht, Utrecht, The Netherlands

Tim Hutchin, Ph.D. Clinical Chemistry Department, Children's Hospital, Birmingham, England

William J. Kimberling, Ph.D. Center for the Study and Treatment of Usher Syndrome, Department of Genetics, Boys Town National Research Hospital, Omaha, Nebraska, U.S.A.

Mary-Claire King, Ph.D. Departments of Medicine and Genome Sciences, University of Washington, Seattle, Washington, U.S.A.

Shrawan Kumar, Ph.D. Department of Genetics, Boys Town National Research Hospital, Omaha, Nebraska, U.S.A.

Anil K. Lalwani, M.D. Division of Otology, Neurotology, and Skull Base Surgery, Department of Otolaryngology–Head and Neck Surgery, New York University, New York, New York, U.S.A.

Philippe P. Lefebvre, M.D., Ph.D. Department of Otorhinolaryngology, University of Liège, Liège, Belgium

P. Kevin Legan, Ph.D. School of Biological Sciences, University of Sussex, Brighton, England

Yan Li, M.D. Division of Otolaryngology, Department of Surgery, University of California–San Diego, La Jolla, California, U.S.A.

Anne C. Madeo, M.S. Hearing Section, National Institute on Deafness and Other Communication Disorder, National Institutes of Health, Rockville, Maryland, U.S.A.

Brigitte Malgrange, Ph.D. Center for Cellular and Molecular Neuroscience, University of Liège, Liège, Belgium

Alessandro Martini, M.D. Audiology Department, Ferrara University, Ferrara, Italy

Wyman T. McGuirt, M.D.   Molecular Otolaryngology Research Laboratories, Department of Otolaryngology–Head and Neck Surgery, University of Iowa, Iowa City, Iowa, U.S.A.

Anand N. Mhatre, Ph.D.   Department of Otolaryngology, New York University, New York, New York, U.S.A.

Gustave Moonen, M.D., Ph.D.   Center for Cellular and Molecular Neuroscience, University of Liège, Liège, Belgium

Robert J. Morell, Ph.D.   Laboratory of Molecular Genetics, National Institute on Deafness and Other Communication Disorders, National Institutes of Health, Rockville, Maryland, U.S.A.

Cynthia C. Morton, Ph.D.   Department of Obstetrics, Gynecology and Reproductive Biology, Brigham and Women's Hospital, and Department of Pathology, Harvard Medical School, Boston, Massachusetts, U.S.A.

Robert Mueller, M.D., F.R.C.P.   Department of Clinical Genetics, St. James's University Hospital, Leeds, England

Lina M. Mullen, Ph.D.   Division of Otolaryngology, Department of Surgery, University of California–San Diego, La Jolla, California, U.S.A.

Kelly N. Owens, Ph.D.   Department of Genome Sciences, University of Washington, Seattle, Washington, U.S.A.

Hong-Joon Park, M.D., Ph.D.   Section on Gene Structure and Function, National Institute on Deafness and Other Communication Disorders, National Institutes of Health, Rockville, Maryland, U.S.A.

Shannon P. Pryor, M.D.   Hearing Section, National Institute on Deafness and Other Communication Disorders, National Institutes of Health, Rockville, Maryland, U.S.A.

Andrew P. Read, Ph.D., R.R.C.Path., F.Med.Sci.   Department of Medical Genetics, St. Mary's Hospital, Manchester, England

Guy P. Richardson, D.Phil.   School of Biological Sciences, University of Sussex, Brighton, England

Nahid G. Robertson, B.S. Department of Obstetrics, Gynecology and Reproductive Biology, Brigham and Women's Hospital and Harvard Medical School, Boston, Massachusetts, U.S.A.

Allen F. Ryan, Ph.D. Division of Otolaryngology, Department of Surgery, University of California–San Diego, La Jolla, California, U.S.A.

Julie M. Schultz, Ph.D. Laboratory of Molecular Genetics, National Institute on Deafness and Other Communication Disorders, National Institutes of Health, Rockville, Maryland, U.S.A.

Hamish S. Scott, Ph.D. Department of Genetics and Bioinformatics Division, the Walter and Eliza Hall Institute of Medical Research, Parkville, Victoria, Australia

Richard J. H. Smith, M.D. Molecular Otolaryngology Research Laboratories, Department of Otolaryngology–Head and Neck Surgery, University of Iowa, Iowa City, Iowa, U.S.A.

Karen Thompson, B.Sc. Molecular Medicine Unit, St. James's University Hospital, Leeds, England

Lisbeth Tranebjærg, M.D., Ph.D. Department of Medical Genetics, Institute of Medical Biochemistry and Genetics, Wilhelm Johannsen Centre of Functional Genomics; Department of Audiology, Bispebjerg Hospital; and University of Copenhagen, Copenhagen, Denmark

Patrizia Trevisi, M.D. Audiology Department, Ferrara University, Ferrara, Italy

Guy Van Camp, Ph.D. Department of Medical Genetics, University of Antwerp, Antwerp, Belgium

Kris Van Den Bogaert, Department of Medical Genetics, University of Antwerp, Antwerp, Belgium

Hilde Van Esch, M.D., Ph.D. Centre for Human Genetics, University of Leuven, Leuven, Belgium

Lut Van Laer, Ph.D. Department of Medical Genetics, University of Antwerp, Antwerp, Belgium

Sigrid Wayne, M.D.   Molecular Otolaryngology Research Laboratories, Department of Otolaryngology–Head and Neck Surgery, University of Iowa, Iowa City, Iowa, U.S.A.

Edward R. Wilcox, Ph.D.   Section on Human Genetics, Laboratory of Molecular Genetics, National Institute on Deafness and Other Communication Disorders, National Institutes of Health, Rockville, Maryland, U.S.A.

Patrick J. Willems, M.D., Ph.D.   GENDIA, Antwerp, Belgium

GENETIC HEARING LOSS

1

Normal Development of the Ear in the Human and Mouse

Lina M. Mullen, Yan Li, and Allen F. Ryan
University of California–San Diego, La Jolla, California, U.S.A.

I. INTRODUCTION

The development of the normal ear is an extremely complex process, owing to the diversity of tissues and cells that are present in the ear compared to some other organs. The outer, middle, and inner ear consist of several different tissues, each of which in turn contains highly diverse cell types. The formation and differentiation of these cell types must occur in a precisely coordinated manner, to result in the intricate structures and complex functional capabilities of the ear. The number of genes that are involved in ear development presumably reflects this tissue and cellular diversity. It is not unreasonable to assume that the coordinated expression of thousands of genes occurs during the development of the ear. Among these, it seems likely that hundreds of genes play a direct role in regulating inner ear development, and the number may be even greater (91,112). These genes provide a major substrate for inherited hearing loss. Indeed, mutations that disturb the normal process of ear development appear to account for the majority of inherited deafness.

To understand inherited hearing loss related to defects in the formation of the ear, it is necessary to first understand the normal process of inner-ear development. This includes the anatomical development of the outer, middle, and inner ears, as well as the appearance and maturation of peripheral auditory function. It is the purpose of this chapter to review this development. Finally, the patterns of gene expression that occur during ear development are ultimately responsible for its anatomical and functional maturation. While a complete review of developmental gene expression in the ear is beyond the scope of this chapter, we describe some general patterns of expression that have implications for the development of the ear and that can provide insights into genetic deafness by highlighting critical molecular events and processes.

While ear development has been studied in a wide variety of species, this review will concentrate on that of the human and mouse. Normal ear development is obviously of critical importance to our understanding of inherited hearing loss in humans. In addition, as the most extensively characterized mammalian animal model for genetics, and the mammalian species in which genetic manipulation is most easily performed, the mouse is the animal model most relevant to inherited hearing loss in humans. The time course of development in these two species is of course very different. Human embryonic development is prolonged, because of the larger size of the species, because human infants arc morc functional at birth, and perhaps because of the higher degree of complexity of the human brain. For example, in man, the embryo progresses from stage 9, at which the inner ear begins development, to stage 23, at which the cochlea has developed 1 1/2 turns, over the period from 3 to 8 postconception weeks (83). Thus the human ear develops over a period of months, and even years, and most of the developmental events that occur in utero are defined by the gestational week in which they occur. In contrast, murine embryonic development is a very rapid process, because the mouse is a small mammal in which the young are born in a very immature state. The mouse embryo undergoes the progression from stages 9 to 23 over the period from 9 to 16 days post-conception (dpc) (115). In this species therefore, the process of ear development occurs in a matter of weeks, and with parturition at around 20 dpc a substantial amount of ear development occurs after birth. Developmental events are thus defined by the gestational day or fraction of a day. These differences must be taken into account when comparing events as they occur in the two species.

II. THE ANATOMICAL DEVELOPMENT OF THE OUTER, MIDDLE, AND INNER EAR

The ear arises during early embryonic development, soon after the central nervous system begins to form, with the temporally coordinated formation of the tissue precursors of the outer, middle, and inner ear. The tissues that make up these three divisions of the ear are derived from a number of different embryonic sources. The divisions of the ear must develop in parallel, and in precise orientation, for normal hearing to arise.

A. Development of the External Ear

1. Human

In humans, the auricle develops from the ectoderm and underlying mesoderm of the first and second branchial arches, beginning as tissue condensations in the fourth fetal week (Fig. 1). Shaping of the external ear begins
with the formation of six distinct hillocks on the first and second arches
located ventrally on the embryo during the fifth week (1,127). Cartilage
formation begins during the sixth week, and the auricle moves dorsolaterally
into its adult position during the seventh week (16,41). The auricle achieves
its mature shape by about 20 weeks of development (43). After birth, the
auricle increases in size, and the underlying cartilage becomes more dense,
until the adult size and consistency is reached by 8–9 years. However, the
auricle increases in length throughout life (89).

The external auditory canal forms from the first branchial groove,
between the first and second arches (44,88,94). During the fourth and fifth
fetal week, this groove deepens to abut the developing tubotympanic cavity for a brief interval (43). However, by the sixth week, proliferating mesenchymal tissue separates the developing middle and external ears again
(80). Whether the transient contact between the developing external and
middle ears serves an inductive purpose is not clear. The meatus deepens
again beginning at the eighth week, but does not remain an entirely open
cavity. As the canal deepens by the proliferation of ectodermal cells, the
cells at the medial end do not cavitate. By the ninth week, a solid cylinder
of ectodermal cells known as the medial ectodermal plate fills the medial
aspect of the deepening meatus (9). This remains intact until the twenty-

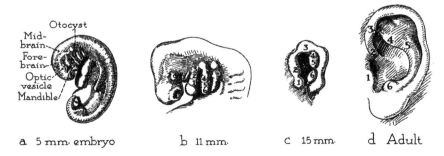

a 5 mm embryo   b 11 mm   c 15 mm   d Adult

Figure 1 Development of the external ear in humans, tracing the development of
adult structures from primordia on the first and second branchial arches. (Adapted
from Ref. 9.)

first week, when its central cells undergo apoptosis to extend the lumen of the meatus to the developing tympanic membrane (44,132). Thus the tympanic membrane can be exposed to airborne sounds as soon as the canal is cleared of fluid after birth. The inner portion of the canal becomes surrounded by bone in the weeks before and after birth, forming the bony auditory meatus (44,49).

2. Mouse

The primordium of the murine auricle first appears at 11.5 dpc with the formation of auditory hillocks similar to those seen in humans. These hillocks amalgamate to form the pinna at 12–12.5 dpc. The external ear remains small and close to the cranium throughout embryonic development (52) and for the first few days of life. The pinna separates from the head and is elevated by approximately 45 degrees at 3 days after birth (dab), 90 degrees by 4 dab, and achieves adult form by 8 dab. The external canal begins to form by 9 dpc. The medial ectodermal plate starts to form at 14.5 dpc (52), and has completely occluded the canal by birth. Recanalization of the canal begins around 7 dab, and is complete by 12 dab, exposing the tympanic membrane to air and to potential acoustic stimulation. (See Table 1.)

Table 1 Morphological Development of the External Ear in the Human and the Mouse

	Developmental age	
	Mouse	Human
External canal appears as cleft between first and second branchial arches	7.5 dpc (53)	3rd fetal week (9,43)
Primordia of the auricle appear	12 dpc (53)	4th fetal week (1)
Meatus deepens to meet tubotympanic space	9.5 dpc (52)	4th–5th fetal week (9,43,122)
Pinna acquires shape, cartilage forms	13 dpc13 (52)	6th fetal week (41)
Ectodermal plug fills medial external canal	14 dpc–birth (52)	8th–20th fetal week (9,122)
Pinna separates from head	3 dab	16th fetal week (9)
Pinna achieves adult shape	7 dab	20th fetal week (9,122)
External meatus recanalizes	8–12 dab	21st fetal week (122)
Pinna achieves adult consistency	15–20 dab	9 years (122)

B. Development of the Middle Ear

1. Human

The middle ear cavity forms from a diverticulum of the first and second pharyngeal pouches, beginning about the third week of human fetal development (29,50). As noted above, it briefly abuts the nascent external canal during the fourth and fifth week. The cavity gradually increases in size to achieve the adult shape by the thirtieth week (43). The embryonic middle ear cavity is completely filled with mesenchymal tissue until the twentieth week. The tympanum becomes largely pneumatized (although fluid filled) through a process of mesenchymal cell apoptosis by the thirty-fourth week, the epitympanum by the thirty-seventh week, and the antrum around birth (9). The epithelium follows the disappearing mesenchyme, until the middle-ear mucosa abuts bone, and the lumen is primarily fluid filled. Fluid clears from the middle ear in the first few postpartum days. The final stages of pneumatization, with loss of mesechymal tissue from the mastoid air spaces and small recesses of the tubotympanum, occur over several years after birth (122).

The auditory ossicles first appear at 6–7 weeks as condensations in the mesenchyme dorsal to the tubotympanic cavity (8,82,85,86). The malleus and incus appear to arise from the cartilage primordia of the first and second branchial arches, with part of each ossicle deriving from two arches (10). In contrast, the stapes appears to originate only from the second arch. The malleus and incus become cartilaginous by the eighth week, and the stapes by the fifteenth week (85). The maleus and incus reach adult size by the fifteenth week, after which they undergo ossification (43). The stapes begins to ossify by the eighteenth week, but does not achieve adult dimensions and complete ossification until the thirthy-second fetal week. The ossicles subsequently lose their marrow spaces, a process completed well after birth (132).

The original connection between the pharyngeal space and the nascent middle ear space is large. This connection persists throughout development, and becomes the eustachian tube through a process of elongation and narrowing. Several cartilaginous elements form around the pharyngeal end of the tube beginning around the fourteenth week. The cartilaginous portion of the tube then grows rapidly, lengthening from approximately 1 mm to 13 mm by the time of birth (111). The eustachian tube continues to undergo substantial developmental change for several years after birth. Ossification of the bony portion of the tube occurs in the perinatal period. However, reorientation and fusion of the cartilaginous elements that surround the tube, allowing adult-like function of the tubotympanic muscles that subserve tubal opening, is not compelte until about the seventh postnatal year (21,58,111).

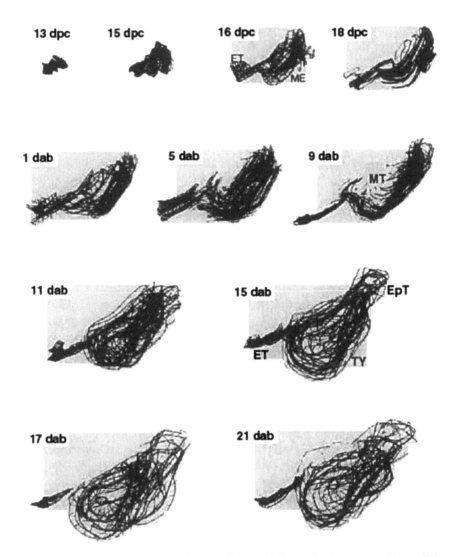

Figure 2 Development of the lumen of the middle ear in the mouse. Up until 9 dab, the lumen of the middle ear is largely filled with mesenchymal tissue (MT). Rapid pneumatization of the tympanum (TY) and epitympanum (EpT) occurs by 15 dab. ET = eustachian tube. (From Ref. 87.)

2. Mouse

The middle-ear cavity begins to form as an extension of the first branchial pouch about 12–12.5 dpc in the mouse (70,87). It remains relatively small throughout embryonic development. The middle-ear cavity begins to expand in the first days after birth, through growth of the bones that define the tympanic bulla. The cavity achieves adult shape and size by 8 dab, at which point it is largely filled with mesenchymal tissue. The bulla then becomes ossified, a process that is largely complete by 14 dab. The pneumatization of the murine middle ear cavity is illustrated in Figure 2. The mesenchyme filling the middle-ear cavity recedes rapidly beginning after 9 dab, through a process of apoptosis (98), until it is largely absorbed by 11 dab, although aeration of the epitympanum does not occur until 15 dab (87). The primordia of the middle-ear ossicles appear as condensations of branchial arch mesenchyme about 12.5–13 dpc, and ossicular cartilage begins to form at 14.5 dpc (52). The ossicles achieve adult size around

Table 2 Morphological Development of the Middle Ear in the Human and the Mouse

	Developmental age	
	Mouse	Human
ME forms as diverticulum of 1st and 2nd branchial pouches	7.5 dpc (70)	3rd fetal week (9,43)
Eustachian tube forms as narrowing of connection from pharynx to ME	11dpc (52)	5th fetal week (50)
Ossicles appear as condensations of 1st and 2nd branchial arch mesenchyme	12 dpc (53)	4th–6th fetal week (122)
First ossicular cartilage	14 dpc (52)	6th fetal week (10)
Ossicles ossify	M + I, 5–12 dab (81)	M + I, 15th fetal week to postnatal 25th week (9,122)
	7–12 dab (S) (81)	S, 18–32 weeks (9,122)
Middle ear achieves adult shape	9 dab	30th fetal week (9,43)
Tympanum pneumatizes	0–11 dab (24,87)	34th fetal week (9)
Antrum pneumatizes	NA	Birth (9)
Epitympanum pneumatizes	3–15 dab (24,87)	37th week (9)
Mastoid air cells pneumatize	NA	Birth to 5–10 years (9,122)

birth. The malleus and incus begin ossification before 5 dab, while the stapes ossification begins around 7 dab. Ossification of the ossicles is largely complete around 12 dab (81). (See Table 2.)

C. Development of the Inner Ear

1. Human

The inner ear originates as a placode on the neuroectoderm of the human embryo adjacent to the rhombencephalic neural groove, at the end of the third fetal week (42,84). The placode invaginates to form the otic pit at 24–26 days, and pinches off to form the otic vesicle, or otocyst, by the end of day 26. At 5 weeks, the otocyst has developed two appendages. A small endolymphatic duct extends dorsally, while a larger cochlear duct extends ventromedially. Shaping of the labyrinth involves the apoptosis of cells, especially in regions of folding (79). Early in the sixth week, the cochlear duct has enlarged and curved to form one half of a turn, and the developing semicircular canals form ridges on the vestibular portion of the otocyst. By the end of the sixth week, the semicircular canals have formed complete loops, and the cochlea has increased in length to a full turn (86). The medial stages of human ear development are illustrated schematically in Figure 3. During the eighth and ninth weeks, the perilymphatic spaces of the cochlea form, near the round and oval windows. They then expand apicalward, following the development of the cochlear duct. By the tenth week, the cochlea has achieved nearly the adult complement of two and one-half turns. By 6 months, the development of the membranous labyrinth is essentially complete, except for the endolymphatic duct and sac, which continue to grow until the cranium achieves adult dimensions during late adolescence (9).

The labyrinthine capsule can first be detected as condensations in the mesenchyme surrounding the otocyst during the fourth fetal week. The first cartilage forms during the seventh week, and ossification begins during the fifteenth week (43). By the twenty-third week, the formation of the cartilaginous capsule is largely complete (13). Ossificiation is not completed until after birth (9).

The sensory epithelium of the cochlea can be observed as a thickening of the cochlear duct epithelium adjacent to the developing scala tympani, and the stria vascularis can be distinguished on the lateral surface of the duct, by the eighth gestational week in the basal turn. The organ of Corti matures in a basal-to-apical manner, and development in the apical turn lags that in the base by several weeks. By 9–10 weeks, the greater and lesser epithelial ridges of the primitive organ of Corti have formed in the base, but

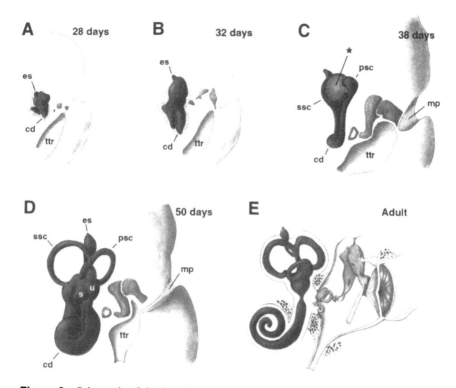

Figure 3 Schematic of the development of the human ear, showing the relationship between the three divisions across age. Asterisk identifies tissue resorption during separation of the SSCs. cd = cochlear duct; es = endolymphatic sac; mp = meatal plug; psc = posterior SSC; s = saccule; ssc = superior SSC; ttr = tubotympanic recess; u = utricle.

hair cells (HCs) are not discernible. By the eleventh week, inner and outer HCs can be distinguished, immature stereociliary bundles are present, but the supporting cells of the organ remain undifferentiated. By 14 weeks, HC morphology is well developed, and stereocilia are more adult-like. Pillar cells are identifiable, and the tunnel of Corti is beginning to form. Supernumerary HCs are often present at this stage, and persist even when the basal turn hair cells achieve adult appearance and the cochlea becomes functional, at around 19 weeks (9,95,63).

As soon as the otocyst forms during the fourth fetal week, cells emerge from its ventromedial epithelium to form the primordium of the stato-acoustic ganglion (84). The auditory and vestibular divisions of the ganglion can be distinguished by the sixth week. The spiral ganglion, which must expand greatly in length, develops in parallel with the elongating cochlea (117). Fibers from the ganglion can be seen entering the cochlear sensory epithelium by the ninth fetal week. Dense accumulations of presumably afferent synapses can be distinguished on developing HCs by the eleventh week. By 15 weeks, the synapses on inner HCs appear at the light micrographic level to be mature. Fibers with the morphological characteristics of efferents can be observed below the inner HCs by the fourteenth week, and below outer HCs by the twenty-second week. Also by the twenty-second week, the afferent synapses on outer HCs are morphologically mature (33,92). The myelination of the axons of the spiral ganglion begins around the fifteenth fetal week, when accumulations of Schwann cells are present on the auditory nerve within the modiolus. These become dense by the twenty-second week, and by the twenty-fourth week light myelin sheaths extend to the glial junction that separates the peripheral from the central nervous system. Myelin sheaths do not appear on the central portions of the exons until the twenty-sixth week (73).

2. Mouse

The murine otic placode forms and begins to invaginate between 8 and 9 dpc. It completes the process of invagination and separation from the surface ectoderm to form the otocyst at around 10 dpc (4,52). The later stages of inner-ear development are illustrated in Figure 4. From the otocyst, the endolyphatic duct forms dorsally as a small, discrete protrusion, while the cochlear duct emerges as a larger protrusion ventrally, at 10.75 dpc. By 11.5 dpc, the semicircular canals form as thin plates. By 12 dpc, the semicircular canals have enlarged and are undergoing cavitation to form free arcs, the utricule has appeared, and the cochlea has extended and begun to coil, consisting of one half turn. By 13 dpc, the canals are freed and considerably thinned, the saccule is apparent, and the cochlea consists of two-thirds of a turn. By 15 dpc the cochlea has one and one-half turns, and by 17 dpc, the membranous labyrinth is fully formed. The cochlea has reached the adult one and three-quarter turns between the base and the apex (104,64,76,52,53). The cochlear capsule appears as a condensation of mesenchyme surrounding the developing otocyst by 12 dpc. Cartilage begins to form by 14 dpc (37). While the otic capsule is one of the first bones to chondrify, it ossifies quite late in development. Ossification has only begun by 5 dab, and is not complete until approximately 12 dab.

The epithelium of the cochlear duct begins to differ between its dorsal and ventral walls at about 12.5 dpc in the base (97,104). The dorsal wall, which will form the organ of Corti, inner sulcus, and spiral limbus, is thicker

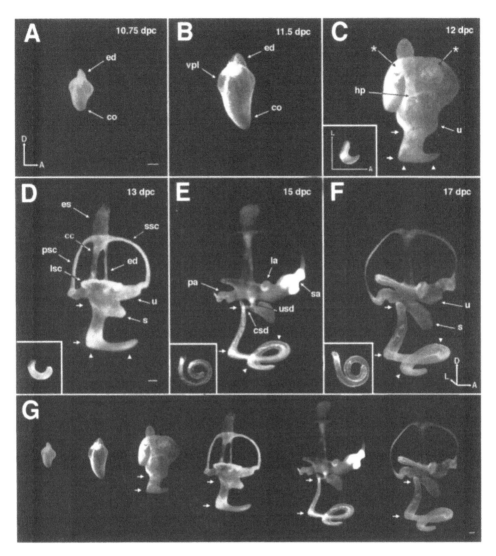

Figure 4 Development of the mouse inner ear. Lateral view of the membranous labyrinth, from 10.75 to 17 dpc, the period during which the adult architecture of the inner ear is achieved. Arrows point to the distal part of the cochlea, while arrowheads point to the proximal part. Asterisks identify regions of tissue resorption during separation of the SSCs. cc = common crus; co = cochlea; csd = cochleasaccular duct; ed = endolymphatic duct; es = endolymphatic sac; hp = horizontal canal plate; la = lateral ampulla; lsc = lateral SSC; pa = posterior ampulla; psc = posterior SSC; s = saccule; sa = superior ampulla; ssc = superior SSC; u = utricle; usd = utriculosaccular duct; vpl = vertical canal plate. Scale bars = 100 μm. (From Ref. 76.)

than the ventral wall, which will develop into the stria vascularis and Reissner's membrane. By 13 dpc, cells that will become HCs and supporting cells in the apical turn are undergoing terminal mitosis. By 14 dpc, the ventral epithelium has developed a greater and lesser epithelial ridge in the basal turn, but the component cells remain undifferentiated. The first cells to possess a specific cellular phenotype are the inner HCs, which separate from the basement membrane and become rounded at the border between the lesser and greater epithelial ridges around 15 dpc in the base. The basal turn outer HCs can first be recognized at 16 dpc. Differentiation of cochlear cells then continues in a wave that progresses along the basal to apical axis of the cochlea. By 17 dpc, all terminal mitoses have occurred. By 18 dpc, a single row of inner hair cells and three rows of outer hair cells are present along most of the cochlear duct. The stereocilia of the HCs first appear at 16 dpc, as tufts of longer microvilli. They appear first on the inner HCs, and then on the outer HCs. The patterns of stereocilia characteristic of the inner and outer HCs are apparent even at these early stages of stereociliary development. However, cochlear HCs possess a true kinocilium during the early formation of the stereociliary array. The stereocilia elongate until they reach adult dimensions about 7 dab in the base and 10 dab in the apex. A period of resorption of supernumerary stereocilia and of microvilli from other regions of the cuticular surface of the HC begins around 3 dab. The resorption of the kinocilia of cochlear HCs occurs between 10 and 14 dab, again progressing from base to apex (64). Cavitation of the space between the pillar cells begins around birth (20 dpc), and is complete by about 7 dab.

The development of the stria vascularis is intimately tied to that of the melanocytes that are derived from neural crest cells, since these melanocytes form the intermediate cells of the stria (109). Neural crest-derived melanocytes occur at many sites, but in the cochlea they are limited to the stria. In the 10-dpc embryo, the melanoblasts have separated from the neural crest, and a few are located under the ectoderm in the region of the otic vesicle. By 12 dpc, melanoblasts are found adjacent to the developing cochlear duct. At 13 dpc, many melanoblasts are clustered near the basal cochlear turn, and a small number are associated with the newly forming apical turn. By 14 dpc, large numbers of melanoblasts are concentrated in the ventral edge of the cochlear duct. In a newborn mouse, the melanocytes are found in the stria vascularis of all cochlear turns (22).

The stria vascularis begins differentiating on 17 dpc, as a condensation of mesenchymal cells adjacent to the cochlear duct. At 19 dpc, the condensation is dense and the wall of the cochlear duct in this area is composed of cuboidal epithelium. On the first dab, the epithelial cells become elongated and are positioned perpendicular to the plane of the lateral mesenchyme. At this stage, they appear to have projections extending into the mesenchyme.

Between the second and third dab, the boundary between the epithelium and mesenchyme becomes indiscernible, and the mesenchymal cells become tightly packed. On the fourth dab, there are two walls of the stria: the inner wall, derived from the otocyst epithelium, and the outer wall, derived from the otic mesenchyme. Between the layers are melanocytes, connective tissue cells, and capillaries. As development proceeds, the connective tissue becomes less cellular, and the three cell types of the stria assume their adult forms by 8 dab (104,109).

Auditory and vestibular neurons of the murine eighth cranial nerve ganglia arise from the otocyst to form the statoacoustic ganglion beginning at 10 dpc. The seventh and eighth cranial nerve ganglia form one cell mass, located medial to the otocyst, in the 11-day embryo. The mass splits into the statoacoustic ganglion and the geniculate ganglion, and fibers from both enter the brain by 12 dpc. Fibers from the statoacoustic ganglion penetrate the otocyst. By 13 dpc, fibers penetrating the lateral wall of the otocyst are deep and numerous, while on the medial side of the rostral portion, fibers are less deep and numerous. The auditory and vestibular divisions of the statoacoustic ganglion can now be recognized. By 14 dpc, spiral ganglion cells are visible under one complete turn of the cochlear duct. By day 18, the vestibular and spiral ganglia are completely separate, the cochlear duct has the full number of coils, and the spiral ganglion extends to the apical coil (99,104). The spiral ganglion dendrites enter the cochlear sensory epithelium around 13 dpc to innervate the region of the inner hair cells. During embryonic development, each fiber may extend collateral fibers to many other inner hair cells; however, in the mature organ, the collateral fibers are lost and each fiber innervates only a single inner HC.

The development of synaptic contacts between spiral ganglion neurons, HCs, and olivocochlear efferents occurs largely after birth. This process has been studied in the mouse, and also in the rat and gerbil, which have similar developmental timetables. Both afferent and efferent synapses are present beneath the inner hair cells (IHCs) at birth. Some of the efferent synapses contact the IHCs directly, but most contact primary afferent dendrites. The presynaptic ribbons that are indicative of afferent synaptic function appear in the IHCs of the mouse during the first week of life (106,107). IHC synaptic maturation is essentially complete by about 12 dab (105). Only afferent fibers contact the outer hair cells (OHCs) at birth, and most of these are type I afferents. The type I afferents withdraw from the OHCs around 6 dab, and are replaced by type II afferent and by efferent synapses. OHC afferent synapses lose their presynaptic specializations (synaptic bodies) before efferent fibers arrived below the OHCs. The efferents subsequently make temporary axodendritic synapses with the afferents, before replacing most of them at the OHC membrane. The first

Table 3 Morphological Development of the Inner Ear in the Human and the Mouse

	Developmental age	
	Mouse	Human
Formation of otic placode	7 dpc (4,64)	End of 3rd fetal week (7,84)
Invagination of the otic pit	8 dpc (4,64,104)	4th fetal week (7)
Separation of the otocyst	8.5–9 dpc (4,70,104)	End of 4th fetal week (7)
Formation of statoacoustic ganglion	9 dpc (104)	End of 4th fetal week (84)
Formation of the cochlear duct and endolymphatic sac buds	10 dpc (70)	5th fetal week (7,11)
Cochlear and vestibular ganglia distinct	11.5–13 dpc (104)	5th fetal week (103)
Formation of SSC buds	10. 5 dpc (53,104)	5th fetal week (9,84)
Separation of SSCs from vestibule	12–13 dpc (53,76)	End of 6th fetal week (7,84)
Cochlea = 1/2 turn	12 dpc (76)	6th fetal week (86)
Cochlea = 1 turn	14 dpc (76)	7th fetal week (86)
Cochlea = 1 1/2 turns	15 dpc (64,76)	End of 7th fetal week (11,86)
Cochlea = adult length	17 dpc (76)	10th fetal week (86)
Birth of HCs (basal turn)	12.5 dpc (99)	Not known
Commitment to HC fate (basal turn)	13.5 dpc (15)	Not known
Differentiation of HCs (basal turn)	15 dpc–7 dab (54,64)	10th–20th fetal week (63,92)

synapses between efferent endings and OHC are seen at 9 dab, but it is not until about 20 dab that OHC efferent synapses are mature. (See Table 3.)

III. FUNCTIONAL DEVELOPMENT OF THE EAR

A. Human

The development of function in the ear has not been extensively studied in humans, primarily because all of the relevant events occur in utero, well before the normal time of birth (44). However, studies of the responsiveness of fetuses to sound delivered to the abdomen of the mother indicate that the ear becomes functional beginning at about the nineteenth week, when reactions to low frequencies are observed (108). Reponses to higher frequencies are observed by 33–35 weeks (47). By birth, the human inner ear functions at essentially an adult level. Although the middle ear is frequently fluid-filled, when this clears in the first days after birth, the middle ear is also fully functional. Reflecting these changes in middle ear fluid status, otoacoustic emissions increase by 5–10 dB in the first 2–3 dab (94).

B. Mouse

The onset of cochlear function has been extensively studied in the mouse and other altricial rodents such as the rat and gerbil. An important determinant of early function is the increased potassium concentration of endolymph, and the appearance of the endocochlear potential (EP). Before birth in the rat and mouse, endolymph and perilymph have similar ionic characteristics. However, beginning at birth the potassium concentration of endolymph increases rapidly, and the sodium concentration falls, to reach adult-like values by about 10 dab. The EP lags this potassium increase, appearing at 3–4 dab in the mouse, reaching adult values by 14 dab (5,6,20,123,102). The maturation of the EP closely follows the morphological development of the stria vascularis.

The cochlear microphonic (CM) can first be recorded from the mouse cochlea in response to very intense stimuli at around 7 dab. CM thresholds improve rapidly until about 15 dab (110). The compound action potential (CAP) shows similar characteristics (45). The maturation of these evoked responses lags EP maturation, suggesting that other factors contribute to the course of their development. Maturation of the HCs themselves is one such factor. In the gerbil the negative EP, observed during anoxia and thought to reflect ion flux through hair cells, develops after the positive EP (123). This and the morphological data reviewed above suggest that HC maturation also lags that of the EP. In the gerbil, direct stimulation of the stapes with a piezoelectric driver elicited CM about 2 days prior to acoustic stimulation, and improved developing thresholds up to 40 dB depending upon frequency (125). This suggests that middle ear immaturity also plays a significant role in delaying the functional development of the cochlea.

While cochlear thresholds appear to mature by 15 dab, the full dynamic range of cochlear responses does not develop until several days later (126). This presumably reflects maturation in the capacity of cochlear cells to produce high levels of output. Also, CAP and VIIIth nerve fibers can respond to higher repetition rates as thresholds and dynamic range improve.

The frequency tuning of the inner ear changes during the period of threshold improvement. The characteristic frequency of tuning curves re-

Table 4 Development of the Auditory Function in the Human and the Mouse

	Developmental age	
	Mouse	Human
Development of endolymph potassium	< 0–7 dab (5)	Not known
Development of endocochlear potential	7–18 dab (109)	Not known
Development of cochlear microphonic	7–15 dab (3)	Not known
Initial behavioral response to sound	8–10 dab (3)	19th fetal week (47)
AP/ABR		
Initial appearance	9–11 dab (19,45)	25th fetal week (61)
Mature	18 dab (19,45)	3 months postnatal (61)
Initial otoacoustic emissions	15 dab (74)	30th fetal week (75)

corded from the same location in the spiral ganglion of the gerbil increases by more than one octave, while tuning curves become dramatically sharper (32). Tonotopy in the cochlear nucleus also shifts, presumably reflecting events in the cochlea (100). This presumably results from a combination of events. The organ of Corti has more mass early in development, which would tend to lower the frequency at which it would be maximally responsive. At the same time, the maturation of the cochlear amplifier acts to shift the best frequency upward.

The development of OHC motility, which is thought to represent the major component of the active cochlear amplifier, has not been studied in the mouse. However, in a similar altricial rodent, the gerbil, it appears by 7–8 dab, and reaches mature levels by 14–17 dab (46). This coincides with the period of OHC synaptic remodeling, and also with the maturation of CAP parameters, such as the "S" shape of the input-output curves and the sharpening of CAP tuning curves (93), that are considered to reflect the activity of the cochlear amplifier. (See Table 4.)

IV. MOLECULAR DEVELOPMENT OF THE EAR

As noted above, the formation of the ear is mediated by the coordinated expression of many developmental genes. A complete review of such expression is beyond the scope of this chapter. Moreover, the developmental expression of a number of genes in which mutations lead to hearing loss will be described in later chapters of this book. However, there are general patterns of gene expression that underlie critical events in the morphogenesis and functional onset of the ear. A brief review of some of these patterns is presented below.

Much of our understanding of the molecular control of ear development is based on information obtained initially in other organs, in which the patterns of gene expression that lead to organogenesis have been explored in some detail. With respect to the general morphogenesis of the outer, middle, and inner ears, the boundary model developed by Meinhardt (72) to explain pattern formation in the vertebrate limb is instructive. According to this model, determination of the limb requires a primary patterning event along the main axis of the embryo. This primary pattern results in areas with different gene expression separated from each other by defined borders. The model proposes that the interaction between at least two differently determined types of cells results in the production of a morphogen that diffuses into the surrounding cells, creating a graded morphogen distribution. This is called positional information. A pattern then becomes determined, and a secondary axis can be formed by interpretation of this positional information. The result of Meinhardt's model is the formation of "organizing regions" that serve to direct development along the different axes in the limb—proximodistal, dorsoventral, and anteroposterior.

As with the inner ear, vertebrate limb initiation takes place in a specific location along the anteroposterior and dorsoventral axes of the developing embryo. This placement appears to rely on the differential and coordinated expression of the *Hox* genes within the lateral plate mesoderm (78). In addition to placement of the limbs, the *Hox* genes are involved in the regulation of later stages of limb development, particularly cartilage proliferation and differentiation.

Limb bud formation is initiated by fibroblast growth factor (FGF) and Wnt signaling, originating in the mesenchyme of the limb-forming region. FGF-10 in the mesenchyme activates expression of FGF-8 in the overlying ectodermal cells, forming the apical ectodermal ridge (AER). This is a thickened rim of ectoderm at the tip of the limb bud that serves as an organizing region for limb outgrowth (116). Furthermore, this ridge arises at a cell lineage-restricted boundary between the Engrailed 1 expressing ventral ectodermal compartment and the radical fringe/Wnt7a expressing dorsal ectodermal compartment (56,62). Radical fringe may in turn interact with the Notch/Delta signaling pathway to maintain the AER, similar to the process in *Drosophila* (18). The interaction of the genes mentioned above may also specify patterning along the dorsoventral axis. Formation of the anteroposterior axis of the limb is mediated by sonic hedgehog (Shh) and bone morphogenic protein (Bmp) expression in the zone of polarizing activity, a small region of mesenchyme cells in the posterior margin of the developing bud (31).

Morphogensis of the ear involves processes of gene expression and pattern formation similar to that of the limb. The normal positioning and development of the ear along the anteroposterior axis of the developing embryo requires the expression of Hox1a and Hox1b in the hindbrain (40). The entire inner ear forms from a simple epithelium that invaginates and separates from the surface ectoderm adjacent to rhombomeres 5 and 6. As in limb bud initiation, studies suggest a role for mesoderm tissue in otic induction, and it has been proposed that FGF-19 expression in the paraxial mesoderm induces Wnt-8c expression in the overlying neural plate, and that both factors act cooperatively in initiating otic development (59). The activity of these two genes results in the expression of some otic placode marker genes like Pax2 Dlx5, Nkx5.1, and SOHo. In addition, these two signals cooperate to induce thickening of the otic placode ectoderm.

The invagination of the otocyst is also induced by the adjacent mesenchymal tissue and neural tissue of the rhombencephalon (120). Based on the expression of FGF-3 in the appropriate region of the rhombencephalon, Represa et al. (96) treated early chick embryos with anti-FGF-3 antisense otligonucleotides and observed repression of otocyst formation. However, when Mansour et al. (68) deleted the *fgf-3* gene in mice, they observed normal otocyst formation. This suggested that FGF-3 was uninvolved, or that functional redundancy existed, presumably with another FGF-family member. Recently Maroon et al. (69) found that FGF-3 and FGF-8 cooperate to induce otocyst formation in the chick, confirming that two members of this gene family participate in otocyst formation.

Specific models for the development of the otocyst into the labyrinth have been developed. Fekete (35) proposed a boundary model for the development and patterning of the otocyst that takes into account the formation of separate gene expression compartments, similar to the boundary model for limb formation. Compartments are defined by broad gene expression domains that will specify different structural parts of the ear such as semicircular canal, saccule, cochlea, utricle, and endolymphatic duct. These compartments arise partly in response to diffusable factors that originate from external sources such as the rhombencephalon and the notochord. According to the model, cells located at the boundary of two or more compartments are induced to secrete a morphogen that will diffuse into the surrounding cells, directing development and pattern formation among the cells that respond to it. The borders may specify location of sensory organs, emigration of neuronal precursors, or endolymphatic duct outgrowth (17). According to the Fekete model, the developing otocyst is divided into eight compartments as a result of the intersection of three boundaries: the dorsoventral boundary, the mediolateral boundary, and the anteroposterior boundary. According to the model, linear structures such as the organ of Corti are the result of the activity at the boundary between two compartments. Punctate structures would arise at the intersection of al least three different compartments, for example the cristae. In support of this model, the development of the endolymphatic duct has been mapped to a putative boundary between medial and lateral zones in the developing mouse ear. In the mouse, the expression of Pax2 and EphA4 has been found in the medial wall of the otic vesicle, including the endolymphatic duct region and the enlarging cochlear duct. Immediately adjacent to this domain is a region of SOHo expression. Work by Brigande et al. (17) has shown that the endolymphatic duct arises in the area of the medial-lateral boundary, defined by the intersection of Pax2/EphA4 and SOHo expression. By labeling individual cells in the developing otocyst and following them by time-lapse photography, Kil and Collazo (25) have found that most otocyst cells move freely between the different regions of the otocyst. This suggests that they may express and be exposed to different morphogens at different times in their development.

The formation of the sensory epithelia has also been studied by Morsli et al. (76), who followed the expression of genes associated with sensory epithelia, HCs, and supporting cells in the developing mouse otocyst. They found that Bmp4 was an early marker of the epithelia of the semicircular canal cristae from 11.5 to 12 dpc, while luntatic fringe was an early marker for developing macular and cochlear epithelia from 12 to 13 dpc.

Once the inner ear is patterned, the development of specific cell types follows templates that are common to many cell types in the body. The development of sensory and neuronal cell types appears to follow patterns similar to those previously delineated in brain. In particular, proneural genes such as the bHLH transcription factor Math1 have been shown to be required for the specification of the neural cell fate in neural progenitor cells. Once a neural fate is established, a number of genes are involved in neuronal differentiation. For example, reciprocal Notch/Delta signaling is important for differentiation of neuronal from nonneuronal cell phenotypes. In addition, members of the Brn-3 family of POU-domain transcription factors are involved in the early differentiation of many different sensory neurons, with different members of the family expressed in different neuronal populations (71).

In the inner ear, Math1 is expressed in the prosensory regions of the inner ear. It is required for HC formation, and exogenous expression can induce HC formation in nonsensory regions of the organ of Corti (15). Math1 expression is observed at 12.5 dpc in vestibular epithelia and 13.5 dpc in the cochlea. The Delta ligand Jagged 2 is expressed in HC precursors following HC fate determination. Deletion of the Jagged 2 gene results in HC duplications (60). The Brn-3 family POU-domain transcription factor

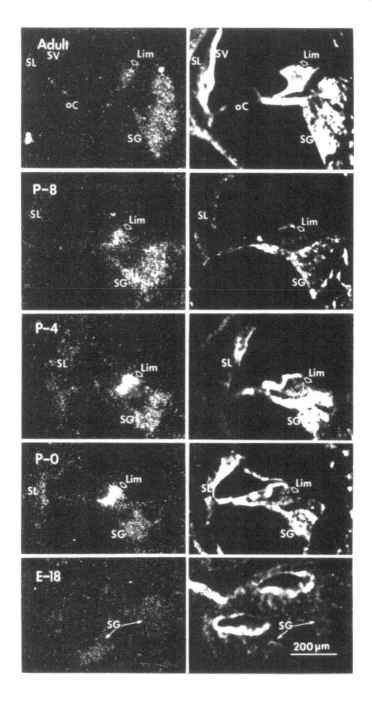

200 µm

Brn-3.1 (Brn-3c, POU4f3) is also expressed in HC precursors immediately after the commitment step occurs, at 12.5 dpc in the vestibular epithelia and 13.5 dpc in the cochlea. Brn-3.1 expression continues throughout life (34,101), and is required for HC differentiation and survival (34,129,118).

Once the cells and tissues of the cochlea are formed, cochlear function depends on the expression of genes that mediate the transduction of sound and the transmission of information into the central auditory system (30,39, 48,128). For example, strong expression of Na,K-ATPase isoforms in the stria vascularis develops in parallel to the appearance of the endocochlear potential (128). The initial expression of the OHC motor protein prestin is correlated with the development of electromotility in these cells (14), while alpha-9 acetylcholine receptor expression precedes efferent innervation of the hair cells (65). The development of glutamate receptor expression in spiral ganglion neurons is related to the functional maturation of the synapse between HCs and spiral ganglion neuron afferent dendrites, as shown in Figure 5 (66).

V. DISCUSSION

The normal development of the external, middle, and inner ears provides the background against which genetic disorders occur. Many forms of inherited hearing loss involve defects in genes that are expressed during development and that are critically involved in regulating the ontogeny of the ear. For this reason, knowledge of normal ear development is helpful in understanding the effects of mutations in genes associated with hearing loss. The reverse relationship is, if anything, more important. The coordination of the development of the components of the ear means that many changes occur in parallel, with the result that temporally related processes are not

---

Figure 5 Expression of mRNA encoding a gene required for inner-ear function, the GluR2 AMPA glutamate receptor, in the developing rat cochlea. Embryonic development of the inner ear in the rat lags that of the mouse by about 4 days. The left panels show autoradiographs corresponding to the tissue illustrated in the right panels. Labeled GluR2 cRNA riboprobes were hybridized to tissue sections from E-18 (17.5 dpc) to adult inner ear. GluR2 mediates neurotransmission between hair cells and the afferent dendrites of spiral ganglion neurons. GluR2 mRNA is expressed in the spiral ganglion well in advance of the onset of auditory function, which occurs at about 10 dab. The function of strong GluR2 expression in the cells of the spiral limbus (Lim) is unknown. P = postnatal day; SL = spiral ligament; SV = stria vascularis; SG = spiral ganglion. (From Ref. 66.)

necessarily causally related. Because virtually everything is changing at the same time, all processes correlate to some degree during development. For this reason, correlational studies in development are often minimally informative regarding causation. More definitive information about causal relationships in development has come from the study of natural and induced mutations, as described in subsequent chapters.

For the purposes of this review, we have concentrated on the human and the mouse. Although ontogeny occurs at a much more rapid rate in the mouse, the development of the ear in the two species appears to occur via very similar processes, This means that the mouse is a good model for molecular research that is targeted at understanding human mutations. Thus we can learn a great deal about genetics in the ear of the human by assessing and manipulating the appropriate genes in the mouse. Of course it is also much easier to obtain information about development in an experimental animal than it is in humans. However, it is important to recognize that there are significant differences between these two species that can influence genetic outcomes. For example, the life span of the mouse is far less than that in the human. Since many mutations in humans develop phenotypes in childhood or even adulthood, it is possible that mice would never live long enough for similar defects to appear. Also, the middle ear of the human is larger and includes structures such as the mastoid air spaces that are not present in the mouse. Genes causing defects in these structures would necessarily have different effects in mice. It should also be noted that almost all of the development of the ear occurs in utero in humans. Virtually all of inner-ear ontogeny including functional onset is complete by the twenty-sixth fetal week, while the middle-ear structures achieve their adult configuration by the thirtieth week. While the initial stages of ear development also occur prior to birth in the mouse, significant development and functional onset occur postnatally. For research purposes this is a benefit. However, middle and external ear maturation in the mouse is likely to be influenced by exposure to the external environment, including air, at a much earlier developmental stage than in the human.

As noted above, the development of the inner ear is an exquisitely coordinated process, involving the precisely timed formation and differentiation of millions of cells. The patterns of gene expression that underlie this process are as yet poorly understood. However, it is clear that thousands of genes are expressed including potentially several hundred that encode developmental regulatory molecules. It is therefore not surprising that mutations can result in abnormal development of the ear and result in inherited hearing loss. In fact, given the complexity of normal ear development, it is perhaps more surprising that the number of genes involved in inherited hearing loss, currently estimated to be a few hundred (90), appears to be relatively small.

This is consistent with the observation that many knockout studies of genes that are expressed in the ear during development and are suspected of an important role in ear ontogeny fail to produce a phenotype (77).

Why do mutations in genes that participate in inner ear development not produce inherited hearing loss? The effects of such mutations may be compensated by redundancy, especially when several genes of the same family are expressed in the ear. Alternatively, mutations may affect the structure of the inner ear, but in relatively minor ways that are not reflected in function. Mutations in still other genes may be lethal during early embryogenesis, so that a potential inner ear phenotype never develops. Genes whose mutations do produce defects in the ear and hearing loss often appear to occupy critical positions in developmental hierarchies. Such genes are sometimes referred to as master regulatory genes. Such genes tend to influence key decisions regarding tissue and cell phenotype, and their alteration has profound influences on subsequent events. Many models of development, examples of which are described above, attempt to characterize critical regulatory events that may be mediated by such master regulatory genes.

The identification of the genes that are involved in inherited hearing loss represents only the beginning of understanding these conditions. Characterization of events downstream from expression of a mutant protein, or lack of expression in null mutations, is required to determine the proximate causes of hearing loss, and to determine means by which such losses might be prevented. Since the majority of deafness genes affect the development of the ear, the events outlined in this chapter are the backdrop against which mutation-induced changes must be viewed.

The fact that many mutations resulting in hearing loss influence inner ear development has profound implications for the development of potential interventions. At present, there are no genetically based treatments for inherited forms of hearing loss. However, there is intense interest in the potential for gene-based therapeutic interventions. A number of experimental studies of gene therapy have been performed in the postnatal rodent ear (51). The formation of the inner ear begins early in human development, during the third week of gestation, and is largely complete by the twenty-sixth week. Therefore, intervention to prevent defects that arise during this period must be effective in utero. Treatment of the gamete or blastocyst is difficult, but allows manipulation of the very earliest stages of the embryo, long before the ear begins to form. However, after implantation intervention becomes much more problematic. Recent developments in the treatment of the human fetus suggest that it may eventually be possible to deliver therapy to the developing inner ear. In this case, a precise understanding of the structural and molecular development of the ear will be critical.

ACKNOWLEDGMENTS

This work was supported by grants from the U.S. National Institutes of Health/NIDCD, DC04233, DC00129 and DC00139, and by the Research Service of the U.S. Veterans Administration.

REFERENCES

1. Aghemo GF, Fortunato G. Observations on the development of the auricle in man. Panminerva Med 1969; 11:10–12.
2. Aletsee C, Beros A, Mullen L, Palacios C, Pak K, Dazert S, Ryan AF. Ras/ MEK but not p38 signaling mediates neurite extension from spiral ganglion neurons. JARO 2001; 2:377–387.
3. Aletsee C, Beros A, Mullen L, Palacios S, Pak K, Dazert S, Ryan AF. The disintegrin kistrin inhibits neurite extension from spiral ganglion explants cultured on laminin. Audiol Neuro Otol 2001; 6:66–78.
4. Anniko M, Wikstrom SO. Pattern formation of the otic placode and morphogenesis of the otocyst. Am J Otolaryngol 1984; 5:373–381.
5. Anniko M, Wroblewski R, Wersall J. Development of endolymph during maturation of the inner ear: a preliminary report. Arch Otorhinolaryngol 1979; 225:133–161.
6. Anniko M, Wroblewski R. Ionic environment of cochlear hair cells. Hearing Res 1986; 22:279–293.
7. Anson B. The early relation of the auditory vesicle to the ectoderm in human embryos. Anat Rec 1934; 58:127–137.
8. Anson B, Bast T. The development of the auditory ossicles and associated structures in man. Ann Otol Rhinol Laryngol 1946; 55:467–493.
9. Anson B, Donaldson J. Surgical Anatomy of the Temporal Bone and Ear. Philadelphia: WB Saunders, 1973.
10. Anson B, Hanson J, Richany S. Early embryology of the auditory ossicles and associated structures in relation to certain anomolies observed clinically. Ann Otol Rhinol Laryngol 1960; 69:427–447.
11. Arnold WH, Lang T. Development of the membranous labyrinth of human embryos and fetuses using computer aided 3D-reconstruction. Ann Anat 2001; 183:61–66.
12. Axelsson A, Ryan AF, Woolf N. The early postnatal development of the cochlear vasculature in the mongolian gerbil. Acta Otolaryngol 1986; 101:75–87.
13. Bast TH. Ossification of capsule in human fetus. Carnegie Contrib Embryol 1930; 21:53–82.
14. Belyantseva IA, Adler HJ, Curi R, Frolenkov GI, Kachar B. Expression and localization of prestin and the sugar transporter GLUT-5 during development of electromotility in cochlear outer hair cells. J Neurosci 2000; 20:RC116.

15. Bermingham N, Hassan B, Price S, Vollrath M, Ben-Arie N, Eatock R, Bellen H, Lysakowski A, Zoghbi H. Math1: an essential gene for the generation of inner ear hair cells. Science 1999; 284:1837–1841.

16. Birnholz JC. The fetal external ear. Radiol 1983; 147:819–821.

17. Brigande J, Kiernan A, Gao X, Iten L, Fekete D. Molecular genetics of pattern formation in the inner ear: do compartment boundaries play a role? PNAS 2000; 97:11700–11706.

18. Brook W, Diaz-Benjumea F, Cohen S. Organizing spatial pattern in limb development. Annu Rev Cell Dev Biol 1996; 12:161–180.

19. Bock G, Steel KP. Inner ear pathology in the deafness mutant mouse. Acta Otolaryngol 1983; 96:39–47.

20. Bosher S, Warren R. A study of the electrochemistry and osmotic relationship of the cochlear fluids in the neonatal rat at the time of development of the endocochlear potential. J Physiol 1971; 212:739–761.

21. Bylander A, Tjernstrom O. Changes in Eustachian tube function with age in children with normal ears: a longitudinal study. Acta Otolaryngol 1983; 96:467–477.

22. Cable J, Jackson IJ, Steel KP. Mutations at the W locus affect survival of neural crest-derived melanocytes in the mouse. Mech Dev 1995; 50:139–150.

23. Chang W, Nunes FD, De Jesus-Escobar JM, Harland R, Wu DK. Ectopic noggin blocks sensory and nonsensory organ morphogenesis in the chicken inner ear. Dev Biol 1999; 216:369–381.

24. Chun YM, Park K, Lim DJ. Development and resorption of murine middle ear mesenchyme. In: Mogi G, Honjo I, Ishii T, Takasaka T, eds. Recent Advances in Otitis Media. Amsterdam: Kugler, 1993:381–387.

25. Kil SH, Collazo A. Origins of inner ear sensory organs revealed by fate map and time-lapse analyses. Dev Biol 2001; 233:365–379.

26. Dazert S, Aletsee C, Brors D, Gravel C, Sendtner M, Ryan AF. In vivo adenoviral transduction of the neonatal rat cochlea and middle ear. Hearing Res 2001; 151:30–40.

27. Dazert S, Kim D, Luo L, Aletsee C, Garfunkel S, Maciag T, Baird A, Ryan AF. Focal delivery of fibroblast growth factor-1 by transfected cells induces spiral ganglion neurite targeting in vitro. J Cell Physiol 1998; 177:123–129.

28. Dechesne CJ, Pujol R. Neuron-specific enolase immunoreactivity in the developing mouse cochlea. Hearing Res 1986; 21:87–90.

29. Declau F, Moeneclaey L, Marquet J. Normal growth pattern of the middle ear cleft in the human fetus. J Laryngol Otol 1989; 103:461–465.

30. Dulon D, Luo L, Zhang C, Ryan AF. Expression of small-conductance calcium-activated potassium channels (SK) in outer hair cells of the rat cochlea. Eur J Neurosci 1998; 10:907–915.

31. Echelard Y, Epstein D, St-Jacques B, Shen L, Mohler J, McMahon J, McMahon A. Sonic hendgehog, a member of a family of putative signaling molecules, is implicated in the regulation of CNS polarity. Cell 1993; 75:1417–1430.

32. Echteler S, Arjmand E, Dallos P. Developmental alterations in the frequency map of the mammalian cochlea. Nature 1989; 341:147–149.

33. Echteler SM. Developmental segregation in the afferent projections to mammalian auditory hair cells. Proc Natl Acad Sci USA 1992; 89:6324–6327.

34. Erkman L, McEvilly RJ, Luo L, Ryan AE, Hoosmand F, O'Connell SM, Keithley EM, Rappaport DH, Ryan AF, Rosenfeld MG. Role of transcription factors Brn-3.1 and Brn-3.2 in auditory and visual system development. Nature 1996; 381:603–606.

35. Fekete D. Cell fate specification in the inner ear. Curr Opin Neurobiol 1996; 6:533–541.

36. Frenz DA, Doan TM, Liu W. Regulation of chondrogenesis in the developing inner ear: a role for sonic hedgehog. Ann NY Acad Sci 1998; 857:252–255.

37. Frenz DA, McPhee J, Van De Water T. Structural and functional development of the ear. In: Jahn A, Santos-Sacchi J, eds. Physiology of the Ear. 2d ed. New York: Raven Press, 2001:191–214.

38. Fritzsch B, Beisel K. Development and maintenance of ear innervation and function: lessons from mutations in mouse and man. Am J Hum Genet 1998; 63:1263–1270.

39. Furuta H, Luo L, Hepler K, Ryan AF. Evidence for differential regulation of calcium by outer versus inner hair cells: plasma membrane Ca-ATPase gene expression. Hearing Res 1998; 123:10–26.

40. Gavalas A, Studer M, Lumsden A, Rijli FM, Krumlauf R, Chambon P. Hoxa1 and Hoxb1 synergize in patterning the hindbrain, cranial nerves and second pharyngeal arch. Development 1998; 125:1123–1136.

41. Gerhardt H, Otto H. The intratemporal course of the facial nerve and its influence on the development of the ossicular chain. Acta Otolaryngol 1981; 91:567–573.

42. Groves AK, Bronner-Fraser M. Competence, specification and commitment in otic placode induction. Development 2000; 127:3489–3499.

43. Gulya J. Anatomy and ebryology of the ear. In: Hughes G, Penshak M, eds. Clinical Otology. 2d ed. New York: Thieme, 1997:3–34.

44. Hall JW. Development of the ear and hearing. J Perinatol 2000; 20:S12–S20.

45. Harvey D, Steel KP. The development and interpretation of the summating potential response. Hearing Res 1992; 61:137–146.

46. He D, Evans B, Dallos P. First appearance and development of electromotility in neonatal gerbil outer hair cells. Hearing Res 1994; 78:77–90.

47. Hepper PG, Shahidullah BS. Development of fetal hearing. Arch Dis Child 1994; 71:F81–F87.

48. Housley G, Luo L, Ryan AF. Localization of mRNA encoding the P2X2 receptor subunit of the adenosine 5′-triphosphate-gated ion channel in the adult and developing rat inner ear by in situ hybridization. J Comp Neurol 1998; 393:403–414.

49. Ikui A, Sando I, Haginomori S, Sudo M. Postnatal development of the tympanic cavity: a computer-aided reconstruction and measurement study. Acta Otolaryngol 2000; 120:375–379.

50. Kanagasuntheram R. A note on the development of the tubotympanic recess in the human embryo. J Anat 1967; 101:731–741.

51. Kanzaki S, Kawamoto K, Oh SH, Stover T, Suzuki M, Ishimoto S, Yagi M, Miller JM, Lomax MI, Raphael Y. From gene identification to gene therapy. Audiol Neurootol 2002; 7:161–164.

52. Kaufman MH. The Atlas of Mouse Development. New York: Academic Press, 1992.

53. Kaufman MH, Bard JBL. The Anatomical Basis of Mouse Development. San Diego, CA: Academic Press, 1999.

54. Kelly M, Bianchi L. Development and neuronal innervation of the organ of Corti. In: Willott J, ed. Handbook of Mouse Auditory Research. New York: CRC Press, 2001:137–156.

55. Khan KM, Marovitz WF. DNA content, mitotic activity, and incorporation of tritiated thymidine in the developing inner ear of the rat. Anat Rec 1982; 202:501–509.

56. Kimmel R, Turnbull D, Blanquet V, Wurst W, Loomis C, Joyner A. Two lineage boundaries coordinate vertebrate apical ectodermal ridge formation. Genes Dev 2000; 14:1377–1389.

57. Kim DW, Aletsee C, Mullen L, Dazert S, Ryan AF. Fibronectin enhances spiral ganglion neurite outgrowth in vitro. Hearing Res 2002. In press.

58. Kitajiri M, Sando I, Takahara T. Postnatal development of the eustachian tube and its surrounding structures: preliminary study. Ann Otol Rhinol Laryngol 1987; 96:191–198.

59. Ladher RK, Anakwe KU, Gurney AL, Schoenwolf GC, Francis-West PH. Identification of synergistic signals initiating inner ear development. Science 2000; 290:1904–1905.

60. Lanford PJ, Lan Y, Jiang R, Lindsell C, Weinmaster G, Gridley T, Kelley MW. Notch signalling pathway mediates hair cell development in mammalian cochlea. Nat Genet 1999; 21:289–292.

61. Lary S, Braissoulis G, de Vries L, Dubowitz L, Dubowitz V. Hearing threshold in preterm and term infants by auditory brainstem response. J Pediatr 1985; 107:593–599.

62. Laufer E, Dahn R, Orozco O, Yeo C, Pisenti J, Henrique D, Abbot U, Fallon J, Tabin C. Expression of radical fringe in limb-bud ectoderm regulates apical ectodermal ridge formation. Nature 1997; 386:366–373.

63. Lavigne-Rebillard M, Pujol R. Development of the auditory hair cell surface in human fetuses: a scanning electron microscopy study. Anat Embryol 1986; 174:369–377.

64. Lim DJ, Anniko M. Developmental morphology of the mouse inner ear: a scanning electron microscopic observation. Acta Otolaryngol Suppl 1985; 422: 1–69.

65. Luo L, Bennett T, Jung HH, Ryan AF. Developmental expression of 9-acetylcholine receptor mRNA in the rat cochlea and vestibular inner ear. J Comp Neurol 1998; 393:320–331.

66. Luo L, Brumm D, Ryan AF. Distribution of non-NMDA glutamate recep-

tor mRNAs in the developing rat cochlea. J Comp Neurol 1995; 361:372–382.

67. Luo L, Koutnouyan H, Baird A, Ryan AF. Expression of mRNA encoding acidic and basic FGF in the adult and developing cochlea. Hearing Res 1993; 69:182–193.

68. Mansour SL, Goddard JM, Capecchi MR. Mice homozygous for a targeted disruption of the proto-oncogene *int-2* have developmental defects in the tail and ear. Development 1993; 117:13–28.

69. Maroon H, Walshe J, Mahmood R, Kiefer P, Dickson C, Mason I. Fgf3 and Fgf8 are required together for formation of the otic placode and vesicle. Development 2002; 29:2099–2108.

70. Masuda Y, Honjo H, Naito M, Ogura Y. Normal development of the middle ear in the mouse: a light microscopic study of serial sections. Acta Med Okayama 1986; 40:201–207.

71. McEvilly R, Erkman L, Luo L, Sawchenko P, Ryan AF, Rosenfeld MG. Requirement for Brn-3.0 in differentiation and survival of sensory and motor neurons. Nature 1996; 384:574–577.

72. Meinhardt H. A boundary model for pattern formation in vertebrate limbs. J Embryol Exp Morph 1983; 76:115–137.

73. Moore J, Linthicum F. Myelination of the human auditory nerve: different tine courses for Schwann cell and glial myelin. Ann Otol Rhinol Laryngol 2001; 110:655–661.

74. Morishita H, Makishima T, Kaneko C, Lee YS, Segil N, Takahashi K, Kuraoka A, Nakagawa T, Nabekura J, Nakayama K, Nakayama KI. Deafness due to degeneration of cochlear neurons in caspase-3-deficient mice. Biochem Biophys Res Commun 2001; 284:142–149.

75. Morlet T, Goforth L, Hood LJ, Ferber C, Duclaux R, Berlin CI. Development of human cochlear active mechanism asymmetry: involvement of the medial olivocochlear system? Hearing Res 1999; 134:153–162.

76. Morsli H, Choo D, Ryan AF, Johnson R, Wu DK. Development of the mouse inner ear and origin of its sensory organs. J Neurosci 1998; 18:3327–3335.

77. Mullen LM, Ryan AF. Transgenic mice: genome manipulation and induced mutations. In: Willott J, ed. Handbook of Mouse Auditory Research: From Molecular Biology to Behavior. New York: CRC Press, 2001:457–474.

78. Ng J, Tamura K, Buscher D, Izpisua-Belmonte J. Molecular and cellular basis of pattern formation during vertebrate limb formation. Curr Top Dev Biol 1999; 41:37–66.

79. Nishikori T, Hatta T, Kawauchi H, Otani H. Apoptosis during inner ear development in human and mouse embryos: an analysis by computer-assisted three-dimensional reconstruction. Anat Embryol 1999; 200:19–26.

80. Nishimura Y, Kumoi T. The embryonic development of the human external auditory meatus. Acta Otolaryngol 1992; 112:496–503.

81. Nishizaki K, Anniko M. Developmental morphology of the middle ear. Auris Nasus Larynx 1997; 24:31–38.

82. Olszewski J. The morphometry of the ear ossicles in humans during development. Anat Anz 1990; 171:187–191.

83. O'Rahilly R. Early human development and the chief source of information on staged human embryos. Eur J Obstet Gynecol Reprod Biol 1979; 9:273–280.

84. O'Rahilly R. The early development of the otic vesicle in staged human embryos. J Embryol Exp Morphol 1963; 11:741–755.

85. O'Rahilly R, Gardner E. The initial appearance of ossification in staged human embryos. Am J Anat 1972; 134:291–301.

86. O'Rahilly R, Muller F. Development of the human ear. In: Ballenger J, Snow J, eds. Otorhinolaryngology: Head and Neck Surgery. Baltimore: Williams & Wilkins, 1996:829–837.

87. Park K, Lim DJ. Luminal development of the eustachian tube and middle ear: murine model. Yonsei Med J 1992; 33:159–167.

88. Peck JE. Development of hearing. Part II. Embryology. J Am Acad Audiol 1994; 5:359–365.

89. Pellnitz D. Über das Wchstum der menschlichen Ohrmusckel. Arch Ohr-Nas-Kehlk-Heilk 1958; 171:334–340.

90. Petit C, Levilliers J, Hardelin JP. Molecular genetics of hearing loss. Annu Rev Genet 2001; 35:589–645.

91. Petit C. Genes responsible for human hereditary deafness: symphony of a thousand. Nature Genet 1996; 14:385–391.

92. Pujol R, Lavigne-Rebillard M. Early stages of innervation and sensory cell differentiation in the human fetal organ of Corti. Acta Otolaryngol 1985; Suppl. 423:43–50.

93. Pujol R. Morphology, synaptology and electrophysiology of the developing cochlea. Acta Otolaryngol 1985; Suppl. 421:5–9.

94. Pujol R, Hilding D. Anatomy and physiology of the onset of auditory function. Acta Otolaryngol 1973; 76:1–11.

95. Pujol R, Lavigne-Rebillard M. Early stages of innervation and sensory cell differentiation in the human fetal organ of Corti. Acta Otolaryngol 1985; Suppl. 423:43–50.

96. Represa J, Leon Y, Miner C, Goraldez F. The *int*-2 proto-oncogene is responsible for induction of the inner ear. Nature 1991; 353:561–563.

97. Retzius G. Das Gehörorgan der Wirbeltiere. II. Das Gehörorgan der Reptilien, der Vögel und Säugetiere. Stockholm: Samson & Wallin, 1884.

98. Roberts DS, Miller SA. Apoptosis in cavitation of middle ear space. Anat Rec 1998; 251:286–289.

99. Ruben RJ. Development of the inner ear of the mouse: a radioautographic study of terminal mitoses. Acta Otolaryngol 1967; 220:1–44.

100. Ryan AF, Woolf N. Development of tonotopic representation in the central auditory system of the mongolian gerbil: a 2-deoxyglucose study. Dev Brain Res 1988; 41:61–70.

101. Ryan AF. Transcription factors and the control of inner ear development. Semin Cell Dev Biol 1997; 8:249–256.

102. Sadanaga M, Morimitsu T. Development of endocochlear potential and its negative component in mouse cochlea. Hearing Res 1995; 89:155–161.

103. Sanchez Del Rey A, Sanchez Fernandez JM, Martinez Ibarguen A, Santaolalla Montoya F. Morphologic and morphometric study of human spiral ganglion development. Acta Otolaryngol 1995; 115:211–217.

104. Sher AE. The embryonic and postnatal development of the inner ear of the mouse. Acta Otolaryngol 1971; Suppl. 285:1–777.

105. Shnerson A, Devigne C, Pujol R. Age-related changes in the C57BL/6J mouse cochlea. II. Ultrastructural findings. Brain Res 1981; 254:77–88.

106. Sobkowicz HM, Rose JE, Scott GE, Slapnick SM. Ribbon synapses in the developing intact and cultured organ of Corti in the mouse. J Neurosci 1982; 2:942–957.

107. Sobkowicz HM, Rose JE, Scott GL, Levenick CV. Distribution of synaptic ribbons in the developing organ of Corti. J Neurocytol 1986; 15:693–714.

108. Sohmer H, Perez R, Sichel JY, Priner R, Freeman S. The pathway enabling external sounds to reach and excite the fetal inner ear. Audiol Neuro-Otol 2001; 6:109–116.

109. Steel KP, Barkway C. Another role for melanocytes: their importance for normal stria vascularis development in the mammalian inner ear. Development 1989; 107:453–463.

110. Steel KP, Harvey D. Development of auditory function in mutant mice. In: Romand R, ed. Development of Auditory and Vestibular Systems. Vol. 2 Amsterdam: Elsevier, 1992:221–242.

111. Swarts JD, Rood SR, Doyle WJ. Fetal development of the auditory tube and paratubal musculature. Cleft Palate J 1986; 23:289–311.

112. Tekin M, Arnos KS, Pandya A. Advances in hereditary deafness. Lancet 2001; 358:1082–1090.

113. Tellier AL, Amiel J, Delezoide AL, Audollent S, Augé J, Esnault D, Encha-Razavi F, Munnich A, Lyonnet S, Vekemans M, Attié-Bitach T. Expression of the PAX2 gene in human embryos and exclusion in the CHARGE syndrome. Am J Med Genet 2001; 93:85–88.

114. Terzic J, Muller C, Gajovic S, Saraga-Babic M. Expression of PAX2 gene during human development. Int J Devel Biol 1998; 42:701–707.

115. Theiler K. The House Mouse; development and normal stages from fertilization to 4 weeks of age. New York: Springer-Verlag, 1972.

116. Tickel C, Munsterberg A. Vertebrate limb development—the early stages in chick and mouse. Curr Opin Genet Dev 2001; 11:478–481.

117. Ulatowska-Blaszyk K, Bruska M. The cochlear ganglion in human embryos of developmental stages 18 and 19. Folia Morphol 1999; 58:29–35.

118. Vahava O, Morell R, Lynch E, Weiss S, Kagan M, Ahituv N, Morrow J, Lee M, Skvorak A, Morton C, Blumenfeld A, Frydman M, Friedman T, King M, Avraham K. Mutation in transcription factor POU4F3 associated with inherited progressive hearing loss in humans. Science 1998; 279:1950–1954.

119. Vega JA, José IS, Cabo R, Rodriguez S, Represa J. Trks and p75 genes are differentially expressed in the inner ear of human embryos: what may Trks and

p75 null mutant mice suggest on human development? Neurosci Lett 1999; 272:103–106.

120. Vendrell V, Carnicero E, Giraldez F, Alonso MT, Schimmang T. Induction of inner ear fate by FGF3. Development 2000; 127:2011–2019.

121. Wayne S, Robertson NG, DeClau F, Chen N, Verhoeven K, Prasad S, Morton CC, Ryan AF, Van Camp G, Smith R. Mutations in the transciptional activator Eya4 cause late-onset deafness at the DFNA10 locus. Hum Mol Genet 2001; 10:195–200.

122. Wong ML. Embryology and developmental anatomy of the ear. In: Bluestone C, Stool S, eds. Pediatric Otolaryngology. Philadelphia: WB Saunders, 1983: 85–111.

123. Woolf N, Harris J, Ryan AF. Development of the endocochlear potential in the gerbil: effects of anoxia. Amer J Physiol 1986; 250:493–498.

124. Woolf N, Koehrn FJ, Ryan AF. Expression of fibronectin in the developing inner ear of the gerbil and rat. Dev Brain Res 1992; 65:21–33.

125. Woolf N, Ryan AF. Contributions of the middle ear to the development of function in the cochlea. Hearing Res 1988; 35:131–142.

126. Woolf N, Ryan AF. The development of auditory function in the cochlea of the mongolian gerbil. Hearing Res 1984; 13:277–283.

127. Wright CG. Development of the human external ear. J Am Acad Audiol 1997; 8:379–382.

128. Xia A, Kikuchi T, Hozawa K, Katori Y, Takasaka T. Expression of connexin 26 and Na,K-ATPase in the developing mouse cochlear lateral wall: functional implications. Brain Res 1999; 846:106–111.

129. Xiang M, Gao WQ, Hasson T, Shin JJ. Requirement for Brn-3c in maturation and survival, but not in fate determination of inner ear hair cells. Development 1998; 125:3935–3946.

130. Yamasaki M, Komune S, Shimozono M, Matsuda K, Haruta A. Development of monovalent ions in the endolymph in mouse cochlea. ORL J Otorhinolaryngol Relat Spec 2000; 62:241–246.

131. Yamashita H, Takahashi M, Bagger-Sjöbäck D. Expression of epidermal growth factor, epidermal growth factor receptor and transforming growth factor-alpha in the human fetal inner ear. Eur Arch Oto-rhino-laryngol 1996; 253:494–497.

132. Yokoyama T, Iino Y, Kakizaki K, Murakami Y. Human temporal bone study on the postnatal ossification process of auditory ossicles. Laryngoscope 1999; 109:927–930.

2

Audiometric Tests and Diagnostic Workup

Paul J. Govaerts
The Eargroup, Antwerp, Belgium

Children with suspected congenital hearing loss are referred for audiological and diagnostic workup. The suspicion is often based on parental anxiety, but more and more children are referred after failing neonatal hearing screening.

The audiological workup aims at establishing the type and degree of hearing loss. Pure tone audiometry is the standard test in daily clinical practice. The technique of pure tone audiometry is explained and some issues that are useful for a good interpretation of audiometric reports are highlighted. Standards are given for age-related deterioration of hearing. In addition, attention is paid to objective tests, such as auditory brainstem responses (ABR), otoacoustic emissions, and tympanometry. These tests play an important role in assessing the hearing of infants or otherwise uncooperative subjects.

The diagnostic workup of hearing loss also aims at refining the diagnosis, excluding associated pathology in case of syndromic hearing loss, and identifying the molecular defect. To exclude associated pathology means looking for syndromes. Typical features such as facial anomalies may be indicative of a syndrome. A thorough clinical examination focusing on any signs of an underlying syndrome is therefore mandatory. In addition, several organs are known to be at risk in case of a congenital hearing problem. These are mainly the kidneys [e.g., branchio-oto-renal syndrome (BOR)], the heart (e.g., long Q-T syndrome), the thyroid (e.g., Pendred syndrome), and the eyes (e.g., Usher syndrome). Special attention should therefore be given to these organs.

I. AUDIOLOGICAL WORKUP

A. Pure Tone Audiometry

Pure tone audiometry is the standard test to assess hearing and hearing loss. It is a way to measure hearing thresholds at different frequencies and at both ears. It is a subjective test as it involves the cooperation of the test person and this is in contrast to objective tests like brainstem evoked audiometry (ABR) or otoacoustic emissions.

1. Technique

The technique of measuring hearing thresholds is standardized (American National Standards Institute, ANSI). The thresholds are expressed in "decibels hearing level" (dBHL), whereby zero dBHL at a given frequency is defined as the lowest sound level that a normal person of 18 years is just able to hear. A hearing loss of, for example, 30 dB means that the intensity of sound has to be 30 dB above the zero level before the subject starts hearing it (the average intensity of conversational speech is 50–60 dB).

In general, hearing is tested in a soundproof room with a calibrated audiometer and earphones that present sounds of varying intensity and frequency to each ear separately. Different test procedures exist. Conventional procedures use attenuation steps of 5 dB or more, thus introducing a minimum error of $\pm$ 5 dB. The test frequencies used are 125, 250, 500, 1000, 2000, 4000, and 8000 Hz. Once the threshold at a given frequency is assessed, it is plotted with a specific symbol on the audiogram. Both the graphic representation and the symbols are defined in international recommendations (1) (Table 1). For unmasked air conduction thresholds the symbols are O for the right ear and X for the left ear (Fig. 1).

Air conduction (AC) audiometry uses earphones to present the different sounds. Bone conduction (BC) audiometry uses a bone-conducting vibrator

Table 1 Common Symbols Used for Audiometric Representation (ASHA 1990)

	Right ear	Left ear
Air conduction (earphones)		
Unmasked	O	X
Masked	Δ	□
Bone conduction (mastoid)		
Unmasked	<	>
Masked	[	]

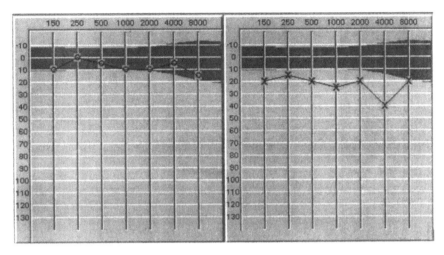

Figure 1 Typical audiogram showing the air-conduction thresholds of the right ear (depicted with the symbol 0 at the left panel) and the left ear (depicted with the symbol X at the right panel). The dark-gray area is the 95% confidence region for an 18-year-old person.

that is positioned on the mastoid of each ear. Air-conducted sound reaches the auditory nerve through the external, the middle, and the inner ear. Bone-conducted sound bypasses the external and the middle ear and reaches the auditory nerve directly through the inner ear. The symbols for unmasked BC thresholds are < for the right and > for the left ear.

2. Conductive, Sensorineural, and Mixed Hearing Loss

Anomalies of the inner ear and/or the central auditory pathways (from the auditory nerve via the brainstem to auditory cortex) result in a "perceptive" or "sensorineural" hearing loss and will affect both AC and BC thresholds (Fig. 2, left ear). Many forms of congenital hearing loss and most types of nonsyndromic hearing loss are sensorineural. Anomalies of the outer and middle ear will affect only AC thresholds. The difference between AC and BC threshold is called the "air-bone gap" and reflects a middle- or outer-ear problem. This is called a "conductive" hearing loss (Fig. 2, right ear). This type of hearing loss is found, for example, in congenital atresias of the outer ear canal, malformations of the middle ear ossicles, and stapedial ankylosis due to otosclerosis.

    Problems at different levels (e.g., middle and inner ear) may result in a "mixed" hearing loss, with a sensorineural component given by a BC loss

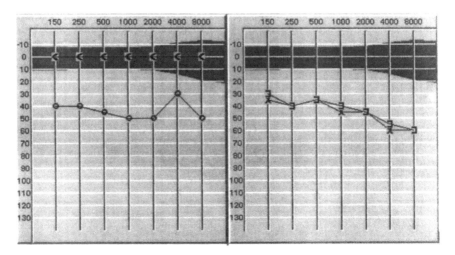

Figure 2 Typical audiograms of a conductive hearing loss at the right ear (left panel) and a senorineural hearing loss at the left ear (right panel). The right ear shows normal bone-conduction thresholds (PTA 0 dBHL) and abnormal air-conduction thresholds (PTA 47 dBHL). The left ear shows abnormal bone- and air-conduction thresholds with a PTA of 40 dBHL and 43 dB, respectively.

and a conductive component given by a superimposed air-bone gap. This type can be found for instance in otosclerosis affecting both the cochlea and the stapes.

3. Masking

Sound that is presented to one ear may also reach the contralateral ear, which should be avoided. The interaural attenuation of AC and BC sound is known for the different test frequencies and in case a risk of crossover exists, the nontest ear should be "masked." Masking is difficult and both the decision whether to mask and the execution of it should not be underestimated and, although strict criteria and guidelines exist, it should be left to audiologists. Masking leads to corrected AC and BC thresholds and special symbols exist to represent these.

4. PTA or Fletcher Index

To summarize the audiometric findings several indices have been introduced, among which the pure tone average (PTA) or "Fletcher index" is the most commonly used. The PTA is the average of the AC thresholds at the frequencies 500, 1000, and 2000 Hz. For instance, the audiogram in Figure 2 has a PTA of 47 dBHL for the right ear and 40 dBHL for the left ear. Hearing losses are often described in a qualitative way that is based on the PTA. Different classifications exist. The WHO recommends the classification of Table 2. In addition one may describe the curve of the audiogram, such as "down-sloping" or U-shaped.

5. Feasibility

Since pure tone audiometry requires a responsive subject, it may be unfeasible in children or in persons who are not able to give reliable responses because of mental or other problems. For small children special observational or conditioning techniques exist that allow fairly reliable audiometric results from the age of approximately 2 years onward. At younger ages, more than one session may be required or alternative techniques, like ABR (see below), may be used.

6. ISO 7029

A special issue of interest is the definition of "normality" in hearing. Zero dBHL is defined as the average threshold in 18-year-old persons with a history free of otological disease. It is, however, known that hearing deteriorates with age and a hearing loss of 25 dBHL at 500 Hz and even 80 dBHL

Table 2 Grades of Hearing Impairment

Grade of impairment	Corresponding audiometric ISO value (average of 500, 1000, 2000, 4000 Hz) of the better ear	Performance
0 No	25 DB or better	No or very slight hearing problems Able to hear whispers.
1 Slight	261–40 DB	Able to hear and repeat words spoken in normal voice at 1 meter
2 Moderate	41–60 dB	Able to hear and repeat words using raised voice at 1 meter
3 Severe	61–80 dB	Able to hear some words when shouted into better ear
4 Profound	81 dB or greater	Unable to hear and understand even a shouted voice

Source: World Health Organization (http://www.who.int/pbd/pdh/Docs/GRADESTable-DEFs.pdf). Adapted from the report of the informal working group on prevention of deafness and hearing impairment programme planning, WHO, Geneva, with adaptations from the report of the first informal consultation on future program developments for the prevention of deafness and hearing impairment, WHO, Geneva.

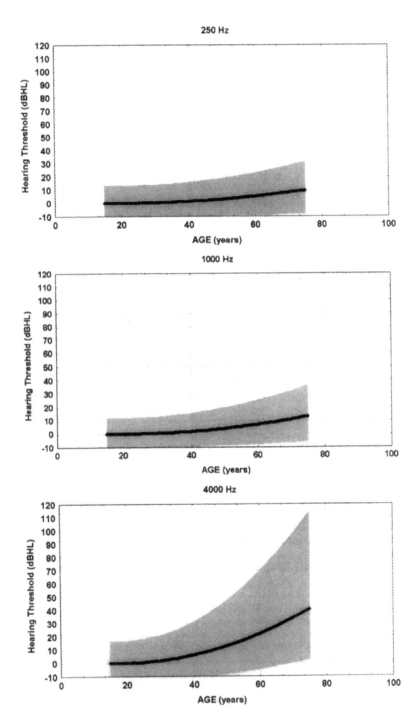

at 8000 Hz is not abnormal for a 70-year-old man. The age- and gender-related distribution of hearing thresholds is defined by the International Organization for Standardization (ISO) 7029 standard [ISO 7029 (1984): "Acoustics—threshold of hearing by air conduction as a function of age and sex for otologically normal persons" (International Organization for Standardization, Geneva)]. The hearing threshold of any given patient can therefore be expressed as the number of standard deviations below or above the median value for the given age and gender. The corresponding percentile can be derived from these data in any table of a normal distribution. For example, the median hearing loss at 500 Hz for a normal 70-year-old man is 8 dBHL according to the ISO 7029 standard with a positive standard deviation of 10 dBHL. A hearing loss of 25 dBHL can be expressed as 1.7 standard deviations (25 dBHL/10 dBHL) above the median and this corresponds to the ninety-sixth percentile (or P96). If normality is defined as the group between P2.5 and P97.5, this is to be considered normal (2) (Fig. 3) Since genetic hearing losses affect different generations in one family, it is important to bear in mind this concept of normality and abnormality.

7. Supraliminal Audiometry

So far only "pure tone" audiometry has been discussed. This is called "liminal" audiometry since it assesses the threshold of hearing. Hearing, however, is far more complex than simply detecting low-level sounds. To understand the sounds one needs to discriminate different sounds. These supraliminal aspects of hearing can be assessed by other tests, such as speech audiometry. Supraliminal tests in general are less standardized than liminal audiometry and they are most often language-dependent. In addition, they assess not only hearing but also higher cognitive and other functions. This renders them less applicable for genetic research.

8. Cochlear Conductive Loss

A rare finding is the so-called "cochlear conductive hearing loss." This is typically found in an enlarged vestibular aqueduct (2) but it may also be found in other types of cochlear anomaly. It shows a conductive hearing loss on audiometry (an air-bone gap). Tympanometry (see below) shows normal

---

Figure 3 Evolution of normal hearing thresholds for 250 Hz (top), 1000 Hz (middle) and 4000 Hz (bottom) in function of age according to the ISO 7029 formula (see text for details). The solid lines are the median hearing thresholds and the gray areas represent the 95% confidence interval.

middle-ear pressure but stapedial reflexes are absent. These audiometric findings are commonly interpreted as an ossicular problem (ossicular malformation or fixation) but exploratory tympanotomy or high-resolution CT scan does not reveal any such condition. Although the underlying mechanism is not quite understood, it is thought that the minor cochlear malformation prevents the traveling wave within the cochlea from proceeding smoothly. Although the sound is well transferred through the middle ear and thus reaches the cochlea without problems, it encounters a mechanical resistance within the fluids of the cochlea itself before arriving at the inner hair cells. This should explain the relatively normal BC thresholds and abnormal AC thresholds.

B. Auditory Brainstem Responses

The evaluation of ABR, also called evoked response audiometry (ERA) or "brainstem evoked response audiometry (BERA), refers to an objective technique of assessing hearing thresholds. It is objective since it does not require the cooperation of the test person. It can even be done under anesthesia. It is based on the recording of electrical responses from the cochlea and the auditory nerve after acoustical stimulation either via AC or via BC. An averaging paradigm is used with a short stimulus (typically a click of 100 μsec) that is presented some 1000–2000 times to allow averaging of the response. Although the test is objective, physical principles allow it merely to assess the thresholds at the higher frequencies (2000 and 4000 Hz). The thresholds at other frequencies are far less reliable. In addition, the confidence interval of the thresholds is higher than the ±5 dB of the pure tone audiometry. This renders ABR a test of second choice that should only be used when regular audiometry is not feasible or reliable, e.g., in infants or mentally disabled persons.

Special devices have been developed to record ABR and to automatically interpret the responses in terms of hearing thresholds. The output is either "pass" or "fail" meaning normal hearing or, respectively, a hearing loss of at least 20–30 dBHL. These are called automated ABRs (AABRs) and are used for screening purposes and especially for neonatal hearing screening.

C. Otoacoustic Emissions

Otoacoustic emissions are acoustic signals that are emitted from the ear (3). Different types exist, but in clinical practice, the so-called transient evoked otoacoustic emissions (TEOAEs) are most commonly used. They are produced by the outer hair cells if they are in good physiological condition and stimulated by an external sound (4,5). The technique and interpretation are well established. If no TEOAEs can be elicited, this is interpreted as a hearing loss of 30 dBHL or more. Presence of TEOAEs means normal or near-normal hearing. The test is fast and no cooperation of the test person is needed. On the other hand, it is rather aspecific, since both sensorineural and conductive hearing loss will result in the absence of TEOAEs and hardly any frequency information can be derived. However, it is a high-quality screening tool and as such it is widely used for neonatal and other hearing screening. Thanks to the many nationwide ("universal") neonatal hearing screening programs, early detection of congenital hearing loss is becoming more and more common practice (6,7).

D. Tympanometry

Tympanometry is a test to register the acoustic impedance of essentially the middle ear. It reflects the pressure within the middle ear cavity and as such it is often used to detect middle ear ventilation problems. A special feature is the possibility to record stapedial reflexes, which are small movements of the stapes, due to a contraction of the stapedial muscle as a response to high-intensity sounds. The movement of the stapes makes the incus, the malleus, and the tympanic membrane move, which can be measured with an external probe. The test is simple and gives information on the mobility of the ossicular chain. An immobile chain fails to give recordable stapedial reflexes. This typically occurs in otosclerosis and also in different types of congenital ossicular malformation with fixation of one of the ossicles.

II. GENERAL WORKUP

A. Blood Examination, Including Connexin 26

Thanks to the universal neonatal hearing screening programs, an increasing number of neonates are referred for diagnostic workup. The amount of blood that is available for laboratory tests is limited. Therefore, not all tests that may contribute to the diagnosis may be done. In the absence of indications for specific underlying pathologies, genetic (connexin 26) and serological examinations may suffice.

Thyroid hormone tests are not useful. Patients with Pendred syndrome are euthyroid at birth. Only half of them become hypothyroid with the development of a goiter after the age of 10 years (8).

B. Genetic Examination

In case of syndromic hearing loss, either karyotyping or specific biochemical and molecular investigations may be useful. Even in the absence of

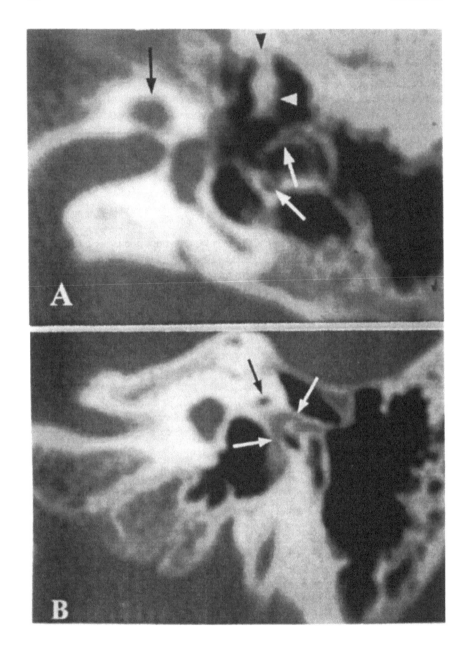

phenotypic indications suggestive of an underlying syndrome, it is recommended to actively exclude the three most frequent syndromes, namely, the autosomal recessive Usher and Pendred syndromes and the X-linked Alport syndrome. The former two syndromes typically have negative familial histories. Ophthalmological examinations with electroretinography (at the age of 5 years), medical imaging, and urine examination are required.

An increasing number of genes causing nonsyndromic hearing loss have been described [see web-page V Camp (9)]. At present it is not possible to routinely search for many of these mutations for practical reasons. Mutations in the connexin 26 gene (GJB2) account for probably 20% of the nonsyndromic congenital hearing losses (10–12). In some populations this figure may even be higher [e.g., 80% in Jewish Ashkenazi children (13,14)]. The most common mutations are the 35delG and the 162delT mutations and these can be routinely found by simple and inexpensive restriction enzyme analysis. Additional mutations should be ruled out by sequencing the gene.

A frequent anomaly found in congenital nonsyndromic hearing loss is an enlarged vestibular aqueduct (2). This may account for over 20% of all congenital hearing losses (15). A number of them [15% (16)] have been shown to be related to mutations in the Pendred syndrome gene (PDS). If an enlarged vestibular aqueduct is found by medical imaging, it may be worthwhile investigating this gene.

C. Serological Examination

Maternal or congenital infections are becoming rare as a cause of congenital deafness in the Western world.

Thanks to widespread vaccination, the rate of confirmed congenital rubella syndrome has decreased to approx 0.05 per 10. 000 life births (17). In

---

Figure 4 CT scan for congenital conductive hearing loss (courtesy J. Casselman). Axial and coronal CT image with bone window through the left middle and inner ear of a patient with congenital conductive hearing loss related to the branchio-oto-renal syndrome. (A) The malleus and incus are fused (white arrowhead) and are fixed against the anterior wall of the middle ear cavity (black arrowhead). The facial nerve descends in an abnormal position through the middle ear cavity and splits in two descending branches (white arrows). Note the hypoplastic cochlea with absence of a normal modiolus. (B) The facial nerve leaves its normal position under the lateral semicircular canal (black arrow) and gives rise to two branches, which are descending, through the middle-ear cavity (white arrows).

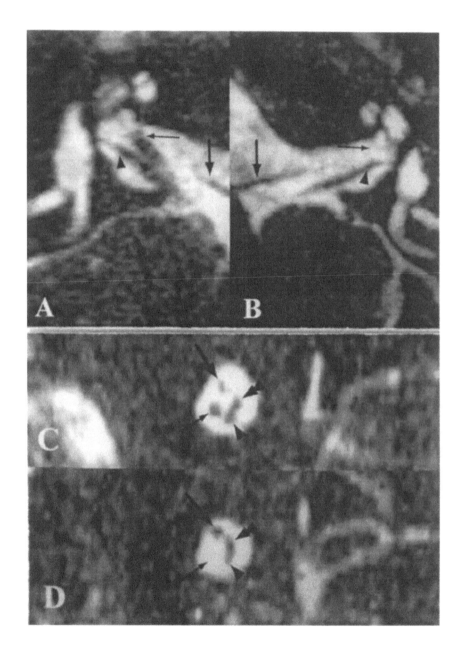

areas where rubella vaccination is not common practice, serological examination is probably justified.

Cytomegalovirus (CMV) is a frequent cause of congenital infections [0.4–2.3% of live births (18)] and may cause congenital hearing loss. Prenatal diagnosis is possible and provides the optimal means for both diagnosing fetal infection and identifying fetuses at risk of severe sequelae (19). Serological evaluation is possible on blood samples and polymerase chain reaction (PCR) diagnosis is possible on urine samples.

D. Imaging

Refining the diagnosis means searching for the etiology.

Middle ear problems often consist of atresia and/or ossicular malformations. In most cases these can be readily seen on high-resolution CT scan (Fig. 4). Therefore, a congenital conductive hearing loss makes a CT scan mandatory. This can be done under sedation or anesthesia if necessary.

Sensorineural hearing losses are mainly caused by cochlear problems (large vestibular aqueduct, Mondini dysplasia, semicircular canal malformations) and to a lesser extent by central auditory lesions, situated in the auditory nerve (aplasia or hypoplasia), the auditory pathways, or the auditory cortex. Magnetic resonance (MR) imaging (Fig. 5) may elucidate the details and is often complementary to CT, especially in the study of inner-ear malformations (20). Routine T2-weighted spin-echo images of the brain are

---

Figure 5 MRI for congenital sensorineural hearing loss (courtesy J. Casselman). Axial 0.7-mm-thick T2-weighted gradient-echo images and sagittal reconstructions perpendicular to the course of the nerves made at the level of the fundus of the internal auditory canal (IAC) through both the right (A, C) and the left (B, D) inner ear in a patient with congenital deafness on the left side. (A) Normal facial nerve (large black arrow), inferior vestibular (black arrowhead), and cochlear (small black arrowhead) branch of the VIIIth nerve can be seen near the floor of the IAC. (B) The facial nerve (large black arrow) and inferior vestibular branch of the VIIIth nerve (black arrowhead) can again be distinguished; however, the cochlear branch of the VIIIth nerve is absent (small black arrow). (C) The facial nerve (large black arrow), superior vestibular (double arrowhead), inferior vestibular (arrowhead), and cochlear (small black arrow) branch of the VIIIth nerve can all be seen on the reconstruction made at the fundus of the right IAC. (D) The facial nerve (large black arrow), superior vestibular (double arrowhead), and inferior vestibular branch (arrowhead) of the VIIIth nerve can again be seen. This image confirms the congenital absence of the cochlear branch of the VIIIth nerve (small black arrow).

ideally suited to exclude white-matter disease or other lesions in the cochlear nuclei and along the auditory pathways. Only MR can demonstrate the abnormal course, hypoplasia, or aplasia of the vestibulocochlear nerve and facial nerve (21). MR techniques have to be adapted for inner-ear malformations. Only heavily T2-weighted gradient-echo sequences, such as three-dimensional Fourier transform constructive interference in steady state (3DFT-CISS), true-fast imaging with steady precession (true-FISP), or 3D-fast spin-echo (3D-FSE) sequences, are suitable for this purpose (22). Moreover, some changes inside the membranous labyrinth can only be seen on submillimetric (0.7 mm thickness) heavily T2-weighted MR images. A CT can be complementary to evaluate the abnormal internal auditory canal or facial nerve canal. Thin CT images (reconstructed 1- or 1.25-mm-thick images every 0.5 or even 0.1 mm) yield detailed information on the bony labyrinth, including modiolus and even the osseous spiral lamina, but they do not give any information on the fluid in the lanyrinthine compartments, which can only be seen on MR images.

E. Ophthalmological Examination with Fundoscopy

One of the most frequent ocular problems linked with congenital hearing loss is retinitis pigmentosa (Usher syndrome). This is seen on fundoscopy. The first signs of retinitis, however, appear no sooner than at the age of a couple of years and often even much later. Therefore, a negative ophthalmological examination is no proof of the absence of Usher syndrome. Electroretinography may provide early diagnosis from the age of 2 years onward and some authors claim that all children with severe to profound, prelingual sensorineural hearing loss should be screened by ophthalmological examination including electroretinogram (23).

Other syndromes may consist of early onset eye problems, such as retinopathy, optic atrophy, or iridal or corneal anomalies.

F. Electrocardiogram

An electrocardiogram is routinely taken to exclude the long Q-T syndrome (Jervell and Lange-Nielsen syndrome).

G. Ultrasound Examination of the Renal System

Ultrasound examination of the kidneys is important to rule out any renal structural malformation, e.g., in the branchio-oto-renal syndrome (BOR).

H. Urine

Urine examination should exclude microscopic hematuria and proteinuria, although the latter is uncommon in children. It is also useful for detecting cytomegalovirus by PCR techniques.

REFERENCES

1. ASHA American Speech-Language-Hearing Association. Guidelines for audiometric symbols. ASHA 1990; 20(suppl 2):25–30.
2. Govaerts PJ, Casselman J, Daemers K, De Ceulaer G, Peeters S, Somers TH, Offeciers FE. Audiological findings in the large vestibular aqueduct syndrome. Int J Pediatr ORL 1999; 51:157–164.
3. Kemp DT. Stimulated acoustic emissions from within the human auditory system. J Acoust Soc Am 1978; 64:1386–1391.
4. Khanna SM, Leonard DG. Measurement of basilar membrane vibrations and evaluation of cochlear condition. Hearing Res 1986; 23:37–53.
5. Sellick PM, Patuzzi R, Johnstone BM. Measurements of basilar membrane motion in the guinea pig using the Mössbauer technique. J Acoust Soc Am 1982; 72:131–141.
6. White KR, Vohr BR, Maxon AB, Behrens TR, McPherson MG, Mauk GW. Screening all newborns for hearing loss using transient evoked otoacoustic emissions. Int J Pediatr Otorhinolaryngol 1994; 29(3):203–217.
7. Govaerts PJ, De Ceulaer G, Yperman M, Van Driessche K, Somers TH, Offeciers FE. A two-stage, bipodal screening model for universal neonatal hearing screening. Otol Neurotol 2001; 22(6):850–854.
8. Reardon W, Coffey R, Chowdhurry T, Grossman A, Jan H, Britton K, Kendall-Taylor P, Trembath R. Prevalence, age of onset, and natural history of thyroid disease in Pendred syndrome. J Med Genet 1999; 36(8):595–598.
9. Van Camp G, Smith RJH. Hereditary Hearing loss Homepage. World Wide Web URL: http://www.uia.ac.be/dnalab/hhh/. (October, 1996).
10. Dahl HH, Saunders K, Kelly TM, Osborn AH, Wilcox S, Cone-Wesson B, Wunderlich JL, Du Sart D, Kamarinos M, Gardner RJ, Dennehy S, Williamson R, Vallance N, Mutton P. Prevalence and nature of connexin 26 mutations in children with non-syndromic deafness. Med J Aust 2001; 175(4): 182–183.
11. Kenna MA, Wu BL, Cotanche DA, Korf BR, Rehm HL. Connexin 26 studies in patients with sensorineural hearing loss. Arch Otolaryngol Head Neck Surg 2001; 127(9):1037–1042.
12. Milunsky JM, Maher TA, Yosunkaya E, Vohr BR. Connexin-26 gene analysis in hearing-impaired newborns. Genet Test 2000; 4(4):345–349.
13. Morell RJ, Kim HJ, Hood LJ, et al. Mutations in the connexin 26 gene (GJB2) among Ashkenazi Jews with nonsyndromic recessive deafness. N Engl J Med 1998; 339:1500–1505.

14. Lerer I, Sagi M, Malamud E, Levi H, Raas-Rothschild A, Abeliovich D. Contribution of connexin 26 mutations to nonsyndromic deafness in Ashkenazi patients and the variable phenotypic effect of the mutation 167delT. Am J Med Genet 2000; 6:53–56.

15. Zhang S, Zhao C, Yu L. Analysis of sensorineural hearing loss in 77 children. Lin Chuang Er Bi Yan Hou Ke Za Zhi 1997; 11(6):252–254.

16. Scott DA, Wang R, Kreman TM, Andrews M, McDonald JM, Bishop JR, Smith RJ, Karniski LP, Sheffield VC. Functional differences of the PDS gene product are asspociated with phenotypic variation in patients with Pendred syndrome and nonsyndromic hearing loss (DFNB4). Hum Mol Genet 2000; 1709–1715.

17. Zimmerman L, Reef SE. Incidence of congenital rubella syndrome at a hospital seving a predominantly Hispanic population. Pediatrics 2001; 107(3):E40.

18. Witters I, Van Ranst M, Fryns JP. Cytomegalovirus reactivation in pregnancy and subsequent isolated bilateral loss in the infant. Genet Couns 2000; 11(4): 375–378.

19. Azam AZ, Vial Y, Fawer CL, Zufferey J, Hohfeld P. Prenatal diagnosis of congenital cytomegalovirus infection. Obstet Gynecol 2001; 97(3):443–448.

20. Casselman JW, Offeciers FE, De Foer B, Govaerts P, Kuhweide R, Somers TH. CT and MR imaging of congenital abnormalities of the inner ear and internal auditory canal. Eur J Radiol 2001; 40(2):94–104.

21. Casselman JW, Offeciers FE, Govaerts PJ, Kuhweide R, Geldof H, Somers TH, D'Hont G. Aplasia and hypoplasia of the vestibulocochlear nerve: Diagnosis with MR Imaging. Radiology 1997; 202:773–781.

22. Casselman JW, Kuhweide R, Deemling M, Ampe W, Dehaene I, Meeus L. Constructive interference in steady state-3DFT MR imaging of the inner ear and cerebellopontine angle. Am J Neuroradiol 1993; 14:47–57.

23. Mets MB, Young NM, Pass A, Lasky JB. Early diagnosis of Usher syndrome in children. Trans Am Ophthalmol Soc 2000; 98:237–242.

3
Classification and Epidemiology

Alessandro Martini and Patrizia Trevisi
Ferrara University, Ferrara, Italy

I. CLASSIFICATION

The American National Standards Institute (ANSI) defined hearing loss (HL) as the difference from the normal ability to detect sounds relative to its established standards.

Hearing impairment is usually classified by site of lesions into two main groups, conductive and sensorineural. More specific definitions of damage localization along the auditory pathway, according to a better diagnostic evaluation, provide a more detailed subdivision of the impairments. The "sensorineural" term is related to disease or deformity of the inner ear/cochlear nerve with an air-bone gap < 15 dB; "neural" refers to pathology of the cochlear nerve; "sensory" means a cochlear disease or deformity. A combined involvement of the outer/middle ears and the inner ear, characterized by >20 dB HL in the bone conduction and associated with >15 dB air-bone gap, is defined as "mixed" impairment. A "central" impairment is due to a disease localized in the central nervous system above the cochlear nerve. This classification appears to be useful in clinical practice. However, a nosological point of view does not fully respect the impact of hearing impairment on individual participation in social life and on quality of life, when health intervention must be planned.

For this reason, several epidemiological studies refer to "permanent" hearing impairment in the better ear and for frequencies ranging from 0.5 to 4 KHz, which are essential for understanding speech. The World Health Organisation (WHO) considers losses of 41 dB or greater in the better ear, for adults, and 31 dB, for children, as disabling impairments.

From a rehabilitative point of view, classifications based on period of acoustic deprivation (permanent/transient), grade of impairment, and age of onset of hearing loss (prenatal, perinatal, postnatal) are adopted.

Grades of hearing impairment (ANSI)
   Mild, 15–30 dB HL
   Moderate, 31–60
   Severe, 61–89
   Profound, 90 or greater
Grades of hearing impairment (WHO)
   No impairment, 25 dB or better
   Slight, 26–40 dB
   Moderate, 41–60 dB
   Severe, 61–80 dB
   Profound, 81 dB or greater
Grades of hearing impairment (EU)
   Mild, over 20 and less than 40 dB
   Moderate, over 40 and less than 70 dB
   Severe, over 70 and less than 95 dB
   Profound, equal to and over 95 dB

Permanent childhood hearing impairments (PCHI) are traditionally classified according to etiology as congenital or acquired (Table 1). Congenital hearing impairment is present at birth, owing to exogenous factors or endogenous-genetic factors, while acquired loss occurs after birth. Based on age of onset and developmental conditions present at the time of hearing deterioration, hearing impairment is classified as pre-, peri-, or postnatal and pre-, peri-, or postverbal.

Global phenotypic expression of the causative factors of hearing loss may involve different systems and organs, with association of signs in recognizable syndromes. Syndromic hearing impairment and isolated non-syndromic hearing impairment are defined. Many syndromes are caused by single gene defects and therefore can be inherited; others, such as Goldenhar's syndrome, are due to exogenous agents and are not hereditable. On the other hand, a hereditary syndrome that includes hearing loss does not necessarily show the defect, owing to the variability of gene expression, but it can be hereditable.

Some misunderstandings between definitions of audiological terms and subdivisions of etiologies still occur. Concerning prenatal causes, "congenital" and "hereditary" mean different conditions. Causes affecting pregnancy, due to exogenous agents, such as rubella, are congenital, not hereditary. Cytomegalovirus infections occur in pregnancy and can cause a delayed hearing damage, defined as progressive hearing loss. In the same

Table 1 Classification of Hearing Impairment by Etiology

Congenital (prenatal)	
Nongenetic	Infections (toxoplasmosis, cytomegalovirus, rubella, AIDS, HSV)
	Ototoxic drugs
	Metabolic disorders
Genetic	Syndromicic
	Non syndromic
Acquired	
Perinatal	Hypoxia
	Hyperbilirubinemia
	Infections
	Prematurity, low weight
Postnatal	Meningitis
	Otitis media
	Viral infections (parotitidis, measles, CMV)
	Noise exposure
	Trauma
Genetic delayed	Progressive hereditary

way, some of the most common types of hereditary hearing impairment are progressive, not present at birth.

II. EPIDEMIOLOGY

A. Prevalence

Prevalence is defined as the total number of subjects with a specific condition in a given population at a specific time. The number of individuals affected by hearing impairment is calculated from population-based national surveys. These data are essential in planning programs for prevention and management of hearing loss. Based on the WHO classification, disabling hearing impairment in children under 15 years of age is defined as a permanent hearing threshold level for the better ear of 31 dB or greater, averaged for the four frequencies 0.5, 1, 2, and 4 kHz. Above this grade of impairment, the WHO recommends hearing aids to preserve communication skills and social integration of these patients. Moreover, a standard classification and an epidemiologically valid methodology are needed to compare data between different countries and to describe the proportion of causes.

In 1995, WHO estimated at least 120 million of hearing impaired people worldwide, with a global prevalence of 2.1%. More than a half of these people were from developing countries.

In a European Economic Community (EEC) study of 1969 cohorts, prevalence estimates for hearing impairment $\geq$ 50 dB in the better ear of 0.9/1000 were found (see Table 2) (1,5,7,8,11–18). In recent studies, the prevalence estimates vary from 0.5 to 4.2/1000 in European countries (2–4).

In Estonia, the estimated prevalence (5) of permanent childhood hearing impairment $\geq$ 40 dB BEHL, birth cohort 1985–1990, was calculated as 172 per 100.000 live births. Concerning the prevalence of profound hearing impairment (4), the overall prevalence was 0.41/1000 and 0.45/1000 live births in Wales and in Denmark, respectively, in the same birth cohort (1975–1980). The proportion of inherited hearing loss is 47–50% in the two countries. A prevalence rate of severe to profound PCHI in 0.24/1000 live birth was found in the Trent region (6).

According to a universal neonatal hearing screening in the United Kingdom, prevalence is 1/1000 live births and increases until the age of 9 years (7); after birth, 50–90% more children are unpredictably diagnosed in the following 10 years. Parving found a prevalence estimate of 1–1.5/1000 live births. The increase in the estimated prevalence of hearing impairment in childhood, reaching at least 3.6–8.2/1000 of live births at 5–9 years of age, was observed (8).

According to a large population study from Great Britain (9), the prevalence of hearing impairments in the adult population is 18% and increases as a function of age, in particular over 70 years. The tendency of the proportion of the elderly to increase in the future has been well known in developed countries (10). Projections of recent studies, in Finnish and English populations, suggest that the number of all hearing-impaired people is expected to increase (9) in the developed countries.

1. Prevalence of Hearing Impairment in Specific Subgroups

The global prevalence of PCHI is low in developed countries; however, in specific subgroups of children, higher prevalence estimates than those reported for the overall population are found (Table 3).

A high prevalence of hearing impairment was found in neonatal intensive care units (NICU). In these studies (9,19,20), hearing impairment was reported to be 20–100 times greater than in the well-baby population. A wide variability between studies was observed, probably depending on different criteria for access to special care units and on the combination of different risk factors.

Particular syndromes with craniofacial malformations, such as Down syndrome, are characterized by inner or middle ear anomalies. In these

Table 2 Prevalence of Hearing Impairment (1,5,7,8,11–18)

Author	Prevalence/1000	Cohorts	Population	Grade dB	Country
Developed countries					
Martin, 1981	0.9	1969	Children	≥50	EEC
Maki Torkko, 1998	1.2	1973–1982		≥40	
		1983–1992			
Parving, 1999 (8)	1–1.5		Newborns	≥40	
	3.6–8.2		5–9 years		
Uus, 2000 (5)	1.72	1985–1990		≥40	Estonia
	0.15 (congenital)				
Streppel, 2000 (12)	0.43		School-aged	≥25	Germany
Dalzell, 2000	2.0		Newborns		NY State, U.S.A.
Neckham, 2001	1.27	1980–1994	Newborns	Moderate	Tyrol
Fortnum, 2001 (7)	0.91	1980–1995	3 years	≥40	UK
	1.65		9–16 years		
Developing countries					
Liu, 2001 (13)	0.67		<15 years		China
	12.8		60 years		
Prasansuk, (14)	3.5	1988–2000	Children		Thailand
Hadjikakou, 2000 (15)	1.19 congenital	1979–1996		≥50	Cyprus
	0.4 acquired				
Elahi, 1998 (16)	7.9		5–15 years	≥31	Pakistan

Table 3 Prevalence of Hearing Impairment in Specific Subgroups

Author	Speech delay, %	NICU, %	VLBW + seizure
Douniadakis, 2001	27.4		
Davis, 1992		3.5	
Salamy, 1989		5.0	
Bergman, 1985			28.6

patients the prevalence of PCHI is high. Hearing impairments are mostly mild, but severe and profound cases are also observed.

The incidence of hearing impairment in children with speech delay was higher than the one found in the general population (21).

2. Risk Factors

Concerning risk factors identified by the Joint Committee of Infant Screening (25) in recent studies, three factors were found to be significant: craniofacial abnormalities, low birth weight (less than 1500 g), and a familial history of hearing loss (22,23). The risk factor associated with the highest incidence of hearing loss was stigmata of syndromes (22). In this study, of 3000 children, a critical review of risk factors was presented. Only a small percentage of infants with a conventional risk indicator for hearing loss actually presented a hearing loss; in contrast, a significant number of hearing impairments without a risk indicator was found. In NICU population the four most common risk factors were ototoxic medications, very low birth weight, assisted ventilation > 5 days, and low APGAR scores. In contrast, in the well-baby nurseries only few risk factors were present: family history, craniofacial abnormalities, low APGAR scores, syndromes, ototoxic drugs, and congenital infections. These data suggest that risk factors, as identified by JCIH raccomendation, reflect the specific condition of the NICU population and do not correspond to actual causes of well-baby population.

B. Age of Identification

Although universal agreement exists about the need of an early identification of hearing impairment (20,26,27), identifying children with significant losses at an early age has proved to be difficult. In an EEC study of deafness on 1970–1980 birth cohorts, only 55% of children affected by 50-dB permanent hearing loss were identified within 3 years of age (1,26).

III. ETIOLOGY

Inherited hearing impairments account for more than 50–70% of PCHI (Table 4).

Acquired causes represent up to 40% of all factors (5,9). In some cases hearing impairment is not isolated, and additional disabilities in 23% are found. In some reports, 32% of all PCHI are progressive (29).

Thirty-five percent of all permanent hearing impairments in Germany are caused genetically and 20% are acquired (28). Causes are unknown in 45%.

Where the cause is known, genetic causes are most common, followed by infections. In these studies, genetic factors appear to be the most important cause of PCHI in developed countries, with greater incidence than was found in the last decade, probably owing to better identification. Mutations of the connexin 26 *GJB2* gene have been found to account for about up to 50% of recessive nonsyndromal prelingual sensorineural hearing impairment (34–40).

About 30% of all genetic syndromes are associated with hearing impairment, characterized by different kinds of anomalies: craniofacial, cardiovascular, musculoskeletal, and others. In these syndromes, the eyes, central nervous system, and musculoskeletal system are often involved (41).

Much sensorineural hearing loss is of unknown cause (2–45% of all cases).

Serous otitis media is the most common cause of mild hearing loss in children, affecting up to two-thirds of preschool children.

Table 4 Relative Prevalence of Causes (1,4,5,30–36)

Author	Genetic	Syndromic, %	Hereditary, isolated, %	Perinatal, %	Unknown, %
Fraser, 1976	40.9			11.8	10.5
Martin, 1981	9			15	41
Parving, 1983	33			14	25
Upfold, 1988	23			4.8	42
Das, 1988	18.7			15.5	35.5
Dias, 1990	22.8			15.9	28.6
Fortnum, 1997	41			10	2
Uus, 2000	36	2		11	34
Gross, 2001	35	8.9			45
Neckham, 2001		8	22	19	36

A. Changes

In longitudinal studies between comparable cohorts (32), born in 1969–1977 and 1979–1987, a significant increase in congenital inherited hearing impairment, from 29% to 43%, was found. The perinatal acquired PCHI have shown a notable change during the last years regarding etiology and prevalence. Congenital rubella has been eliminated in developed countries and in those where national vaccination campaigns have been implemented.

In contrast, other infections, such as cytomegalovirus (CMV) and toxoplasmosis, and alcoholic fetal syndrom tend to increase, probably owing to an increased number of survivors in neonatal intensive care units (NICU) and better identification.

The age of identification of PCHI has improved over the years; in developed countries, the expansion of audiological services and implementation of universal screening have produced a significant reduction of age of diagnosis of moderate, severe, or profound bilateral hearing impairments. However, the age of identification of those children with unilateral hearing loss or with bilateral PCHI of mild degree remains over 5 years.

B. Perinatal Causes

1. Aminoglycosidis

Ototoxic drugs have been identified as causative factors of PCHI. In recent studies these do not appear to be strictly related to hearing damage, compared to previous reports. Among very preterm babies, the coexistence of risk factors for hearing loss may be more important than the individual factors themselves (42). Sensorineural (SNHL) was more likely if bilirubin levels coexisted with netilmicin use or if acidosis occurred when bilirubin levels were high. Aminoglycosidis is not an important risk factor when serum levels are monitored (26).

2. Prematurity

Many children born as extremely preterm (< 25 weeks) have neurological and developmental disabilities (43). Prematurity causes a high risk of hearing impairment, often associated with additional handicaps; severe disability is common among children born as "fragile infant." In a longitudinal study (44) on very preterm and very low-birth-weight babies (VLBW), the prevalence of sensorineural hearing loss present at 5 years of age was 15 times as high as in normal children of the same age. Birth weight between 1000 and 1500 g and gestational age <31 weeks, in particular the NICU population, are predictive indicators for hearing impairment (25). On the other hand, improved medical treatment in a NICU reduces the probability of hearing impairment.

3. CMV and Other Viral Infections

CMV infection is the most frequent cause of congenital infection in both phenotypes, symptomatic and asymptomatic, occurring in 0.4–2.3% of live births (45). In developed countries, CMV infection is the only relevant viral agent of sensorineural hearing loss, because of vaccination campaigns for rubella, measles, and mumps in the last decade (43). Hearing loss consequent to this infection can show a delayed onset or progressive deterioration of hearing, necessitating long-term clinical follow-up. Less than half of all congenital SNHL, CMV infection is present at birth (46). Late-onset hearing loss occurs throughout the first 6 years of life, with a cumulative incidence of 15.4%. Both asymptomatic and symptomatic infection develop SNHL, in 7.4% and 40.7% of cases, respectively (47,48). In the symptomatic group, CT scan abnormalities are present in 70% of cases, usually developing at least one neurological sequela, also associated with SNHL (46,49).

C. Meningitis

Meningitis is responsible in 4–10% of all cases of sensorineural hearing loss, 37% of perinatal cases (50–52) (4%, Newton, 1885; 4.2%, Drake, 2000, 7%, Parving, 1985; 10%, Derekoy, 2000; 37% among perinatal hearing losses in Martin, 1982), also depending on collection criteria (overall or selected population, date of reports, and timing of clinical evaluation). The infection causes hearing loss by affecting the labyrinth, spreading from the meninges through aqueductus cochleae, or damaging the cochlear nerve as in crypto-coccal meningitis (53). Common agents are *Streptococcus pneumoniae*, *Hemophilus influenzae*, *Escherichia coli*, viral agents (mumps and measles), and rarely tuberculosis (54); 10–28% of patients with bacterial meningitis develop sensorineural hearing loss as a sequela (55). Hearing loss is usually bilateral and severe (55,57; 63% in Yeat, 58); there have been cases of unilateral and mild hearing loss. Negative prognostic indicators for hearing are considered coma and cranial computerized tomography alterations (52).

Labyrinthus ossificans is described as a sequela of meningitis and needs early intervention for cochlear implant. On the other hand, cases of sponta-neous recovery of sensorineural hearing loss have been observed (59), with partial or complete recovery, suggesting the need for repeated audiological assessments in children affected by bacterial meningitis. Deafness may be progressive, causing a long-term deterioration of hearing (60). Dexamethasone may be beneficial in some cases of bacterial meningitis in adults; neurological complications with hearing loss are less frequent in patients treated with dexamethasone (61,62). Steroids play a role in preventing the development of labyrinthus ossificans even in children with pneumococcal meningitis. Recently the antipneumococcal vaccine has effectively prevented this infection.

In "meningitis belt" countries, in middle, west, and central Africa, meningococcal infection represents the most common cause of severe to profound hearing loss (63–65). Epidemic meningitis is frequent in the overall population, causing death and neurological damage; *Hemophilus influenzae* is most dangerous in children under 12 months of age, causing up to 50% of death in a long-term period. In sub-Saharan Africa, many thousands of survivors annually suffer severe to profound hearing loss. In Gambia, endemic childhood meningitis has many severe sequelae, including hearing loss, in 29% of pneumococcal survivors and 9% of *Hemophilus* survivors (65).

D. Unilateral Hearing Loss

Permanent unilateral hearing impairment is considered a risk factor concerning speech and learning acquisition. An early-onset, severe unilateral hearing loss in children may be associated with academic or behavioral problems in school (31%, Omaha study, 67). It may represent one-third of all PCHI (66) > 25 dB HL. Unilateral defect is often found to be severe or profound (10% in Brookhouser, 67). It is characterized by a delayed diagnosis (> 5 years) and a difficult identification of causes (34–60% unknown).

IV. EPIDEMIOLOGY AND ETIOLOGY OF HEARING IMPAIRMENT IN DEVELOPING COUNTRIES

The proportion of hearing impairment is estimated to be wider in developing countries than in developed countries (15–18). However, the number of people affected in these countries is not yet known, because of a lack of valid epidemiological surveys. Little information is available about prevalence estimates and proportion of causes. In most cases, applied criteria for classification and diagnosis of hearing loss are not standard. WHO estimated that at least 78 million people have disabling hearing impairment in the developing countries (63). In a recent survey, conducted on a randomly selected sample of the WHO protocol in four developing countries, the prevalences are more than twice as great as the global result of 2.1% in the world. This result points out that prevalences of hearing impairment in the world could be largely underestimated. A total of 12–17% of children under 5 years of age were estimated to be affected by permanent hearing loss, owing to poor conditions of life and lack of availability of ear care services. It has been estimated that 50% of the causes of hearing impairment, such as chronic otitis media (COM), could be fully prevented. Some causes of deafness are due to poor health intervention; other causes vary by region. In some regions meningitis is an endemic infection; in other regions consanguineous marriages are common, increasing the occurrence of inherited deafness. In the Indian school population inhertited deafness was found in up to 80%, owing to common marriage between first cousins. In Pakistan 70% of severe PCHI was the result of marriage between cousins. COM probably represents the major cause of mild to moderate hearing impairment, related to poverty in developing countries and to disadvantaged ethnic groups in developed countries. Congenital exogenous and perinatal problems, such as rubella, asphyxia, and use of ototoxic drugs, show a high to moderate frequency and are considered preventable causes. In the majority of undeveloped countries, vaccination has not been undertaken and rubella remains a significant cause of congenital problems. Syphilis is present in several part of the world and it is associated with a high risk of congenital hearing impairment. The lack of preventive care during pregnancy and delivery causes a globally high mortality and morbidity in newborns. Infections, birth trauma, and rhesus incompatibility remain frequent causes of perinatal hearing loss.

REFERENCES

1. Martin J. Childhood deafness in the European Community. Scan Audio 1981; 10:165–174.
2. Davidson J, Hyde ML, Alberti PW. Epidemiology of hearing impairment in childhood. Scand Audiol Suppl 1988; 30:13–20.
3. Parving A. Hearing International and the promotion of ear care programs: Baltic countries and Eastern Europe. Scand Audiol Suppl 1997; 45:33–34.
4. Uus K, Davis AC. Epidemiology of permanent childhood hearing impairment in Estonia, 1985-1990. Audiolgy 2000 Jul-Aug; 39(4):192–197.
5. Parving A, Stephens D. Profound permanent hearing impairment in childhood: causative factors in two European countries. Acta Otolaryngol 1997 Mar; 117(2):158–160.
6. Fortnum H, Davis A. Epidemiology of permanent childhood hearing impairment in Trent Region, 1985–1993. Br J Audiol 1997 Dec; 31(6):409–446.
7. Fortnum HM, Summerfield AQ, Marshall DH, Davis AC, Bamford JM. Prevalence of permanent childhood hearing impairment in the United Kingdom and implications for universal neonatal hearing screening: questionnaire based ascertainment study. BMJ 2001 Sep; 323(7312):536–540.

8. Parving A. Hearing screening—aspects of epidemiology and identification of hearing impaired children. Int J Pediatr Otorhinolaryngol 1999 Oct 5; 49(suppl 1):S287–S292.

9. Davis A, Wood S. The epidemiology of childhood hearing impairment: factor relevant to planning of services. Br J Audiol 1992 Apr; 26(2):77–90.

10. Uimonen S, Huttunen K, Jounio-Ervasti K, Sorri M. Do we know the real need for hearing rehabilitation at the population level? Hearing impairments in the 5- to 75-year-old cross-sectional Finnish population. Br J Audiol 1999 Feb; 33 (1):53–59.

11. Maki-Torkko EM, Jarvelin MR, Sorri MJ, Muhli AA, Oja HF. Aetiology and risk indicators of hearing impairments in a one-year birth cohort for 1985-86 in northern Finland. Scand Audiol 1998; 27(4):237–247.

12. Streppel M, Richling F, Walger M, von Wedel H, Eckel HE. Epidemiology of hereditary hearing disorders in childhood: a retrospective study in Germany with special regard to ethnic factors. Scand Audiol 2000; 29(1):3–9.

13. Dalzell L, Orlando M, MacDonald M, Berg A, Bradley M, Cacace A, Campbell D, DeCristofaro J, Gravel J, Greenberg E, Gross S, Pinheiro J, Regan J, Spivak L, Stevens F, Prieve B. The New York State universal newborn hearing screening demonstration project: ages of hearing loss identification, hearing aid fitting, and enrollment in early intervention. Ear Hear 2000 Apr; 21(2):118–130.

14. Nekahm D, Weichbold V, Welzl Mueller K, Hirst-Stadlmann A. Improvement in early detection of congenital hearing impairment due to universal newborn hearing screening. Int J Pediatr Otorhinolaryngol 2001 May 31; 59(1): 23–28.

15. Liu XZ, Xu LR, Hu Y, Nance WE, Sismanis A, Zhang SL, Xu Y. Epidemiological studies on hearing impairment with reference to genetic factors in Sichuan, China. Ann Otol Rhinol Laryngol 2001 Apr; 110(4):356–363.

16. Prasansuk S. Incidence/prevalence of sensorineural hearing impairment in Thailand and Southeast Asia. Audiology 2000 Jul-Aug; 39(4):207–211.

17. Hadjikakou K, Bamford J. Prevalence and age of identification of permanent childhood hearing impairment in Cyprus. Audiology 2000 Jul–Aug; 39(4):198–201.

18. Elahi MM, Elahi F, Elahi A, Elahi SB. Paediatric hearing loss in rural Pakistan. J Otolaryngol 1998 Dec; 27(6):348–353.

19. Bergman I, Hirsch RP, Fria TJ, Shapiro SM, Holzman I, Painter MJ. Cause of hearing loss in the high-risk premature infant. J Pediatr 1985 Jan; 106(1):95–101.

20. Salamy A, Eldredge L, Tooley WH. Neonatal status and hearing loss in high-risk infants. J Pediatr 1989 May; 114(5):847–852.

21. Douniadakis DE, Kalli KI, Psarommatis IM, Tsakanikos MD, Apostolopoulos NK. Incidence of hearing loss among children presented with speech-language delay. Scand Audiol Suppl 2001; (52):204–205.

22. Ayache S, Kolski C, Stramandinoli E, Leke A, Krim G, Strunski V. Neonatal deafness screening with the evoked otoacoustic emissions technique. Study of 320 newborns at the neonatal resuscitation service of the Amiens neonatal care unit. Ann Otolaryngol Chir Cervicofac 2001 Apr; 118(2):89–94.

23. Cone-Wesson B, Vohr BR, Sininger YS, Widen JE, Folsom RC, Gorga MP, Norton SJ. Identificatoin of neonatal hearing impairment: infants with hearing loss. Ear Hear 2000 Oct; 21(5):488–507.

24. Vohr BR, Widen JE, Cone-Wesson B, Sininger YS, Gorga MP, Folsom RC, Norton SJ. Identification of neonatal hearing impairment: characteristics of infants in the neonatal intensive care unit and well-baby nursery. Ear Hear 2000 Oct; 21(5):373–382.

25. Joint Committee of Infant Hearing. Position statement. Pediatrics 1995; 100: 152–156.

26. Yoshinaga-Itano C, Apuzzo ML. Identification of hearing loss after age 18 months is not early enough. Am Ann Deaf 1998 Dec; 143(5):380–387.

27. Yoshinaga-Itano C, Sedey AL, Coulter DK, Mehl AL. Language of early- and later-identified children with hearing loss. Pediatrics 1998 Nov; 102(5): 1161–1171.

28. Finckh-Kramer U, Spormann-Lagodzinski M, Gross M. German registry for hearing loss in children results after 4 years. Int J Pediatr Otorhinolaryngol 2000 Dec; 56(2):113–127.

29. Walch C, Anderhuber W, Kole W, Berghold A. Bilateral sensorineural hearing disorders in children: etiology of deafness and evaluation of hearing tests. Int J Pediatr Otorhinolaryngol 2000 Jun 9; 53(1):31–38.

30. Gross M, Finckh-Kramer U, Spormann-Lagodzinski M. Congenital hearing disorders in children. 1: Acquired hearing disorders. HNO 2000 Dec; 48(12):879–886. Review. German.

31. Fraser G. The causes of profound deafness in childhood, Ballière Tindall, 1976.

32. Parving A, Hauch AM. The causes of profound hearing impairment in a school for the deaf-a longitudinal study. Br J Audiol 1994 Apr; 28(2):63–69.

33. Holten A, Parving A. Aetiology of hearing disorders in children at the schools for the deaf. Int J Pediatr Otorhinolaryngol 1985 Dec; 10(3):229–236.

34. Upfold LJ. Children with hearing aids in the 1980s: etiologies and severity of impairment. Ear Hear 1988 Apr; 9(2):75–80.

35. Das V. Bilateral sensorineural deafness in children. J Laryngol Otol 1988; 102: 975–980.

36. Dias O. Surdez infantil: estudo clìnico e epidemiologico, Lisboa: Eurolitho Ed.

37. Estiviel X, Fortina P, Surrey S, Rabionet R, Melchionda S, D'Agruma L, Mansfield E, Rappaport E, Govea N, Mila M, Zelante L, Gasparini P. Connexin-26 mutations in sporadic and inherited sensorineural deafness. Lancet 1998 Feb 7; 351(9100):394–398.

38. Denoyelle F, Marlin S, Weil D, Moatti L, Chauvin P, Garabedian EN, Petit C. Clinical features of the prevalent form of childhood deafness, DFNB1, due to a connexin-26 gene defect: implications for genetic counselling. Lancet 1999 Apr 17; 353(9161):1298–1303.

39. Orzan E, Polli R, Martella M, Vinanzi C, Leonardi M, Murgia A. Molecular genetics applied to clinical practice: the Cx26 hearing impairment. Br J Audiol 1999 Oct; 33(5):291–295.

40. Tekin M, Akar N, Cin S, Blanton SH, Xia XJ, Liu XZ, Nance WE, Pandya A. Connexin 26 (GJB2) mutations in the Turkish population: implications for the

origin and high frequency of the 35delG mutation in Caucasians. Hum Genet 2001 May; 108(5):385–389.

41. Gorlin RJ, Toriello HV, Cohen MM. Hereditary hearing loss and its syndromes. New York: Oxford University Press, 1995.

42. Marlow ES, Hunt LP, Marlow N. Sensorineural hearing loss and prematurity. Arch Dis Child Fetal Neonatal Ed 2000 Mar; 82(2):F141–F144.

43. Wood NS, Marlow N, Costeloe K, Gibson AT, Wilkinson AR. Neurologic and developmental disability after extremely pretern birth. EPICure Study Group. N Engl J Med. 2000 Aug 10; 343(6):378–384.

44. Veen S, Sassen ML, Schreuder AM, Ens-Dokkum MH, Verloove-Vanhorick SP, Brand R, Grote JJ, Ruys JH. Hearing loss in very preterm and very low birhtweight infants at the age of 5 years in a nationwide cohort. Int J Pediatr Otorhinolaryngol 1993 Feb; 26(1):11–28.

45. Witters I, Van Ranst M, Fryns JP. Cytomegalovirus reactivation in pregrnancy and subsequent isolated bilateral hearing loss in the infant. Genet Couns 2000; 11:375–378.

46. Lagasse N, Dhooge I, Govaert P. Congenital CMV-infection and hearing loss. Acta Otorhinolaryngol Belg 2000; 54(4):431–436 (Review).

47. Fowler KB, Dahle AJ, Boppana SB, Pass RF. Newborn hearing screening: will children with hearing loss caused by congenital cytomegalovirus infection be missed? Pediatr 1999 Jul; 135(1):60–64.

48. Dahle AJ, Fowler KB, Wright JD, Boppana SB, Britt WJ, Pass RF. Longitudinal investigation of hearing disorders in children with congenital cytomegalovirus. J Am Acad Audiol 2000 May; 11(5):283–290.

49. Boppana SB, Fowler KB, Vaid Y, Hedlund G, Stagno S, Britt WJ, Pass RF. Neuroradiographic findings in the newborn period and long-term outcome in children with symptomatic congenital cytomegalovirus infection. Pediatrics 1997 Mar; 99(3):409–414.

50. Newton VE. Aetiology of bilateral sensori-neural hearing loss in young children. J Laryngol Otol 1985; 10:1–57.

51. Drake R, Dravitski J, Voss L. Hearing in children after meningococcal meningitis. J Paediatr Child Health 2000 Jun; 36(3):240–243.

52. Derekoy FS. Etiology of deafness in Afyon school for the deaf in Turkey. Int J Pediatr Otorhinolaryngol 2000 Sep; 55(2):125–131.

53. Low WK. Cryptococcal meningitis: implications for the otologists. ORL J Otorhinolaryngol Relat Spec 2002 Jan-Feb; 64(1):35–37.

54. Kotnis R, Simo R. Tuberculous meningitis presenting as sensorineural hearing loss. J Laryngol Otol 2001 Jun; 115(6):491–492.

55. Couto MI, Monteiro SR, Lichtig I, Casella EB, Carvallo RM, de Navarro JM. Audiological assessment and follow-up after bacterial meningitis. Arq Neurosiquiatr 1999 Sep; 57(3B):808–812.

56. Mencia Bartolome S, Casado Flores J, Marin Barba C, Gonzalez-Vicent M, Ruiz Lopez MJ. Pneumococcal meningitis in children. Review of 28 cases. An Esp Pediatr 2000 Aug; 53(2):94–99.

57. Neuman A, Molinelli P, Hochberg I. Post-meningitic hearing loss: report on three cases. J Commun Disord 1981 Mar; 14(2):105–111.

58. Yeat SW, Mukari SZ, Said H, Motilal R. Post meningitic sensori-neural hearing loss in children—alterations in hearing level. Med J Malaysia 1997 Sep; 285–290.

59. Marx RD, Baer ST. Spontaneous recovery of profound post-meningitic hearing loss. J Laryngol Otol 2001 May; 115(5):412–414.

60. Jayarajan V, Rangan S. Delayed deterioration of hearing following bacterial meningitis. J Laryngol Otol 1999 Nov; 113(11):1011–1014.

61. Gijwani D, Kumhar MR, Singh VB, Chadda VS, Soni PK, Nayak KC, Gupta BK. Dexamethasone therapy for bacterial meningitis in adults: a double blind placebo control study. Neurol India 2002 Mar; 50(1):63–67.

62. Hartnick CJ, Kim HY, Chute PM, Parisier SC. Preventing labyrinthitis ossificans: the role of steroids. Arch Otolaryngol Head Neck Surg 2001 Feb; 127(2):180–183.

63. Smith AW. WHO activities for prevention of deafness and hearing impairment in children. Scan Audiol Suppl 2001; (53):93–100.

64. Salih MA. Childhood acute bacterial meningitis in the Sudan: and epidemiological, clinical and laboratory study. Scand J Infect Dis Suppl 1990; 66:1–103.

65. Hodgson A, Smith T, Gagneux S, Akumah I, Adjuik M, Pluschke G, Binka F, Genton B. Survival and sequelae of meningococcal meningitis in Ghana. Int J Epidemiol 2001 Dec; 30(6):1440–1446.

66. Kiese-Himmel C, Kruse E. Unilateral hearing loss in childhood. An empirical analysis comparing bilateral hearing loss. Laryngorhinootologie 2001 Jan; 80(1):18–22.

67. Brookhouser PE, Worthington DW, Kelly WJ. Unilateral hearing loss in children. Laryngoscope 1991 Dec; 101(12 Pt 1):1264–1272.

4

Usher Syndrome

William J. Kimberling
Boys Town National Research Hospital, Omaha, Nebraska, U.S.A.

I. INTRODUCTION

Usher syndrome is the most common cause of combined neurosensory loss in the developed world. The hearing impairment is usually prelingual but the vision loss, due to retinitis pigmentosa, is gradual. The result is that more than 50% of all adults who are deaf and blind have Usher syndrome. Research into the causes of Usher syndrome has resulted in the recognition that at least 11 different genes are involved, of which six have been specifically identified. This knowledge is now proving helpful in the diagnosis of this interesting group of disorders. More important, the Usher syndromes are providing a window into the commonalities of the neurosensory processes of vision and hearing.

Usher syndrome is defined as an autosomal recessive hereditary disorder characterized by hearing loss and retinitis pigmentosa. It is clinically and genetically heterogeneous. There are three clinical types, I, II, and III: type I has a prelingual, profound hearing loss, prepubertal onset of the retinitis pigmentosa, and a vestibular areflexia; type II is has a milder hearing that which is more severe in the high frequencies than in the lower; type III has a progressive hearing loss (34). Type I individuals consider themselves deaf and typically grow up in the deaf culture relying on sign language as the main mode of communication while type II individuals consider themselves to be "hard of hearing" and typically use oral communication. Also, Usher type II persons do not have vestibular problems. Usher type I and II comprise over 90% of all Usher cases in the United States and most of Europe (except Finland). Usher type III has a progressive hearing loss, with an onset usually in childhood, progressing more rapidly in the high frequencies (21,31). As children or young adults, the audiograms of Usher III persons look like those of type II but as they age, the hearing deteriorates into the severe-to-profound range typical of Usher type I; it is believed that Usher III individuals also develop vestibular areflexia over time. These distinctions between type I, II, and III are not perfect and there are a few cases that are intermediate (5,24,25). A subset of atypical type I cases have profound prelingual hearing loss and walk at a normal age showing a normal vestibular response (30). Some atypical type II individuals have been reported to have subnormal vestibular responses and others have demonstrated a progressive hearing loss (24,37,40).

At least 11 different genes have been identified, each responsible for a different subtype. For the most, mutations in each gene produce a fairly consistent phenotype, but there are interesting exceptions, discussed below. Usher type I has been found to be associated with four different mutations at genes *MYO7A*(11q), *HARM*(11p), *CDH23*(10q), and *PCDH15*(10q) (2,11,38,43). The *USH2A* and *USH3* genes have also been identified (13,19). These six genes harbor mutations that cause each of the three clinical Usher types. About one-third of all Usher cases are due to genes that remain to be identified. The locations of four of these have been found: 3p (Usher IIb), 5q (Usher IIc), 14q (Usher Ia), 21q (Usher If), and 17q (Usher Ig) (12,16,20,29,32). Usher IId has been tentatively recognized by virtue of its lack of linkage to the regions know to contain the other Usher genes (32). The appears to be a certain degree of phenotypic specificity for the molecular subtypes (5,17), but there is also considerable overlap.

II. USHER TYPES

A. Usher Type Ib

Usher type Ib is due to mutations in the gene *MYO7A* on chromosome 11q (43). *MYO7A* encodes the protein myosin VIIa, a molecular motor that moves along actin filaments using energy obtained from the hydrolysis of ATP. The myosin VIIa molecular consists of three major sections, the head, neck, and tail. The head is the motor domain and possesses the actin binding site as well as a site to catalyze ATP hydrolysis. The head region is highly conserved across different myosins. The neck region is composed of five isoleucine-glutamine (IQ) motifs, which are predicted to bind calmodulin. The tail differs from one type of myosin to another and is believed to confer binding specificity through its protein-protein interacting domains. Myosin VIIa has a motility that is calmodulin dependent and is mediated through an interaction with an actin filament (36).

Mutations throughout the Usher gene have been observed to produce Usher syndrome type I. The mouse model, sh-1, has been shown to also have mutations in the *myo7a* murine homolog (15,28). There are nine different mutant strains showing variable hearing deficit with vestibular disturbance. Interestingly, retinal dystrophy, to the degree seen in humans is lacking, although there is a reduction of ERG amplitudes in five strains (23). This suggested that some mutations in *MYO7A* might result in a nonsyndromic hearing loss, *DFNB2* (44). A few families with apparent *DFNB2* have been described (26,44), though one has since developed a retinal dystrophy in some of the family members (45). There is no pattern to the mutations that would suggest that certain domains are more critical to one sense organ rather than the other. Also, a few cases with Usher type II and III phenotypes have been reported with *MYO7A* mutations. However, it is unlikely that mutations in *MYO7A* cause a very high proportion of nonsyndromic deafness and there is the possibility that "*DFNB2*" may be Usher type I cases where the diagnosis of retinitis pigmentosa has been missed, because of mild expression (6). The most curious observation was that of a family of Japanese origin with a mutation in the coiled-coil domain with a dominantly inherited hearing loss (27). No other mutations causing frank Usher syndrome type I have been observed in the coiled-coil domain, which has the function of mediating the formation of homodimers. Still, there seem to be a good possibility that there is variation in the severity of expression of the retinal phenotype. If so, then the study of the origin of such variation could highlight environmental or background genetic factors that might be useful in the development of preventive therapies for the retinitis pigmentosa.

B. Usher Type Id

At least two Usher genes have been shown to be on chromosome 10q, and there is the possibility for a third (7,41,42). One of these genes has been identified as cadherin 23 (*CDH23*) and mutations in *CDH23* have been associated with a wide rang of phenotypes (5,10,11,39). In general, the tendency is that the more severe the mutation, the more severe the disorder. All nonsyndromic cases with mutations in *CDH23* had missense mutations, whereas the typical Usher I case had a higher proportion of nonsense mutations; milder atypical Usher I cases had an intermediate frequency of nonsense mutations . The data suggest severity of both the retinal and cochlear phenotypes is modulated by the severity of the mutation (5,10).

The gene consists of 69 coding exons that code for a predicted protein of 3354 amino acids (10,11). The cadherin 23 protein consists of a small intracellular domain, a long extracellular domain, and, of course, a transmembrane domain. The extracellular domain is composed of 27 extracellular cadherin (EC) repeats, most of which possess Ca2C-binding motifs characteristic of cadherins. These motifs may be responsible for mediating cell-cell adhesion through a calcium-dependent interaction with other. The single transmembrane domain is followed by a short 268-amino-acid cytoplasmic region. This cytoplasmic domain contains two PDZ-binding interfaces (PDI), which have been shown to interact with PDZ1 and PDZ2 domains of harmonin (33). There is alternative splicing, which allows for the inclusion of an additional 68 amino acids in the cochlear form vis-a-vis the retinal form. The added amino acids are believed to reduce the strength of the interaction of cadherin 23 internal PDI with PDZ1 of harmonin in the cochlea freeing the PDZ1 for other protein-protein interactions (33).

C. Usher Type If

Usher type If is due to mutation in the protocadherin 15 gene (2,4). These mutations produce a phenotype in both mouse and human that is similar to that produced by mutations in cadherin 23. The *PCDH15* gene is located close to the *CDH23* gene on chromosome 10q. Protocadherin 15 is a novel member of the cadherin superfamily. It has the same basic overall structure seen with cadherin 23, in that it possesses a large extracellular domain, a transmembrane domain, and a unique cytoplasmic domain with two highly conserved proline-rich regions. Proline-rich regions are known to serve as binding sites for several protein, among which are profilin, which regulates polymerization of actin filaments, and proteins containing SH3 and WW motifs, which participate in the assembly of signaling complexes (4). The pattern of expression in the inner ear indicates that protocadherin 15 protein lies in the stereocilia, suggesting. that it may participate in the cadherin 23/ harmonin complex (4).

Observation of stereociliary disruption of the Ames waltzer mouse suggests that protocadherin may play a role in the regulation of planar polarity, specifically in the orientation of the stereociliary bundle. Though also expressed in other areas of the cochlea, namely the supporting cells and outer sulcus cells as well as the spiral ganglion, the early morphological defect in the mouse appears to affect only the stereocilia, with preservation of the inner and outer cell bodies. The function in the retina is not well understood. But, it is expressed in human adult and fetal inner outer synaptic layers, in the nerve fiber layer, and, in just the adult, in the outer limiting membrane of photoreceptor inner segments (3,4).

D. Usher Type Ic

French Acadians have been known to have a high frequency of Usher type I, thought to be due to a founder effect (22). That type of Usher syndrome was found to genetically different from the Usher syndrome due to *MYO7A* mutations, and has been labeled Usher type Ic (35). A PDZ-containing protein coded for by a gene on chromosome 11p has been shown to be responsible for this type of Usher syndrome and the Acadian mutation has been identified as a 2916G > A affecting splicing (9,38). While mutations in *USH1C* are frequent in the French Acadians, Usher type Ic is not limited to that population. One mutation, 238insC, was detected in several European individuals (38) who shared a common haplotype, suggesting a common origin for that allele (46). Several other mutations have also been observed. The *USH1C* gene codes for several alternatively spliced transcripts. In the mouse, these transcripts correspond to at least eight harmonin isoforms, ranging from 420 to 910 amino acids in length (38). The protein consists of two or three PDZ domains, one or two coiled-coil domains, a PST (proline-serine-threonine) domain, and a PBI domain at the carboxy terminus.

E. Usher Type IIa

Usher type IIa is the mildest of the Usher syndromes identified to date. The hearing loss ranges from mild to moderate in the low frequencies to severe to profound in the higher frequencies. About 10% of patients with Usher II experience a progressive hearing loss, but the progression is slower than that seen with Usher type III. The retinitis pigmentosa is reported to be milder. Usher type II is probably the most common form of Usher syndrome, being twice as frequent as Usher type I in some patient series.

The *USH2A* gene is located on chromosome 1q41 and has been identified as encoding a novel protein with partial homology to the laminin protein group (13). The gene has 21 exons and the protein has 1546 amino acids. The protein has a signal peptide at the amino end, a thrombospondin domain, a laminin N-terminal module (LN) followed by a series of laminin-EGF-like domains, and four fibonectin modules. The protein has been given the name usherin. Usherin is found in association with collagen in basement membranes of the inner ear and retina and is believed to act either as a structural component of the basement membrane or as part of a signaling system between that and cells it supports. Missense mutations in the LE domain have been found to disrupt the binding of usherin to type IV collagen, demonstrating one mechanism whereby *USH2A* mutations can cause the Usher II phenotype (8).

F. Usher Type III

Usher syndrome type III (USH3) is unique among the three clinical subtypes of Usher syndrome in that it shows postlingual, progressive hearing
loss and late onset of retinitis pigmentosa, along with a progressive loss
of vestibular function. A relatively small, compared to the other Usher
genes, and novel gene was identified that was reported to have a limited
homology to stargazen, a four-transmembrane-domain protein present in
cerebellar synapses (1,18). Thus, it was postulated that clarin-1 may
function at the level of hair cell and photoreceptor synapses. The gene is
expressed in the retina, skeletal muscle, testis, and olfactory epithelium.
Specific expression of clarin-1 was also observed in the inner and outer hair
cells (1).

   Usher type II is common in the Finnish population. One mutation,
Y100X, was found to account for most of the Finnish cases (19). 144T > G
mutation was found to be responsible for the majority of cases of Usher III
seen in individuals of Askenazi descent (1,14). Overall, USH3 mutations
appear to be responsible for no more than 3% of all Usher cases.

G. Other Usher Types

Fives types of Usher syndrome are still unidentified. Usher type I loci are
know to exist on chromosomes 14q, 21q, and 17q (12,20,29). Two additional
Usher II loci are located on chromosome 3p and 5q (16,32).

III. CONCLUSIONS

Usher syndrome is the most common form of combined hearing and visual
impairment in Europe and the United States. As such, it causes a considerable
burden to society as well as to the individuals and families involved. Research
into the causes of this disorder is progressing at a rapid pace with identification of six of the 11 genes know to be involved. The identification of the
leads has led directly toward a better understanding of the underlying
mechanisms by which changes in these proteins cause this combined sensory
defect. Four of the proteins, usherin, harmonin, protocadherin 15, and clarin
1, are novel and the discovery of their very existence was predicated on
research into this rare disorder. The two other proteins, myosin VIIA and
cadherin 23, were know but their function in the ear and eye was not realized
until the discovery of the link between those genes and Usher syndrome.
Unraveling the roles of genes that impact on the two most important human
senses not only serves to push us further toward the development of effective

therapies but also provides new insights into the basic cell biology of vision and hearing.

REFERENCES

1. Adato A, et al. USH3A transcripts encode clarin-1, a four-transmembrane-domain protein with a possible role in sensory synapses. Eur J Hum Genet 2002; 10(6):339–350.
2. Ahmed ZM, et al. Mutations of the protocadherin gene PCDH15 cause Usher syndrome type 1F. Am J Hum Genet 2001; 69(1):25–34.
3. Alagramam KN, et al. The mouse Ames waltzer hearing-loss mutant is caused by mutation of Pcdh15, a novel protocadherin gene. Nat Genet 2001; 27(1):99–102.
4. Alagramam KN, et al. Mutations in the novel protocadherin PCDH15 cause Usher syndrome type 1F. Hum Mol Genet 2001; 10(16):1709–1718.
5. Astuto LM, et al. CDH23 Mutation and phenotype heterogeneity: a profile of 107 diverse families with Usher syndrome and nonsyndromic deafness ASTUTO2002. Am J Hum Genet 2002; 71(2):262–275.
6. Astuto LM, et al. Searching for evidence of DFNB2. Am J Med Genet 2002; 109(4):291–297.
7. Astuto LM, et al. Genetic heterogeneity of Usher syndrome: analysis of 151 families with Usher type I. Am J Hum Genet 2000; 67(6):1569–1574.
8. Bhattacharya G, et al. Localization and expression of usherin: a novel basement membrane protein defective in people with Usher's syndrome type IIa. Hearing Res 2002; 163(1–2):1–11.
9. Bitner-Glindzicz M, et al. A recessive contiguous gene deletion causing infantile hyperinsulinism, enteropathy and deafness identifies the Usher type 1C gene. Nat Genet 2000; 26(1):56–60.
10. Bolz H, et al. Mutation of CDH23, encoding a new member of the cadherin gene family, causes Usher syndrome type 1D. Nat Genet 2001; 27(1):108–112.
11. Bork JM, et al. Usher syndrome 1D and nonsyndromic autosomal recessive deafness DFNB12 are caused by allelic mutations of the novel cadherin-like gene CDH23. Am J Hum Genet 2001; 68(1):26–37.
12. Chaib H, et al. A newly identified locus for Usher syndrome type I, USH1E, maps to chromosome 21q21. Hum Mol Genet 1997; 6(1):27–31.
13. Eudy JD, et al. Mutation of a gene encoding a protein with extracellular matrix motifs in Usher syndrome type IIa. Science 1998; 280(5370):1753–1757.
14. Fields RR, et al. Usher syndrome type III: revised genomic structure of the USH3 gene and identification of novel mutations. Am J Hum Genet 2002; 71(3):607–617.
15. Gibson F, et al. A type VII myosin encoded by the mouse deafness gene shaker-1. Nature 1995; 374(6517):62–64.
16. Hmani M, et al. A novel locus for Usher syndrome type II, USH2B, maps to chromosome 3 at p23-24.2. Eur J Hum Genet 1999; 7(3):363–367.

17. Hmani-Aifa M, et al. Distinctive audiometric features between USH2A and USH2B subtypes of Usher syndrome. J Med Genet 2002; 39(4):281–283.

18. Joensuu T, et al. A sequence-ready map of the Usher syndrome type III critical region on chromosome 3q. Genomics 2000; 63(3):409–416.

19. Joensuu T, et al. Mutations in a novel gene with transmembrane domains underlie Usher syndrome type 3. Am J Hum Genet 2001; 63(3):673–684.

20. Kaplan J, et al. A gene for Usher syndrome type I (USH1A) maps to chromosome 14q. Genomics 1992; 14(4):979–987.

21. Karjalainen S, et al. Progressive hearing loss in Usher's syndrome. Ann Otol Rhinol Laryngol 1989; 98:863–866.

22. Kloepfer HW, Laguaite JK, McLaurin JW. The hereditary syndrome of congenital deafness and retinitis pigmentosa (Usher's syndrome). Laryngoscope 1966; 76:850–862.

23. Libby RT, Steel KP. Electroretinographic anomalies in mice with mutations in Myo7a, the gene involved in human Usher syndrome type 1B. Invest Ophthalmol Vis Sci 2001; 42(3):770–778.

24. Liu XZ, et al. A mutation (2314delG) in the Usher syndrome type IIA gene: high prevalence and phenotypic variation. Am J Hum Genet 1999; 64(4):1221–1225.

25. Liu XZ, et al. Mutations in the myosin VIIA gene cause a wide phenotypic spectrum, including atypical usher syndrome. Am J Hum Genet 1998; 63(3):909–912.

26. Liu XZ, et al. Mutations in the myosin VIIA gene cause non-syndromic recessive deafness. Nat Genet 1997; 16(2):188–190.

27. Liu XZ, et al. Autosomal dominant non-syndromic deafness caused by mutation in the myosin VIIA gene. Nat Genet 1997; 17:268–269.

28. Mburu P, et al. Mutation analysis of the mouse myosin VIIA deafness gene. Genes Funct 1997; 1(3):191–203.

29. Mustapha M, et al. A novel locus for Usher syndrome type I, USH1G, maps to chromosome 17q24-25. Hum Genet 2002; 110(4):348–350.

30. Otterstedde CR, et al. A new clinical classification for Usher's syndrome based on a new subtype of Usher's syndrome type I. Laryngoscope 2001; 110(4):84–86.

31. Pakarinen L, et al. Usher's syndrome type 3 in Finland. Laryngoscope 1995; 105(6):613–617.

32. Pieke-Dahl SA, et al. Genetic heterogeneity of Usher syndrome type II: localisation to chromosome 5q. J Med Genet 2000; 37(4):256–262.

33. Siemens J, et al. The Usher syndrome proteins cadherin 23 and harmonin form a complex by means of PDZ-domain interactions. Proc Natl Acad Sci USA 2002.

34. Smith RJ, et al. Clinical diagnosis of the Usher syndromes. Usher Syndrome Consortium. Am J Med Genet 1994; 50(1):32–38.

35. Smith RJ, et al. Localization of two genes for Usher syndrome type I to chromosome 11. Genomics 1992; 14(4):995–1002.

36. Udovichenko IP, Gibbs D, Williams DS. Actin-based motor properties of native myosin VIIa. J Cell Sci 2002; 115(Pt 2):445–450.

37. van Aarem A, et al. Stable and progressive hearing loss in type 2A Usher's syndrome. Ann Otol Rhinol Laryngol 1996; 105(12):962–967.

38. Verpy E, et al. A defect in harmonin, a PDZ domain-containing protein expressed in the inner ear sensory hair cells, underlies Usher syndrome type 1C. Nat Genet 2000; 26(1):51–55.

39. von Brederlow B, et al. Identification and in vitro expression of novel CDH23 mutations of patients with Usher syndrome type 1D. Hum Mutat 2002; 19(3): 268–273.

40. Wagenaar M, et al. Hearing impairment related to age in Usher syndrome types 1B and 2A. Arch Otolaryngol Head Neck Surg 1999; 125(4):441–445.

41. Wayne S, et al. Localization of the Usher syndrome type ID gene (Ush1D) to chromosome 10. Hum Mol Genet 1996; 5:1689–1692.

42. Wayne S, Lowry RB, McLeod DR, Knaus R, Farr C, Smith RJH. Localization of the Usher syndrome type IF to chromosome 10. Am J Hum Genet 1997; 61:A300.

43. Weil D, et al. Defective myosin VIIa gene responsible for Usher syndrome type 1B. Nature 1995; 374(6517):60–61.

44. Weil D, et al. The autosomal recessive isolated deafness, DFNB2, and the Usher 1B syndrome are allelic defects of the myosin-VIIA gene. Nat Genet 1997; 16(2):191–193.

45. Zina ZB, et al. From DFNB2 to Usher syndrome: variable expressivity of the same disease. Am J Med Genet 2001; 101(2):181–183.

46. Zwaenepoel I, et al. Identification of three novel mutations in the USH1C gene and detection of thirty-one polymorphisms used for haplotype analysis. Hum Mutat 2001; 17(1):34–41.

5
Pendred Syndrome

Shannon P. Pryor, Hong-Joon Park, Anne C. Madeo, and Andrew J. Griffith
National Institute on Deafness and Other Communication Disorders, National Institutes of Health, Rockville, Maryland, U.S.A.

John A. Butman
Warren G. Magnuson Clinical Center, National Institutes of Health, Bethesda, Maryland, U.S.A.

I. HISTORY AND EPIDEMIOLOGY

Pendred syndrome is named for Vaughan Pendred, who in 1896 described two siblings who were both goitrous and deaf (1). In 1927, Brain reported 12 similarly affected individuals in five families, and suggested an autosomal recessive pattern of inheritance (2). The sensivity for detection of the thyroid phenotype was significantly increased with the introduction of the perchlorate discharge test by Morgans and Trotter in 1958 (3). Fraser subsequently published his landmark epidemiological study in which he described the clinical features of 207 U.K. families with 334 cases of Pendred syndrome (4). He estimated the prevalence at 7.5–10 cases per 100,000 population and indicated that Pendred syndrome may be responsible for up to 10% of hereditary hearing impairment. Subsequent epidemiological estimates based on clinical diagnosis in diverse ethnic populations confirm that the syndrome comprises approximately 4–10% of prelingual deafness (5).

II. ETIOLOGY: PDS AND PENDRIN

In 1996, two independent studies demonstrated linkage of Pendred syndrome to short tandem repeat markers on chromosome 7q22-31.1 (6–8),

75

within the interval previously defined for the nonsyndromic recessive deafness locus *DFNB4*. Everett et al. used a positional cloning strategy to identify the *PDS/SLC26A4* gene at 7q31, and demonstrated that *PDS* mutations underlie most, if not all, cases of Pendred syndrome (9). *PDS* comprises 21 exons that encode an open reading frame of 2343 base pairs. Northern blot analysis of multiple tissues detected *PDS* mRNA in thyroid and kidney, and cochlear expression was inferred from detection of *PDS* by PCR analysis of a fetal cochlear cDNA library. The polypeptide product, pendrin, is 86 kDa and contains 780 amino acids. Li and colleagues subsequently reported a large, consanguineous Indian pedigree cosegregating homozygosity for a mutant *PDS* allele and nonsyndromic deafness (without goiter) at the *DFNB4* locus (10). Interestingly, reascertainment of the kindred originally used to map the DFNB4 locus revealed that the mutant phenotype included thyroid goiter (10).

III. PENDRIN FUNCTION

Pendrin appears to be a transmembrane protein with a long carboxy terminus, although the precise topology has yet to be experimentally determined. Whereas the computational algorithm PHDhtm predicts 11 transmembrane domains with an intracellular amino terminus and extracellular carboxy terminus (9), other programs predict 12 transmembrane domains with cytoplasmic termini (11), and at least one prediction algorithm (TMHMM 2.0) predicts only nine transmembrane domains. A cytoplasmic location of the carboxy terminus is supported by the results of immunofluorescence studies of permeabilized cells with antibodies to the carboxy terminus (12).

Pendrin was initially noted to have sequence similarity to a family of sulfate transporters (9), but subsequent electrophysiological studies of heterologously expressed pendrin have not detected sulfate transport activity (13–15). Similar heterologous expression studies have shown that it can transport iodide, chloride, formate, bicarbonate, and nitrate across plasma membranes in an energy- and sodium-independent manner (13,14,16,17). Scott and Karniski extended these conclusions, demonstrating that pendrin is thus capable of mediating chloride-formate exchange, an important step in the regulation of pH by the kidney (16).

A. Pendrin Function: Thyroid

In the thyroid, antipendrin antibodies specifically bind to the apical aspect of follicular thyrocytes (11,18). Pendrin was thus proposed to mediate the transport of iodide from folliculocytes across their apical membranes into the colloid where it is conjugated with thyroglobulin in the biosynthesis of thyroxine (8,11,19). Transport of iodide across the basolateral membrane into the folliculocyte is mediated in an energy-dependent fashion by the sodium-iodide symporter. The immunolocalization and observed iodide transport activity of pendrin strongly support a model in which *PDS* mutations reduce or prevent the transport of iodine into the thyroid follicle, thus inhibiting the efficient biosynthesis of thyroxine. Goiter is thought to result from compensatory hypertrophy of the thyroid follicles (4).

B. Pendrin Function: Kidney

In the kidney, a combination of immunolocalization and physiological studies utilizing isolated nephron preparations from *pds* knockout mice indicate that pendrin mediates bicarbonate secretion by non-alpha intercalated cells in the renal cortical collecting ducts (20–23). Although an abnormal renal phenotype has not been reported for humans or mice with *PDS* mutations, reduced base secretion capacity in the kidney may only be revealed with a metabolic alkali load that is so large that it exceeds the compensatory capacity of the respiratory system (20,24). It is also possible that there is functional redundancy for secretion of bicarbonate within the kidney itself. This role for base/anion exchange in the kidney raises the possibility that pendrin underlies a similar role in pH homeostasis in the inner ear (16).

C. Pendrin Function: Ear

A critical role for *PDS* within the auditory system was initially established by the demonstration of its specific expression in distinct regions of nonsensory inner ear epithelia thought to be important for homeostasis of endolymph (25). In situ hybridization analyses of mouse inner ears detected *pds* mRNA expression beginning at embryonic day 13 (E13), first in the endolymphatic duct and sac, then in the cochlea and vestibule at E15. *pds* mRNA is eventually expressed throughout the endolymphatic duct and sac, in the external sulcus below the spiral prominence of the cochlea, and in specific nonsensory portions of the utricle and saccule, adjacent to the maculae. This localization pattern suggested that pendrin may play a crucial role in endolymph homeostasis; the endolymphatic duct and sac are believed to be involved in endolymph resorption (25). More specifically, Kitano et al. had previously suggested that luminal chloride/bicarbonate exchange is crucial both for the production of endolymph and for the maintenance of the endolymphatic potential (26).

It is also possible that defective iodide transport by pendrin in the inner ear could cause the observed mutant *PDS* auditory phenotypes. Inactive thyroid hormone T4 is converted to its active form, T3, by high levels of type 2 deiodinase activity within the postnatal cochlea (27). Removal of liberated iodide ions from the inner ear might require pendrin, and *PDS* mutations could thus result in iodide accumulation. End product inhibition of the deiodination reaction could result in decreased production of T3, which is required for physiological and structural maturation of the organ of Corti. Iodide (or chloride) retention may lead to an osmotic imbalance with abnormal endolymphatic fluid resorption. A resorption defect with resulting osmotic imbalance might thus lead to the observed dilation of the endolymphatic system and sensory cell damage (25). *PDS* mutations could therefore cause sensorineural hearing loss through impairment of endolymph ionic and osmotic homeostasis, pH regulation, thyroid hormone biosynthesis, or any combination of these mechanisms.

IV. *pds* KNOCKOUT MOUSE

A $pds^{-/-}$ knockout mouse generated and characterized by Everett et al. has provided fascinating insights into the function of pendrin in the inner ear and the pathogenesis of hearing loss in Pendred syndrome (24). Homozygous $pds^{-/-}$ mice manifest variable degrees of vestibular dysfunction as evidenced by gait unsteadiness, circling behavior, head tilting, and abnormal performance in rotarod balance testing. Auditory brainstem response analyses demonstrated that $pds^{-/-}$ mice are deaf, whereas $pds^{+/-}$ heterozygotes have normal hearing.

The inner ears of $pds^{-/-}$ mice are anatomically normal until E15, at which time the endolymphatic duct and sac begin to enlarge in comparison with control mice. Shortly thereafter, the cochlea and saccule of $pds^{-/-}$ mice also become grossly enlarged and dysmorphic owing to dilatation of all of the endolymph-containing spaces. The semicircular canals become enlarged in 16% of the $pds^{-/-}$ mice. Scanning electron microscopic studies of auditory and vestibular end organs demonstrated variable, irregular inner and outer hair cell degeneration that was sometimes associated with enlarged stereocilia. Although the vestibular organs appeared normal until postnatal day 7 (P7), the maculae degenerated and the otoconia were observed to be absent or abnormally enlarged between p7 and p15, and these changes progressed as the mice aged. Interestingly, no thyroid abnormalities were detected in the $pds^{-/-}$ mice.

Although serum thyroid function tests and macroscopic and histological studies could not detect any abnormalities, it is possible that a subtle iodination defect is still present. Since these phenotypic features are also incompletely penetrant in Pendred syndrome, and the auditory/vestibular phenotype is so similar to those observed in human patients, the *pds* knockout mouse should continue to provide an outstanding mouse model for further studies of pendrin and hearing loss in Pendred syndrome. One possible line of investigation would be analysis of endolymph pH and ionic composition in the knockout inner ear. The results of such analyses may elucidate how *PDS* mutations affect endolymph pH and ionic composition. Rational pharmacological therapies might eventually be available to reverse such effects and the progression or fluctuation of hearing loss and vestibular dysfunction that is often observed in Pendred syndrome. The *pds* knockout mouse could provide an animal model for preclinical testing of potential therapies.

V. *PDS* MUTATIONS

Mutations have been found throughout *PDS*; at the time of this writing, over 60 mutations have been reported (9,10,17,28–44). Thus far, mutations have been identified in nearly every coding exon. They occur in predicted transmembrane domains, extracellular and intracellular loops, and both amino and carboxy termini. Missense, splice site, and frameshift/truncation mutations have all been reported (Table 1) and occur in individuals of all ethnic backgrounds. While some mutations appear to be more common than others, no single predominant *PDS* mutation has been identified. An early report by Van Hauwe et al. described 14 different mutations in 14 unrelated families with Pendred syndrome (37). Two of these mutations, L236P and T416P, were observed in seven and five of the families, respectively, with the remainder of the identified mutations each found in only one of the 14 families. Haplotype analysis of the L236P families, which were all Western European or North American in origin, was consistent with a founder effect. The results of a similar analysis of T416P were also consistent with a common founder. Two additional mutations, IVS8 + 1G > A and E384G, have also emerged as common *PDS* mutations among families of Western European origin.

Our recent genetic epidemiological study of *PDS* deafness in Asian populations has demonstrated that, while the prevalence of *PDS* mutations and DFNB4 deafness in Asian populations is similar to that in Western ethnic groups, the mutations are distinctly different (44b). Moreover, within each Asian ethnic group there is a similar degree of allelic diversity with a few predominant founder mutations. One of these founder mutations, H723R, appears to be a particularly common cause of deafness in Korea and Japan (44b).

Table 1 Reported PDS Mutations

Exon	Type	Mutation	Missense	Ref.
IVS1	Splice site	IVS1-2A > G		35
2	Missense	85G > C	E29Q	30
IVS2	Splice site	IVS2-1G > A		33
3	Frameshift	279delT		39
4	Missense	314A > G	Y105C	30
4	Missense	317C > A	A106D	30
4	Missense	349C > T	L117F	38
4	Frameshift	406delTCTCA*		35
4	Frameshift	336-337insT		32
4	Missense	395C > T	T132I	35
4/IVS4	Complex	412-IVS4 + 21del5/ins5	V138X	33
4	Missense	412G > T	V138F	32,37
4	Splice site	IVS4 + 7 A > G		44
5	Missense	416G > C	G139A	37
5	Missense	801C > T*	T193I	43
6	Missense	826G > T	G209V	37
6	Missense	707T > C	L236P	32,37
6	Frameshift	783–784insT		30
6	Frameshift	753–756delCTCT		32
7	Missense	811G > C	D271H	37
7	Frameshift	917delT		41
IVS8	Splice site	IVS8 + 1G > A		32
IVS8	Splice site	IVS8-2A > G		44a
9	Missense	1008T > C	F335L	30
9	Missense	1105A > G	K369E	41
9	Missense	1115C > T	A372V	41
9	Frameshift	1146delC		37
10	Missense	1151A > G	E384G	32
10	Deletion	1181–1183delTCT		44a
10	Frameshift	1197delT		9
10	Missense	1226G > A	R409H	37
10	Missense	1229C > T	T410M	32
10	Missense	1231G > C	A411P	33
10	Missense	1246A > C	T416P	32,37
11	Deletion	1284–1286delTGC	A429del	32
11	Missense	1334T > G	L445W	37
11	Missense	1337A > G	Q446R	38
12	Frameshift	1334–1335insAGTC		32
12	Frameshift	1341delG	FS 446 X454	9
13	Missense	1440T > A*	V480D	30
13	Missense	1468A > C	1490L	10

Table 1 Continued

Exon	Type	Mutation	Missense	Ref.
13	Missense	1489G > A	G497S	10
13	Missense	1523C > A	T508N	13
13	Frameshift	1536–1537delAG		32
IVS13	Splice site	IVS13 + 9C > G (1544 + 9)		44a
14	Missense	1588T > C	Y530H	32
15	Frameshift	1652insT*		· 36
15	Missense	1667A > G	Y556C	37
15	Missense	1666T > C	Y556H	35
15	Missense	1694G > A	C565Y	37
16	Missense	1790T > C	L597S	30
17	Frameshift	1898delA		37
17	Missense	1958T > C	V653A	30
17	Missense	2000T > G	F667C	9
17	Missense	2015 G > A*	G672E	32
19	Frameshift	2111insGCTGG		41
19	Frameshift	2127delT		32
19	Missense	2162C > T	T721M	41
19	Missense	2168A > G	H723R	37
19	Frameshift	2182–2183insG		42
21	Missense/ elongation	2343A > G	X871W	35

Whenever possible, mutations are listed in format consistent with the recommendations of the Nomenclature Working Group (76): nucleotide 1 is defined here as the A of the initiator ATG codon of *PDS* cDNA. Those mutations marked with an asterisk (*) could not be reconciled and are listed as originally published.

Two important conclusions arise from these molecular studies: First, *PDS* mutations are a common worldwide cause of hereditary deafness, providing molecular confirmation of clinical epidemiological estimates in Western populations. Second, the degree of allelic diversity within and among ethnic groups will significantly reduce any utility of screening approaches for *PDS* mutations that include only selected exons or that screen for specific mutations, especially in ethnically heterogeneous individuals.

PDS mutations are not found in every patient with an apparent clinical diagnosis of Pendred syndrome, though. Numerous groups have reported sizable series of Pendred and nonsyndromic deafness with enlarged vestibular equeduct families analyzed with SSCP and/or sequencing analysis of all coding regions (30,32,42). In many cases, only one copy of a mutation or no mutations at all have been detected. The presence of identifiable mutations in *PDS* appears to be more frequent in multiplex families; in one such series reported by Campbell et al. in 2001, *PDS* mutations were found in 82% (9/11) of multiplex families and in 30% (14/47) of simplex families (30). Similarly, the incidence of only one mutant allele in affected individuals seems to be more common in isolated cases; in the Campbell study, only one mutant allele was identified in 11 of the 14 simplex cases but in only three of the nine multiplex families. It thus cannot be said with certainty that *PDS* mutations are responsible for all cases of Pendred syndrome. However, most linkage analyses have found inheritance consistent with a monogenic etiology (6–9,45), and many groups have postulated that those patients in whom two mutated alleles cannot be identified may have undetected intronic or regulatory region mutations (32,46). Other possible explanations include multigenic inheritance in some cases or the existence of modifying environmental factors. Campbell et al. suggested that most simplex cases of deafness with EVA are of nongenetic origin (30), but thus far no environmental etiological or contributive agent has been identified.

VI. PHENOTYPE: OTOLOGICAL

Deafness in individuals with Pendred syndrome is usually prelingual in onset, although it is not always congenital. Pure tone audiometry generally reveals downsloping or flat, severe to profound sensorineural hearing loss (4,47,48). Milder hearing impairments and other audiometric configurations have been reported. Whie bilateral hearing loss is the rule, it is sometimes not symmetrical. Many affected individuals have a stable degree of hearing impairment, but progression and fluctuation are well documented and progression may be stepwise (often associated with minor head trauma or barotrauma) or gradual (45,47). Permanent improvement in hearing levels has not been reported.

These audiological characteristics of patients with classic Pendred syndrome are strikingly similar to those of a clinical entity that had been independently referred to as the large vestibular aqueduct syndrome (LVAS) in the otolaryngological, audiological, and radiological literature (49). Multiple studies of patients with LVAS have revealed that unilateral losses do occur, and the degree of hearing impairment does not correlate with the size of the vestibular aqueduct (49). In addition, a small 5–10-decibel conductive hearing loss component in the lower frequencies is commonly observed (50). Although the cause(s) of LVAS was (were) previously unknown, familial cases were consistent with recessive inheritance (51). Subsequent molecular studies of LVAS confirmed that it is often associated with biallelic or monoallelic *PDS* mutations (10), although there are also cases with no detectable *PDS* mutations. It is currently not clear whether LVAS and Pendred syndrome are distinct entities or represent the extremes of a continuum of manifestations of a single disorder.

Patients with more severe inner ear malformations such as the Mondini deformity (incomplete partition of adjacent cochlear turns with variable malformations of the vestibular labyrinth) may also have increased susceptibility to leakage of inner ear perilymph into the middle ear through the oval or round windows (perilymph fistulae). Perilymph fistulae are associated with sudden hearing loss, severe rotatory vertigo, and may occasionally lead to meningitis. Vestibular dysfunction is an inconsistent and variable finding in Pendred syndrome; severity ranges from subclinical caloric hyporeflexia to severe vertiginous attacks (52,53).

VII. PHENOTYPE: GOITER

Goiter is the other clinical manifestation of Pendred syndrome (1,4). Patients are nearly always euthyroid, though mild hypothyroidism does occur and TSH levels are often at the higher end of the normal range (3–5,54). The goiter is often multinodular and occasionally requires surgical extirpation for cosmetic concerns or local mass effects. While thyroid carcinoma has been reported in a few Pendred syndrome patients, it is not clear whether the risk is any higher than that for unaffected individuals (29).

The onset of goiter typically occurs around adolescence but may occur earlier in some patients (4,55). The distinction between Pendred syndrome and nonsyndromic hearing loss (with EVA) can therefore be difficult to make during childhood. This problem is exacerbated by the subjective nature of a physical examination. While ultrasound examination with volume determinations may be helpful, normal gland size varies with age and, typically, volume determinations have not been reported in a normalized fashion. Finally, goiter due to other causes is common in some regions and populations, and can thus lead to phenocopies and the potential for misdiagnosis (39). Goiter is therefore neither a sensitive nor a specific diagnostic criterion for Pendred syndrome.

The goiter usually found in Pendred syndrome is not universal (5,8,56). *PDS* mutations also cause nonsyndromic deafness DFNB4 (10,57). Although the affected members of the family originally used to define the DFNB4 region were later found to have goiter (10), Li et al. reported in 1998 on a large family with 10 affected individuals ranging from 5 to 38 years of age (10). Affected individuals had deafness, but no goiter. Thyroid function studies were normal, but the perchlorate test was not administered so it is uncertain whether these individuals possessed a subclinical thyroid organ-

ification defect. Computed tomography (CT) scanning of the temporal bones
was performed on 3 affected family members and one unaffected member; the
affected individuals all were found to have enlarged vestibular aqueducts and
normal cochleae, while the unaffected member had no anatomical abnormalities. Affected family members were homozygous for two missense mutations
in *PDS* exon 13, G497S and I490L. Scott et al. found *PDS* mutations in 3 of
20 (15%) patients with enlarged vestibular aqueducts and nonsyndromic
deafness (17).

VIII. PERCHLORATE TEST

Owing to the lack of sensitivity and specificity of goiter or thyroid function
tests as diagnostic criteria for Pendred syndrome, the perchlorate discharge
test has emerged as the evaluation of choice to detect the underlying iodine
organification defect (3,58). The thyroid glands of affected individuals show
normal uptake of orally administered radioiodine from the bloodstream, but
fail to organify iodine at a normal rate. The perchlorate discharge test is
used to measure this defect (3). A dose of radiolabeled iodine is administered
and the radioactivity over the thyroid is measured and used as a baseline.
Potassium perchlorate is then administered. This allows unincorporated
iodide to diffuse back into the circulatory system. Serial measurements of
thyroid radioactivity are used to calculate the percentage of iodine that is
discharged from the gland. In a normal thyroid, organification is rapid and
less than 10–15% of the radioiodine is washed out, whereas a greater
amount (usually more than 20–30%) of radioiodine is released from the
glands of Pendred syndrome patients.

Although the perchlorate test has been a useful adjunct to the clinical
and molecular diagnosis of Pendred syndrome, there are problems with its
use. First, there are no well-established normative data and the criterion for
a positive discharge result varies among investigators. Most investigators
consider any discharge above 10% as abnormal (32,42,55,59,60), but other
studies have used 15% (17,30,39,61,62) or even 20% (37) as the upper limit
of normal. Another problem is that a positive discharge result is not specific
for Pendred syndrome: abnormally high discharge is also observed in
Hashimoto's thyroiditis, thyrotoxicosis treated with ^{131}I, cretinism, and
peroxidase deficiency (3,39,61,63). Rigorous medical histories, physical
examinations, and the appropriate laboratory evaluations must rule out
these potential causes of an abnormally high discharge result. Furthermore,
false negative results may occur when initial thyroid uptake is low (61).
Finally, potential effects of differences in perchlorate dosage or the size of
patients (especially children) on the discharge response have not been

systematically analyzed. In toto, these caveats and potential pitfalls dictate that perchlorate discharge studies be interpreted cautiously.

It is not clear that deafness and goiter associated with *PDS* mutations are always associated with a positive perchlorate test result. Masmoudi et al. reported two large families cosegregating Pendred syndrome and the L445W mutation, but all of the affected homozygotes that were tested had negative (< 3%) perchlorate tests, while goiter varied (56). Other studies have concluded that the perchlorate discharge phenotype does not correlate with the size or presence of goiter, underlying *PDS* genotype, or temporal bone anatomy. The results may also vary with time; Stinckens et al. reported two perchlorate discharge tests performed 5 years apart on the same patient (at ages 9 and 14) in which the results were 27% and 63% discharge (64). This apparent variability of the perchlorate discharge test may reflect one or more of the confounding factors discussed above, especially since few medical centers routinely administer the test (5) and variations in technique and interpretation are almost certainly a problem. Other obstacles to performing the perchlorate test include the difficulty of administration in young children and the necessity to discontinue any thyroid medications 4–6 weeks before testing (3).

IX. PHENOTYPIC VARIABILITY

Thyroid phenotypic variability in Pendred syndrome is significant and might be due to any one or a combination of environmental factors (e.g., long-term thyroid hormone replacement therapy, dietary iodine intake), con-comitant thyroid disorders, genetic background, stochastic variation, under-lying *PDS* mutant genotypes, or differences in ascertainment. The last factor is especially problematic in evaluating and comparing the results of different studies of goiter or perchlorate discharge test results for the reasons previously discussed. The literature indicates that there is wide intra- and interfamilial variability of the thyroid phenotype, whether the phenotype is defined as goiter or as an abnormal perchlorate discharge result. Some of this variability may be attributed to undetected phenocopies or differences in the administration and interpretation of the perchlorate discharge test. If the criterion of 10 or 15% for an abnormal discharge is too low (which is very likely), many of the individuals with a reported abnormal perchlorate discharge will be false positives. Unfortunately, few published studies report actual percent discharge, thus prohibiting a critical retrospective analysis of their results.

Some splice site mutations or mutations that create cryptic splice sites have been reported to be associated with wide variability in both the thyroid and auditory phenotypes, suggesting that the observed variability is not simply due to differences in ascertainment of the thyroid phenotype. Lopez-Bigas et al. hypothesized that variability in processing of mutant *PDS* mRNA transcripts among different individuals may account for the observed phenotypic variability (44).

While numerous authors have suggested the possibility of a genotype-phenotype correlation in Pendred syndrome (10,30,45,65), the significant inter- and intrafamilial variability of the thyroid phenotype among individuals segregating the same mutations (including those that do not affect splice sites) indicates that any such correlation will be extremely difficult to demonstrate (30,37,39,44,48). As alluded to earlier, correlation of *PDS* genotype with the auditory phenotype may be more straightforward since auditory status is not as complicated by phenocopies and a lack of normative data. However, there are still no data to suggest that the hearing loss phenotype is correlated with the underlying *PDS* mutation, as any potential correlation may be obscured by intrafamilial variation of both auditory functional and radiological phenotypes.

A functional study of anion transport by *PDS* mutant allele products has been valuable toward confirming the pathogenic nature of a few *PDS* mutations. These investigators extrapolated their data to hypothesize a correlation of the anion transport phenotype with the thyroid phenotype (17). Scott et al. used a *Xenopus* oocyte expression system to evaluate the iodide and chloride transport function of various mutant pendrin products modeled on known human mutations. T416P, L236P, and E384G were considered to be mutations associated with classic Pendred syndrome (with goiter), while I490L, G497S, V480D, and V653A were considered to be associated with nonsyndromic deafness. The authors observed that the former group of mutations abolished anion transport, whereas the latter group of mutations reduced, but did not eliminate, activity. They concluded that functional null alleles cause deafness plus goiter, whereas hypomorphic alleles cause deafness without goiter.

However, the pathogenic nature of at least one of the putative non-syndromic alleles (e.g., V653A) is unclear since it is a nonconservative substitution observed in a single heterozygote, and may simply be a benign polymorphism. Furthermore, reduced but detectable transport activity is not proof of pathogenicity and may reflect normal polymorphic variation of functional activity (66). The high degree of variation of thyroid phenotype and the problems associated with its ascertainment currently prevent any conclusions to be drawn about its correlation with the underlying *PDS* genotype and anion transport function. Attempts to correlate thyroid phenotype with *PDS* genotype should only be made if and when specific mutant alleles are rigorously shown to be uniformly and commonly associated with either Pendred syndrome or nonsyndromic deafness.

X. PHENOTYPE: INNER EAR ANATOMY

Gross malformations of the inner ear have long been known to be associated with Pendred syndrome. Hvidberg-Hansen and Jorgensen, in their 1968 case report of a patient with Pendred syndrome (67) described the histological findings of enlarged vestibular aqueduct, enlarged endolymphatic duct and sac, incomplete partition of the apical turn of the cochlea, deficient modiolus, and vestibular malformation in a patient with Pendred syndrome. This constellation of abnormalities is often referred to as a "Mondini deformity," and it is essentially identical to the combination of malformations originally described by Mondini in 1791. Some authors use the Mondini eponym to describe any inner ear with an incomplete partition of the cochlea. A larger series of histological findings in five Pendred patients was published by Johnsen et al. in 1986; all were found to have Mondini malformations (68). Similarly, Illum et al. found that seven of 15 Pendred syndrome patients had cochlear partition defects on conventional tomographic examination (61). In 1989, Johnsen et al. demonstrated that CT scanning is more sensitive than conventional tomography at detecting the Mondini malformation, and found Mondini malformations in all of five Pendred syndrome patients imaged by CT scan (69).

While the full Mondini defect is observed in the ears of many Pendred syndrome patients, it is not universally present. Enlargement of the vestibular aqueducts (EVA) is a much more sensitive radiological marker for Pendred syndrome that can be detected by CT scanning or MRI scanning (38,41,47,48), although it is actually the soft tissue and fluid contents of the vestibular aqueduct (the endolymphatic duct and sac) that are visualized by MRI (Fig. 1). The vestibular aqueduct is considered enlarged when its diameter exceeds 1.5 mm at the midpoint between the posterior cranial fossa and the vestibule of the inner ear (49). Of a series of 40 Pendred syndrome patients examined by CT and MRI, Phelps et al. identified enlarged vestibular aqueducts in 31 of 40 imaged by CT and enlarged endolymphatic sacs and ducts in all of 20 imaged by MRI (48). The identification of EVA as a highly penetrant radiological marker for Pendred syndrome was an important observation since it identified temporal bone imaging as a much more sensitive modality for the ascertainment of Pendred syndrome.

Reardon et al. evaluated a series of 57 patients with enlarged vestibular aqueducts and found *PDS* mutations in 86% (38). Although EVA is a reliable

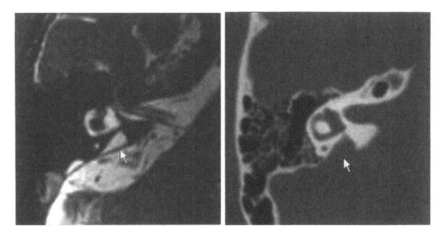

Figure 1 Images of right temporal bone demonstrating enlarged vestibular aqueduct (arrows). (left panel) MRI scan showing enlarged endolymphatic sac and duct. Fluid-filled spaces are light and bone and soft tissues dark. (right panel) CT scan showing enlarged vestibular aqueduct. Bone is white and fluid and air-filled spaces are black.

marker for *PDS*-related deafness, it is not pathognomonic. In addition to its occurrence in nonsyndromic deafness and Pendred syndrome, EVA has been reported for a few patients with branchio-oto-renal syndrome (70) caused by mutations in the EYA1 locus, deafness-oligodontia syndrome (71), and deafness associated with the recessive form of distal renal tubular acidosis (72). Although there are no reports of nonsyndromic deafness phenotypes allelic with any of these three syndromes (36), it is possible that mutant alleles at these loci may contribute to some cases of nonsyndromic hearing loss associated with EVA.

A causal relationship of EVA to hearing impairment has not been established; initially it was believed that the enlarged endolymphatic system transmits otherwise benign pressure fluctuations with reflux of endolymphatic sac contents from the posterior fossa to the inner ear (73). However, there is little evidence to support this theory, as obliteration of the endolymphatic sac and duct do not reverse or even prevent further hearing loss in patients with EVA (74). It is more likely that hearing loss is due to a defect in endolymph homeostasis or, in some cases associated with classical Mondini deformities, perilymph fistulae. Sudden drops and fluctuation of hearing may also be caused by intrascalar fistulae with mixing of endolymph and perilymph, a hypothesis that is suggested by the high degree of endolymphatic hydrops observed in $pds^{-/-}$ mice (24). Finally, some have suggested that EVA may represent an arrest in normal development at about 7 weeks of human gestation (61) but this is not likely to be the case. The size of the vestibular aqueduct in EVA is larger than a normal VA at any stage of its development. Anatomical evidence from the $pds^{-/-}$ mice further argues against the theory of arrested development, as $pds^{-/-}$ mice initially have a normal inner ear anatomy, and then develop dilatation (24). This indicates that other causes of EVA may also be due to perturbations of endolymph pH, ionic, or osmotic homeostasis. Identification of these other etiologies, especially mutant genetic loci, may further elucidate the molecular pathways of homeostasis in the auditory system.

XI. DIAGNOSIS AND MANAGEMENT

The diagnosis of Pendred syndrome is not always straightforward. History and physical examination can be very suggestive, but not diagnostic. When a patient presents with prelingual sensorineural hearing loss with or without goiter, CT or MRI scanning should be included whenever possible as part of the initial evaluation. The presence of EVA or a Mondini malformation should trigger further investigation into the possibility of Pendred syndrome.

Ultrasound measurement of thyroid volume can be helpful in the detection of subtle goiters. Although problems exist with its interpretation, the perchlorate discharge test, when positive, can be a useful adjunct in detecting a thyroid organification defect before goiter appears. Molecular testing of *PDS* is currently available; any *PDS* screening should ideally include all coding regions, given the lack of a single predominant mutation or mutated exon and the ethnic variability of *PDS* mutations. Vestibular testing should be performed when clinically indicated, but is not often useful in distinguishing Pendred syndrome from other entities.

Management of patients with Pendred syndrome should focus first on rehabilitation. Amplification can be helpful when deafness is not profound. Patients should be cautioned to avoid minor head injuries and barotrauma, which may cause additional hearing loss. Those with Mondini malformations should also be informed of the possible increased susceptibility to meningitis. Patients with EVA have undergone cochlear implantation with good results (75). Ears with EVA may have a higher risk of mild CSF leaks upon cochleostomy, but these seem to be easily controlled without long-term sequelae (75). Endolymphatic sac obliteration and shunting have led to worsened hearing and are contraindicated in these patients (73,74).

Treatment of the thyroid manifestations of Pendred syndrome is primarily symptomatic. Thyroid function monitoring is appropriate and function may be treated pharmacologically when clinically indicated. Goiter may be treated surgically when symptomatic.

XII. CONCLUSIONS

The introduction of the perchlorate discharge test, positional cloning of the *PDS* gene, and the generation of a knockout mouse model have significantly advanced our understanding of Pendred syndrome. Avenues for future research include elucidating the pathogenesis of hearing loss in the significantly high proportion of patients with hearing loss and EVA who appear to be heterozygous carriers of *PDS* mutations. Are there unidentified *trans* mutant *PDS* alleles in these individuals or mutant alleles of other genes, or do environmental factors cause hearing loss in *PDS* carriers? Rigorous correlation of auditory and thyroid phenotypes with *PDS* molecular test results is needed to define more precise diagnostic criteria for Pendred syndrome. Finally, the *pds* knockout mouse model may be used to delineate the endolymph homestatic defect that presumably leads to hearing loss in this disorder. Newborn hearing screening and early diagnosis of Pendred syndrome may provide an opportunity to pharmacologically reverse such a defect, thus preventing or retarding further postnatal deterioration of hearing that occurs in many of these patients (76).

REFERENCES

1. Pendred V. Deaf-mutism and goitre. Lancet 1896; 2:532.
2. Brain WR. Heredity in simple goitre. Q J Med 1927; 20:303.
3. Morgans ME, Trotter WR. Association of congenital deafness with goitre: the nature of the thyroid defect. Lancet 1958; I:607–609.
4. Fraser GR. Association of congenital deafness with goitre (Pendred's syndrome): a study of 207 families. Ann Hum Genet 1965; 28:201–249.
5. Reardon W, Coffey R, Phelps PD, Luxon LM, Stephens D, Kendall-Taylor P, Britton KE, Grossman A, Trembath R. Pendred syndrome—100 years of underascertainment? Q J Med 1997; 90:443–447.
6. Coucke P, Van Camp G, Demirhan O, Kabakkaya Y, Balemans W, Van Hauwe P, Van Agtmael T, Smith RJ, Parving A, Bolder CH, Cremers CW, Willems PJ. The gene for Pendred syndrome is located between D7S501 and D7S692 in a 1.7-cM region on chromosome 7q. Genomics 1997; 40:48–54.
7. Coyle B, Coffey R, Armour JA, Gausden E, Hochberg Z, Grossman A, Britton

K, Pembrey M, Reardon W, Trembath R. Pendred syndrome (goitre and sensorineural hearing loss) maps to chromosome 7 in the region containing the nonsyndromic deafness gene DFNB4. Nat Genet 1996; 12:421–423.

8. Sheffield VC, Kraiem Z, Beck JC, Nishimura D, Stone EM, Salameh M, Sadeh O, Glaser B. Pendred syndrome maps to chromosome 7q21-34 and is caused by an intrinsic defect in thyroid iodine organification. Nat Genet 1996; 12:424–426.

9. Everett LA, Glaser B, Beck JC, Idol JR, Buchs A, Heyman M, Adawi F, Hazani E, Nassir E, Baxevanis AD, Sheffield VC, Green ED. Pendred syndrome is caused by mutations in a putative sulphate transporter gene (*PDS*). Nat Genet 1997; 17:411–422.

10. Li XC, Everett LA, Lalwani AK, Desmukh D, Friedman TB, Green ED, Wilcox ER. A mutation in *PDS* causes non-syndromic recessive deafness. Nat Genet 1998; 18:215–217.

11. Royaux IE, Suzuki K, Mori A, Katoh R, Everett LA, Kohn LD, Green ED. Pendrin, the protein encoded by the Pendred syndrome gene (*PDS*), is an apical porter of iodide in the thyroid and is regulated by thyroglobulin in FRTL-5 cells. Endocrinology 2000; 141:839–845.

12. Zheng J, Long KB, Shen W, Madison LD, Dallos P. Prestin topology: localization of protein epitopes in relation to the plasma membrane. Neuroreport 2001; 12:1929–1935.

13. Bogazzi F, Bartalena L, Raggi F, Ultimieri F, Martino E. Pendrin does not increase sulfate uptake in mammalian COS-7 cells. J Endocrinol Invest 2000; 23:170–172.

14. Scott DA, Wang R, Kreman TM, Sheffield VC, Karniski LP. The Pendred syndrome gene encodes a chloride-iodide transport protein. Nat Genet 1999; 21:440–443.

15. Kraiem Z, Heinrich R, Sadeh O, Shiloni E, Nassir E, Hazani E, Glaser B. Sulfate transport is not impaired in pendred syndrome thyrocytes. J Clin Endocrinol Metab 1999; 84:2574–2576.

16. Scott DA, Karniski LP. Human pendrin expression in *Xenopus laevis* oocytes mediates chloride/formate exchange. Am J Physiol Cell Physiol 2000; 278: C207–C211.

17. Scott DA, Wang R, Kreman TM, Andrews M, McDonald JM, Bishop JR, Smith RJ, Karniski LP, Sheffield VC. Functional differences of the *PDS* gene product are associated with phenotypic variation in patients with Pendred syndrome and non-syndromic hearing loss (DFNB4). Hum Mol Genet 2000; 9:1709–1715.

18. Bidart JM, Mian C, Lazar V, Russo D, Filetti S, Caillou B, Schlumberger M. Expression of pendrin and the Pendred syndrome (*PDS*) gene in human thyroid tissues. J Clin Endocrinol Metab 2000; 85:2028–2033.

19. Kohn LD, Suzuki K, Nakazato M, Royaux I, Green ED. Effects of thyroglobulin and pendrin on iodide flux through the thyrocyte. Trends Endocrinol Metab 2001; 12:10–16.

20. Royaux IE, Wall SM, Karniski LP, Everett LA, Suzuki K, Knepper MA, Green ED. Pendrin, encoded by the Pendred syndrome gene, resides in the

apical region of renal intercalated cells and mediates bicarbonate secretion. Proc Natl Acad Sci USA 2001; 98:4221–4226.

21. Soleimani M, Greeley T, Petrovic S, Wang Z, Amlal H, Kopp P, Burnham CE. Pendrin: an apical Cl-/OH-/HCO3-exchanger in the kidney cortex. Am J Physiol Renal Physiol 2001; 280:F356–F364.

22. Soleimani M. Molecular physiology of the renal chloride-formate exchanger. Curr Opin Nephrol Hypertens 2001; 10:677–683.

23. Knauf F, Yang CL, Thomson RB, Mentone SA, Giebisch G, Aronson PS. Identification of a chloride-formate exchanger expressed on the brush border membrane of renal proximal tubule cells. Proc Natl Acad Sci USA 2001; 98: 9425–9430.

24. Everett LA, Belyantseva IA, Noben-Trauth K, Cantos R, Chen A, Thakkar SI, Hoogstraten-Miller SL, Kachar B, Wu DK, Green ED. Targeted disruption of mouse Pds provides insight about the inner-ear defects encountered in Pendred syndrome. Hum Mol Genet 2001; 10:153–161.

25. Everett LA, Morsli H, Wu DK, Green ED. Expression pattern of the mouse ortholog of the Pendred's syndrome gene (Pds) suggests a key role for pendrin in the inner ear. Proc Natl Acad Sci USA 1999; 96:9727–9732.

26. Kitano I, Mori N, Matsunaga T. Role of endolymphatic anion transport in forskolin-induced Cl-activity increase of scala media. Hearing Res 1995; 83: 37–42.

27. Campos-Barros A, Amma LL, Faris JS, Shailam R, Kelley MW, Forrest D. Type 2 iodothyronine deiodinase expression in the cochlea before the onset of hearing. Proc Natl Acad Sci USA 2000; 97:1287–1292.

28. Bogazzi F, Raggi F, Ultimieri F, Campomori A, Cosci C, Berrettini S, Neri E, La Rocca R, Ronca G, Martino E, Bartalena L. A novel mutation in the pendrin gene associated with Pendred's syndrome. Clin Endocrinol (Oxf) 2000; 52: 279–285.

29. Camargo R, Limbert E, Gillam M, Henriques MM, Fernandes C, Catarino AL, Soares J, Alves VA, Kopp P, Medeiros-Neto G. Aggressive metastatic follicular thyroid carcinoma with anaplastic transformation arising from a long-standing goiter in a patient with Pendred's syndrome. Thyroid 2001; 11: 981–988.

30. Campbell C, Cucci RA, Prasad S, Green GE, Edeal JB, Galer CE, Karniski LP, Sheffield VC, Smith RJ. Pendred syndrome, DFNB4, and PDS/SLC26A4 identification of eight novel mutations and possible genotype-phenotype correlations. Hum Mutat 2001; 17:403–411.

31. Coucke PJ, Van Hauwe P, Everett LA, Demirhan O, Kabakkaya Y, Dietrich NL, Smith RJ, Coyle E, Reardon W, Trembath R, Willems PJ, Green ED, Van Camp G. Identifications of two different mutations in the *PDS* gene in an inbred family with Pendred syndrome. J Med Genet 1999; 36:475–477.

32. Coyle B, Reardon W, Herbrick JA, Tsui LC, Gausden E, Lee J, Coffey R, Grueters A, Grossman A, Phelps PD, Luxon L, Kendall-Taylor P, Scherer SW, Trembath RC. Molecular analysis of the *PDS* gene in Pendred syndrome. Hum Mol Genet 1998; 7:1105–1112.

33. Gonzalez Trevino O, Karamanoglu Arseven O, Ceballos CJ, Vives VI, Ramirez RC, Gomez VV, Medeiros-Neto G, Kopp P. Clinical and molecular analysis of three Mexican families with Pendred's syndrome. Eur J Endocrinol 2001; 144:585-593.

34. Kitamura K, Takahashi K, Noguchi Y, Kuroishikawa Y, Tamagawa Y, Ishikawa K, Ichimura K, Hagiwara H. Mutations of the Pendred syndrome gene (*PDS*) in patients with large vestibular aqueduct. Acta Otolaryngol 2000; 120:137-141.

35. Lopez-Bigas N, Melchionda S, de Cid R, Grifa A, Zelante L, Govea N, Arbones ML, Gasparini P, Estivill X. Identification of five new mutations of PDS/SLC26A4 in Mediterranean families with hearing impairment. Hum Mutat 2001; 18:548.

36. Namba A, Abe S, Shinkawa H, Kimberling WJ, Usami SI. Genetic features of hearing loss associated with ear anomalies: *PDS* and *EYA1* mutation analysis. J Hum Genet 2001; 46:518-521.

37. Van Hauwe P, Everett LA, Coucke P, Scott DA, Kraft ML, Ris-Stalpers C, Bolder C, Otten B, de Vijlder JJ, Dietrich NL, Ramesh A, Srisailapathy SC, Parving A, Cremers CW, Willems PJ, Smith RJ, Green ED, Van Camp G. Two frequent missense mutations in Pendred syndrome. Hum Mol Genet 1998; 7:1099-1104.

38. Reardon W, CF OM, Trembath R, Jan H, Phelps PD. Enlarged vestibular aqueduct: a radiological marker of pendred syndrome, and mutation of the PDS gene. Q J Med 2000; 93:99-104.

39. Kopp P, Arseven OK, Sabacan L, Kotlar T, Dupuis J, Cavaliere H, Santos CL, Jameson JL, Medeiros-Neto G. Phenocopies for deafness and goiter development in a large inbred Brazilian kindred with Pendred's syndrome associated with a novel mutation in the *PDS* gene. J Clin Endocrinol Metab 1999; 84:336-341.

40. Cremers WR, Bolder C, Admiraal RJ, Everett LA, Joosten FB, van Hauwe P, Green ED, Otten BJ. Progressive sensorineural hearing loss and a widened vestibular aqueduct in Pendred syndrome. Arch Otolaryngol Head Neck Surg 1998; 124:501-505.

41. Usami S, Abe S, Weston MD, Shinkawa H, Van Camp G, Kimberling WJ. Non-syndromic hearing loss associated with enlarged vestibular aqueduct is caused by *PDS* mutations. Hum Genet 1999; 104:188-192.

42. Fugazzola L, Mannavola D, Cerutti N, Maghnie M, Pagella F, Bianchi P, Weber G, Persani L, Beck-Peccoz P. Molecular analysis of the Pendred's syndrome gene and magnetic resonance imaging studies of the inner ear are essential for the diagnosis of true Pendred's syndrome. J Clin Endocrinol Metab 2000; 85:2469-2475.

43. Adato A, Raskin L, Petit C, Bonne-Tamir B. Deafness heterogeneity in a Druze isolate from the Middle East: novel OTOF and PDS mutations, low prevalence of GJB2 35delG mutation and indication for a new DFNB locus. Eur J Hum Genet 2000; 8:437-442.

44. Lopez-Bigas N, Rabionet R, de Cid R, Govea N, Gasparini P, Zelante L,

Arbones ML, Estivill X. Splice-site mutation in the *PDS* gene may result in intrafamilial variability for deafness in Pendred syndrome. Hum Mutat 1999; 14:520–526.

44a. Yong AM, Goh SS, Zhao Y, Eng PH, Koh LK, Khoo DH. Two Chinese families with Pendred's syndrome—radiological imaging of the ear and molecular analysis of the pendrin gene. J Clin Endocrinol Metab 2001; 86:3907–3911.

44b. Park H-J, Shautak S, Liu XZ, Hahn S, Naz S, Ghosh M, Riazuddin S, Kim HN, Moon SK, Abe S, Tukamoto K, Erdenetungalag R, Radnaabazar J, Pandya A, Nance WE, Usami S, Wilcox ER, Griffith AJ. Origins and frequencies of *SLC26A4 (PDS)* mutations in East and South Asians: global implications for the epidemiology of deafness. J Med Genet 2003; 40:242–248.

45. Abe S, Usami S, Hoover DM, Cohn E, Shinkawa H, Kimberling WJ. Fluctuating sensorineural hearing loss associated with enlarged vestibular aqueduct maps to 7q31, the region containing the Pendred gene. Am J Med Genet 1999; 82:322–328.

46. Kopp P. Pendred's syndrome: identification of the genetic defect a century after its recognition. Thyroid 1999; 9:65–69.

47. Cremers CW, Admiraal RJ, Huygen PL, Bolder C, Everett LA, Joosten FB, Green ED, van Camp G, Otten BJ. Progressive hearing loss, hypoplasia of the cochlea and widened vestibular aqueducts are very common features in Pendred's syndrome. Int J Pediatr Otorhinolaryngol 1998; 45:113–123.

48. Phelps PD, Coffey RA, Trembath RC, Luxon LM, Grossman AB, Britton KE, Kendall-Taylor P, Graham JM, Cadge BC, Stephens SG, Pembrey ME, Reardon W. Radiological malformations of the ear in Pendred syndrome. Clin Radiol 1998; 53:268–273.

49. Valvassori GE, Clemis JD. The large vestibular aqueduct syndrome. Laryngoscope 1978; 88:723–728.

50. Nakashima T, Ueda H, Furuhashi A, Sato E, Asahi K, Naganawa S, Beppu R. Air-bone gap and resonant frequency in large vestibular aqueduct syndrome. Am J Otol 2000; 21:671–674.

51. Griffith AJ, Arts A, Downs C, Innis JW, Shepard NT, Sheldon S, Gebarski SS. Familial large vestibular aqueduct syndrome. Laryngoscope 1996; 106:960–965.

52. Bergstrom L. Pendred's syndrome with atypical features. Ann Otol Rhinol Laryngol 1980; 89:135–139.

53. Das VK. Pendred's syndrome with episodic vertigo, tinnitus and vomiting and normal bithermal caloric responses. J Laryngol Otol 1987; 101:721–722.

54. Johnsen T, Larsen C, Friis J, Hougaard-Jensen F. Pendred's syndrome: acoustic, vestibular and radiological findings in 17 unrelated patients. J Laryngol Otol 1987; 101:1187–1192.

55. Reardon W, Coffey R, Chowdhury T, Grossman A, Jan H, Britton K, Kendall-Taylor P, Trembath R. Prevalence, age of onset, and natural history of thyroid disease in Pendred syndrome. J Med Genet 1999; 36:595–598.

56. Masmoudi S, Charfedine I, Hmani M, Grati M, Ghorbel AM, Elgaied-Boulila

A, Drira M, Hardelin JP, Ayadi H. Pendred syndrome: phenotypic variability in two families carrying the same *PDS* missense mutation. Am J Med Genet 2000; 90:38–44.

57. Wilcox ER, Everett LA, Li XC, Lalwani AK, Green ED. The *PDS* gene, Pendred syndrome and non-syndromic deafness DFNB4. Adv Otorhinolaryngol 2000; 56:145–151.

58. Niepomniszcze H, Coleoni AH, Degrossi OJ, Scavini LM, Curutchet HP. Biochemical studies on the iodine organification defect of Pendred's syndrome. Acta Endocrinol (Copenh) 1978; 89:70–79.

59. Sato E, Nakashima T, Miura Y, Furuhashi A, Nakayama A, Mori N; Murakami H, Naganawa S, Tadokoro M. Phenotypes associated with replacement of His by Arg in the Pendred syndrome gene. Eur J Endocrinol 2001; 145:697–703.

60. Jamal MN, Arnaout MA, Jarrar R. Pendred's syndrome: a study of patients and relatives. Ann Otol Rhinol Laryngol 1995; 104:957–962.

61. Illum P, Kiaer HW, Hvidberg-Hansen J, Sondergaard G. Fifteen cases of Pendred's syndrome: congenital deafness and sporadic goiter. Arch Otolaryngol 1972; 96:297–304.

62. Kopp P. Pendred's syndrome and genetic defects in thyroid hormone synthesis. Rev Endocr Metab Disord 2000; 1:109–121.

63. Suzuki H, Mashimo K. Significance of the iodide-perchlorate discharge test in patients with 131 I-treated and untreated hyperthyroidism. J Clin Endocrinol Metab 1972; 34:332–338.

64. Stinckens C, Huygen PL, Joosten FB, Van Camp G, Otten B, Cremers CW. Fluctuant, progressive hearing loss associated with Meniere like vertigo in three patients with the Pendred syndrome. Int J Pediatr Otorhinolaryngol 2001; 61: 207–215.

65. Everett LA, Green ED. A family of mammalian anion transporters and their involvement in human genetic diseases. Hum Mol Genet 1999; 8:1883–1891.

66. Griffith AJ, Chowdhry AA, Kurima K, Hood LJ, Keats B, Berlin CI, Morell RJ, Friedman TB. Autosomal recessive nonsyndromic neurosensory deafness at *DFNB1* not associated with the compound-heterozygous GJB2 (connexin 26) genotype M34T/167delT. Am J Hum Genet 2000; 67:745–749.

67. Hvidberg-Hansen J, Jorgensen MB. The inner ear in Pendred's syndrome. Acta Otolaryngol 1968; 66:129–135.

68. Johnsen T, Jorgensen MB, Johnsen S. Mondini cochlea in Pendred's syndrome: a histological study. Acta Otolaryngol 1986; 102:239–247.

69. Johnsen T, Sorensen MS, Feldt-Rasmussen U, Friis J. The variable intrafamiliar expressivity in Pendred's syndrome. Clin Otolaryngol 1989; 14:395–399.

70. Chen A, Francis M, Ni L, Cremers CW, Kimberling WJ, Sato Y, Phelps PD, Bellman SC, Wagner MJ, Pembrey M, et al. Phenotypic manifestations of branchio-oto-renal syndrome. Am J Med Genet 1995; 58:365–370.

71. Marlin S, Denoyelle F, Busquet D, Garabedian N, Petit C. A particular case of deafness-oligodontia syndrome. Int J Pediatr Otorhinolaryngol 1998; 44: 63–69.

72. Berrettini S, Neri E, Forli F, Panconi M, Massimetti M, Ravecca F, Sellari-Franceschini S, Bartolozzi C. Large vestibular aqueduct in distal renal tubular acidosis: high-resolution MR in three cases. Acta Radiol 2001; 42:320–322.

73. Jackler RK, De La Cruz A. The large vestibular aqueduct syndrome. Laryngoscope 1989; 99:1238–1242; discussion 1242–3.

74. Wilson DF, Hodgson RS, Talbot JM. Endolymphatic sac obliteration for large vestibular aqueduct syndrome. Am J Otol 1997; 18:101–106; discussion 106–7.

75. Fahy CP, Carney AS, Nikolopoulos TP, Ludman CN, Gibbin KP. Cochlear implantation in children with large vestibular aqueduct syndrome and a review of the syndrome. Int J Pediatr Otorhinolaryngol 2001; 59:207–215.

76. Antonarakis SE. Recommendations for a nomenclature system for human gene mutations. Nomenclature Working Group. Hum Mutat 1998; 11:1–3.

6
Waardenburg Syndrome

Andrew P. Read
St. Mary's Hospital, Manchester, England

I. HISTORY

Waardenburg syndrome is named for the Dutch ophthalmologist and geneticist Petrus Waardenburg (1886–1979) whose monumental 1951 paper (1) contains the first systematic clinical description of what we now call Type 1 Waardenburg syndrome (WS1). In fact, auditory-pigmentary syndromes have a long history and are known in many mammalian species, reviewed by Steel and Barkway (2). The combination of hearing loss with white spotting, white coat, and/or pale eyes has been noted in mice, rats, hamsters, dogs, cats, horses, and cattle, and probably other species too. In humans, sporadic reports of auditory-pigmentary phenotypes have appeared over many years. Waardenburg himself first became interested in the condition through ophthalmology. He had reported in 1947 on dystopia canthorum in a Dutch tailor who was deaf, and remarked that a similar eye abnormality had been described in twins who were "coincidentally" also deaf. Later, on a visit to David Klein in Geneva he saw a 10-year-old girl who had a remarkably severe auditory-pigmentary syndrome, in which the features he had noted in his tailor were present to an extreme degree, combined with severe limb amyoplasia. No longer confident that the hearing loss was coincidental, he conducted a major study of residents of a Dutch institution for the deaf, looking for inherited dystopia canthorum. He ascertained 14 unrelated probands, whose families included 161 affected individuals.

In 1971 Sergio Arias (3) pointed out that dystopia was not a universal feature of Waardenburg syndrome, but was characteristic of particular families. Within those families dystopia was highly penetrant (98–99%), but in other families none of the affected people had dystopia. Thus Arias distinguished Type 1 WS (with dystopia; MIM 193500) from Type 2 (without dystopia; MIM 193510). Except for the facial build, the features were the same in both types. Perhaps because his primary interest was in ophthalmology, Waardenburg had noted absence of dystopia in only two of his 161 cases, but in fact Type 2 WS is at least as common as Type 1.

Klein's patient, with very extreme features of WS combined with amyoplasia, was the subject of some controversy. In his 1951 paper (1) Waardenburg speculated that she might be a homozygote (family details were unclear); later he came to feel she represented a different syndrome. This came to be known as Klein-Waardenburg syndrome, or Type 3 WS (MIM 148820). Later, other cases with features of WS1 plus muscular hypoplasia or joint contractures were also gathered under the Klein-Waardenburg label, although none of them was nearly so severely affected as Klein's original patient. Klein himself regarded all these cases as part of the spectrum of a unitary Waardenburg syndrome, and felt that the name Klein-Waardenburg syndrome should apply to everybody.

Type 4 WS (MIM 277580) is often called Shah-Waardenburg syndrome, after a report by Shah et al. (4) of 12 Indian babies with Hirschsprung disease (HSCR) and white forelocks. Contrary to common belief, they did not have Waardenburg eye coloration—Shah reported that they had "isochromia irides, light brown irides with mosaic pattern...a common inherited condition in our population." All 12 died before their hearing was assessed. Thus it is far from clear that these babies had the WS-HSCR combination that characterizes WS4.

II. THE DEVELOPMENTAL BASIS OF WAARDENBURG SYNDROME

The reason why pigmentary anomalies and hearing loss are frequently associated is that melanocytes are required for both processes. In the inner ear, the intermediate cells of the stria vascularis are melanocytes, and in their absence the stria fails to perform its function of maintaining the unusual ionic composition of the cochlear endolymph. The consequence is a loss of hearing. Melanin pigment is not itself necessary for this function, because albinos have grossly normal hearing; auditory pigmentary syndromes result from a physical absence of melanocytes in the affected tissues.

All melanocytes, except those of the retinal pigment epithelium, originate in the embryonic neural crest. During embryogenesis, between days 9 and 12 in the mouse, melanocyte precursors migrate out of the neural crest to their final locations in the skin, hair, eyes, and inner ear. Thus

Waardenburg syndrome can result either from a defect restricted to melanocytes or their direct precursors, or from a more general disturbance of
neural crest function. Type 2 WS is a purely auditory-pigmentary syndrome
(or rather a collection of diverse syndromes with those features, see below)
and is caused by melanocyte-specific problems. The other types of WS all
involve other neural crest derivatives (the facial bones, limb muscles, and
enteric ganglia) and are thus neurocristopathies.

Many other auditory-pigmentary syndromes are distinguished from
WS. The standard text by Gorlin et al. (5) lists 16 human syndromes involving hearing loss and pigmentary abnormalities. Neural crest differentiation is so complex, and gives rise to so many different adult tissues,
that there must be many different neurocristopathies that produce features of
Waardenburg syndrome combined with other abnormalities. A distinction is
often made on the basis of the distribution of pigment. The pigmentary
anomalies in Waardenburg syndrome are typically patchy, with areas of
normal pigmentation and others lacking melanocytes. In some deaf patients
there is a uniform dilution of pigmentation. This is usually labeled Tietz or
Tietz-Smith syndrome (MIM 103500). In fact, the distinction between patchy
and diluted pigmentation may not be very fundamental. In the *microphthalmia* mouse, an important animal model of WS2 (see below), some *mi*
alleles produce spotting and others produce uniform dilution.

III. CLINICAL FINDINGS

A. Type 1 WS

Diagnostic criteria for WS1 were suggested by the International Waardenburg Consortium (6) (Table 1). The key feature is dystopia canthorum, an
outward displacement of the inner canthi of the eyes, with the inferior
lacrimal puncta opening opposite the iris rather than the sclera. Dystopia is
not the same as hypertelorism (an outward displacement of the entire globe),
but there is considerable confusion between the two in descriptions of WS
patients, not least because most WS1 patients have both dystopia and
hypertelorism. Dystopia is best assessed by measuring the inner canthal,
interpupillary, and outer canthal distances, in millimeters, using a rigid ruler
held against the forehead, and then applying the formula in Figure 1. As a
quick check, when a WS1 patient looks straight ahead, typically far less
white is visible on the inner side of the iris than on the outer side. Despite the
rather Byzantine numbers in the formula (produced by a discriminant
analysis), the resulting W index has proved a highly reliable predictor of
WS1. Figure 2 shows the average and extreme W values from 51 families
studied by the Waardenburg Consortium (7). Linkage analysis divided the

Table 1 Diagnostic Criteria for Waardenburg Syndrome as Proposed by the Waardenburg Consortium (6)

To be counted as affected an individual must have two major or one major plus two minor criteria, from the following list:

Major criteria

    Congenital sensorineural hearing loss

    Pigmentary disturbances of iris: (a) complete heterochromia iridum—two eyes of different color; (b) partial or segmental heterochromia: segments of blue or brown pigmentation in one or both eyes; or (c) hypoplastic blue eyes—characteristic brilliant blue in both eyes

    Hair hypopigmentation—white forelock

    Dystopia canthorum—W > 1.95 averaged over affected family members (this was modified from the original proposal of W > 2.07 in the light of experience)

    Affected first-degree relative

Minor criteria

    Congenital leukoderma—several areas of hypopigmented skin

    Synophrys or medial eyebrow flare

    Broad and high nasal root

    Hypoplasia of alae nasi

    Premature graying of hair—scalp hair predominantly white before age 30

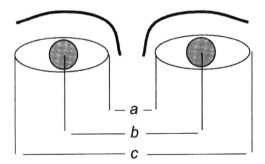

Figure 1 Method of calculating the W index for dystopia canthorum. (1) Measure a (inner canthal distance), b (interpupillary distance), and c (outer canthal distance) in millimeters using a rigid ruler held against the forehead. (2) Calculate X = (2a − 0.2119c − 3.909)/c. (3) Calculate Y = (2a − 0.2479b − 3.909)/b. (4) Calculate W = X + Y + a/b. Dystopia is present when W > 1.95.

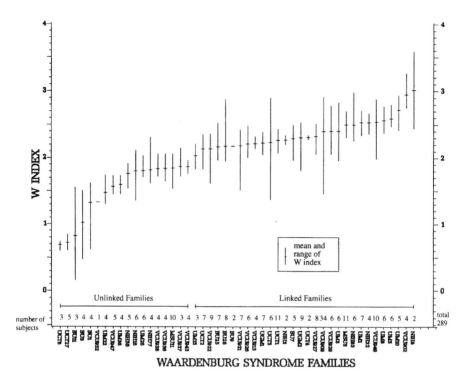

Figure 2 W index as a means of discriminating Types 1 and 2 WS. Each vertical line represents the mean and range of W values among affected people in one family. Data are shown from 51 families studied by the Waardenburg Consortium that had been tested for linkage to the *PAX3* locus on chromosome 2q35. The families are arranged from left to right in order of increasing mean W value. All families with mean W > 1.95 showed linkage to *PAX3* (Type 1 WS); no family with W < 1.95 showed linkage (Type 2 WS). (Data from Farrer et al. Am J Hum Genet 55:728-737, 1994, reproduced with permission.)

families into those linked to 2q35 (the locus for WS1, see below) and those not linked. It can be seen that a family average W value of 1.95 cleanly separates linked and unlinked families, although individual affected family members may lie either side of the threshold. Clearly, larger series are likely to include the occasional family where the average of affected members happens to lie on the wrong side of the threshold, but the averaged W index remains by far the best discriminator of Types 1 and 2 WS. Other common facial features of WS1 are a high nasal bridge, broad square jaw, hypoplastic alae nasi, and synophrys, although none of these is reliable on its own.

Dystopia is the most penetrant feature of WS1, and is seen in >95% of cases (3). All the other features are extremely variable, both between families and within families. Table 2 lists the penetrances seen for a number of features in the study of Liu et al. (8), with for comparison figures for Type 2 Waardenburg syndrome.

The hearing loss of WS1 is congenital, sensorineural and nonprogressive, at least after the first month. There have been suggestions that functional hearing is lost as the cochlea degenerates in response to the abnormal ionic composition of the endolymph, but clear evidence of this is lacking. The loss can be of any degree, and unilateral or bilateral. Audiogram configurations are extremely variable (9), presumably reflecting the random patchy absences of melanocytes. Vestibular problems are not reported. There is only a single report of temporal bone histology of a patient with mutation-confirmed WS1 (10). The patient had typical features of WS1 including dystopia, heterochromia, and white hair, and a confirmed *PAX3* mutation. She had a low-frequency loss on the right side, which had been stable for many years, though with gradually increasing thresholds, and normal hearing on the left side. After her death from cancer at the age of 76, temporal bone histology showed an entirely normal inner ear on the left, while on the right only the lower turn of the cochlea was normal, consistent with her retained high-frequency hearing. In the more apical parts there was absence of melanocytes, absence of the stria, missing hair cells, dysmorphogenesis of the tectorial membrane, and lack of peripheral processes on the spiral ganglion cells. This case nicely confirms the observations on mice (2) showing a clean correlation between hearing loss and the absence of melanocytes in the stria, and shows that the hearing loss is a downstream consequence of malfunction of the stria vascularis caused by absence of intermediate cells.

Table 2 Penetrance (%) of Clinical Features of Type I and Type II Waardenburg Syndrome

Type	Source	n	SNHL	HetI	HypE	WF	EG	Skin	HNR	Eyb
WS1	Liu et al.	60	58	15	15	48	38	36	100	63
	Literature	210	57	31	18	43	23	30	52	70
WS2	Liu et al.	81	78	42	3	23	30	5	0	7
	Literature	43	77	54	23	16	14	12	14	7

Source: Data from Liu et al. (8). The data comprise a personally examined series and a series taken from the literature. SNHL, sensorineural hearing loss; HetI, heterochromia irides; HypE, hypoplastic blue eyes; WF, white forelock; EG, early graying; Skin, white skin patches; HNR, high nasal root; Eyb, medial eyebrow flare.

Heterochromia may present either as different-colored eyes (typically one blue and one brown eye) or as different colors within a single eye. Usually this takes the form of sharply demarcated radial sectors of different colors; circular frills or fringes of color are not a good indicator. In some patients both eyes are a striking pale-blue color, and the iris stroma is hypoplastic. This should not be confused with the pale eye coloration in some newborn babies of dark-skinned parents, where the normal brown eye color develops gradually after birth.

A white central forelock is often present from birth, varying from a few white hairs to an extensive blaze (patients may disguise it by dyeing). Alternatively it may first appear some time after birth as the first sign of the early graying that is a common feature of the syndrome. Forelocks of different colors (black, red) or colored locks in different positions are sometimes reported, though it is not clear how many of these patients have proven WS1. White skin patches are an occasional feature; if depigmentation is extensive, the alternative diagnosis of piebaldism (MIM 172800) should be considered.

Many other features have been described in WS1 patients, summarised by da-Silva (11), but it is not clear how many of these are truly part of WS1. There is unquestionably a small increased risk of spina bifida, probably also of cleft palate and Sprengel shoulder. A risk of Hirschsprung disease is often mentioned, but this is based on confusing WS1 with the genetically different condition of WS4, where HSCR is a defining feature.

B.   Other Subtypes of Waardenburg Syndrome

Apart from the absence of dystopia canthorum and the associated facial features, WS2 is identical to WS1. Many series report a higher incidence of hearing loss, but this is likely to be a bias of ascertainment—without dystopia as a guide, it is difficult to report a WS2 family member as affected unless there is hearing loss. WS2 is a clinical label rather than a unitary genetic condition, and it is best to restrict that label to cases where abnormalities are restricted to melanocytes, in which case by definition one would not expect other complications. This rather circular argument does not answer the concern of a WS2 patient about the risk of a child being more severely affected, but it does correspond to the reality, that WS2 is not associated with other abnormalities, once cases with Hirschsprung disease are reclassified as WS4. In particular, there is no evidence of an increased risk of neural tube defects or limb abnormalities. Of course, homozygotes might well be severely affected. No definite human WS2 homozygote has been reported, but in an animal model, the *microphthalmia* mouse, homozygotes are totally depigmented and may have microphthalmia, mast cell defects, osteopetrosis, and abnormal teeth.

WS3 (Klein-Waardenburg syndrome) has the features of WS1, including dystopia, plus limb abnormalities. There are two very different sets of cases. It was recently demonstrated (12) that Waardenburg was correct in his original hypothesis about Klein's patient: she is homozygous for WS1 (in fact, a compound heterozygote for two *PAX3* mutations, G99S/R270C), although the family history is still unresolved. Two other proven homozygotes have been reported. One (13) closely resembles Klein's patient; the other (14; our unpublished data) was a grossly abnormal fetus, conceived by incest between brother and sister with WS1 and aborted because of exencephaly detected on scan. Apart from these three cases, all other reported "WS3" patients had a much milder phenotype. Several had relatives with typical WS1, and some were shown to be heterozygous for *PAX3* mutations typical of WS1. Thus these mild "WS3" patients simply represent part of the range of expression of WS1, and do not merit a separate label. Conversely, they suggest that there is always a small risk of such relatively mild limb problems in any WS1 family.

For WS4 the label Shah-Waardenburg syndrome is probably best discarded in favor of the more descriptive "Waardenburg-Hirschsprung syndrome." Most cases described do not have dystopia canthorum, although there seems to be no a priori reason why some patients might not have a disturbance of development affecting both the precursors of the enteric ganglia and the cell lineages affected by WS1 mutations. The range of phenotypes to be expected can only be discussed once the underlying genetic defect has been defined.

IV. FORMAL GENETICS OF WAARDENBURG SYNDROME

WS1 and WS2 are autosomal dominant conditions with very variable expression. For WS1 the penetrance is very high (98–99%) because dystopia is a near-universal feature. For WS2, there are some families where penetrance is high, and a large penumbra of families with a much more vague pattern of hearing loss and/or minor pigmentary anomalies. Whether these latter families should be described as WS2 is questionable. Minor disturbances of melanocyte function (whether due to defective migration from the embryonic neural crest or a failure of proliferation or survival) are common in the general population, and these may occur as low-penetrance dominant phenotypes in families. WS2 is unquestionably genetically heterogeneous. Mutations in the only gene defined to date, *MITF* (see below), are largely confined to families with a pronounced dominant history, but operationally, we have been unable to define clinical criteria that separate all MITF families from the "penumbra" families.

WS3, as described above, is a purely clinical description of a set of WS1 homozygotes or heterozygotes, and is not a genetic entity. WS4 includes several different genetic conditions. Some, caused by mutations in endothelin 3 and its receptor, are recessive; others, caused by mutations in *SOX10*, are dominant (but often new mutations), while yet others are at present undefined. Occasional patients homozygous for mutations in *EDNRB* or *EDN3* have pigmentary features but not Hirschsprung disease, and are describable clinically as WS2.

V. IDENTIFICATION OF GENES UNDERLYING WAARDENBURG SYNDROME

Five genes, *PAX3*, *MITF*, *EDN3*, *EDNRB,* and *SOX10*, have been implicated in Waardenburg syndrome, and others remain to be defined. The relation of genotypes to phenotypes is summarized in Table 3.

Table 3 Phenotypes and Genotypes in Human Auditory-Pigmentary Syndromes

Condition	Phenotype	Genotype(s)
Type 1 WS	Auditory-pigmentary features plus dystopia	Heterozygous for loss of function mutations in *PAX3*
Type 2 WS ·	As Type 1, but without dystopia	10–15% of families heterozygous for loss-of-function mutations in *MITF*
		Rarely, homozygous for loss of function mutations in *EDNRB* or *EDN3*
		Most families without known cause
Type 3 WS	As Type 1, but with limb abnormalities	Loss of function mutations in *PAX3*
		Homozygous in rare severe cases; heterozygous in others
Type 4 WS	As Type 2, but with Hirschsprung disease	(a) Homozygous for loss-of-function mutations in *EDNRB*
		(b) Homozygous for loss-of-function mutations in *EDN3*
		(c) Heterozygous for loss-of-function (?) mutations in *SOX10*
		(d) Many cases without known cause
Tietz syndrome	Dominant severe hearing loss with uniform pigmentary dilution	2 families heterozygous for dominant negative (?) mutations in *MITF*
		Most cases without known cause

A. Identification of *PAX3*

Linkage analysis mapped a WS1 locus to distal 2q in 1990 (15,16). This region shows strongly conserved synteny with the distal part of mouse chromosome 1. A mouse mutant, *Splotch*, mapped to the same area. *Sp* heterozygous mice have a white belly spot, while homozygotes die with lethal neural tube defects (17) or (it was later discovered) conotruncal heart defects (18). *Splotch* was not an obvious candidate for a WS1 homolog because the heterozygous mice had no apparent hearing defect [confirmed in later detailed work (19)], while homozygotes had inner ear malformations, placing *Splotch* in the morphogenetic rather than cochleosaccular category in Steel's classification of hearing defects (20). However, an interesting candidate gene for a neurocristopathy mapped to the approximate candidate region in the mouse. This was *Pax-3*, a gene encoding a transcription factor expressed in the embryonic neural crest. Part of the likely human homolog of *Pax-3* had been cloned by Burri et al. (21) and named HuP2. Simultaneous analysis of mouse and human DNA revealed mutations in *Pax-3* in *Sp* and in HuP2, now renamed *PAX3*, in WS1 patients (22–24).

B. Identification of *MITF*

A promising mouse model for WS2, the *microphthalmia* mouse (25), mapped to mouse chromosome 6, but synteny is poorly conserved between mouse and human in this region, and attempts to use the mouse map to predict the map location of human WS2 genes were unsuccessful. A whole genome search in a large WS2 family mapped the locus to the proximal short arm of chromosome 3, at 3p14-p21 (26). Eventually *mi* was cloned, and the human homolog was then identified and physically mapped (27). Since the human gene, *MITF*, mapped to precisely the location on 3p defined by our linkage studies, *MITF* became a strong candidate for this WS2 gene, and mutations were soon identified (28).

C. Identification of *EDNRB* and *EDN3*

Disruption of *Ednrb*, encoding the endothelin receptor B, in mice unexpectedly identified that gene as the cause of a much-studied WS4 model, *piebald-lethal* (s^l) (29). A variable Waardenburg-Hirschsprung phenotype had been mapped to human chromosome 13 in a very large Mennonite family, and a number of other case reports also suggested the presence on chromosome 13 of a gene implicated in Waardenburg-Hirschsprung disease (30). The human *EDNRB* gene mapped within the chromosome 13 WS-HSCR candidate region, and so was tested for mutations. These were soon detected in the Mennonite family, and subsequently in other WS4 families (31,32). The ligand of the *ENDRB* receptor is endothelin 3, encoded by the *EDN3* gene located on chromosome 20. In the mouse, disruption of *Edn3* produced another WS-HSCR phenotype, *lethal-spotting* (*ls*), and homozygous *EDN3* mutations were identified in a few WS4 patients (33,34).

D. Identification of *SOX10*

A third mouse model of WS-HSCR is *Dominant megacolon* (*Dom*). The gene underlying this phenotype was identified by positional cloning as *Sox10* (35,36). Waardenburg, Hirschsprung, and Waardenburg-Hirschsprung patients were tested for mutations in the human homolog, *SOX10*, and these were found in a small number of WS-HSCR patients (37). *SOX10* is located on human chromosome 22q13, but because of the severity of the phenotype, most cases are new mutations, and linkage analysis played no part in identifying the human gene.

VI. MOLECULAR PATHOLOGY OF WAARDENBURG SYNDROME

PAX3, *MITF*, and *SOX10* all encode transcription factors. In common with many other transcription factors, the genes are dosage sensitive—a half dose of the gene product is not enough for completely normal development (haploinsufficiency). Conditions caused by haploinsufficiency are typically very variable, even within families, and Waardenburg syndrome is typical in this respect. Presumably there is a fairly fine balance within the cell, and the final outcome will reflect both variations in the interacting partners and chance events.

    PAX3 is a member of the paired box family of genes, which comprises nine genes, *PAX1–PAX9*, in mice and humans. Their common feature is a paired box, encoding a 128- or 129-amino-acid bipartite DNA-binding domain first characterized in the *Drosophila paired* gene (38). The *PAX3*, *-4*, *-6*, and *-7* genes additionally encode a 60-amino-acid homeodomain. Thus the PAX3 protein contains three DNA-binding elements, the N-terminal and C-terminal parts of the paired domain, and the paired-type homeodomain. Additionally there is a typical serine-threonine-rich transactivation domain toward the C-terminal part of the protein, and a conserved octapeptide, HSIDGILS, of unknown function located between the paired and homeo domains. The three DNA-binding elements interact, allowing a rich and subtle repertoire of interactions that are far from fully understood. Additionally there must be protein-protein interactions, which may involve the homeodomain and octapeptide as well as the transactivation domain.

The *PAX3* gene comprises 10 exons, covering almost 100 kb of genomic DNA at chromosome 2q35. Exons 2–4 contain the paired box, and exons 5 and 6 the homeobox. Alternative splicing at the 3' end produces isoforms terminating in exon 8, 9, or 10, and other forms have been reported that terminate after exon 4. It is not known whether any of these differences are functionally important. Alternative splice acceptors at the start of exon 3 produces forms with (+Q) or without (−Q) glutamine at amino acid 108. These variants show differential patterns of transcriptional activation in an in vitro assay (39). *PAX3* is expressed, as expected, in the embryonic neural crest and in some of the populations of cells migrating out of this tissue.

As is usually the case with transcription factors, identifying the downstream targets has been difficult. The DNA-binding sequences are not tightly enough specified to allow database searching to define target genes, and experimental approaches have an uncertain relation to the reality in the cell. An ambitious attempt to define targets by an in vitro cyclical DNA amplification and selection method (40) has produced a long list of possible targets, which will need painstaking validation. Known targets include *MITF* (41), *MET* (42), *RET* (43), and (perhaps indirectly) *MyoD* and/or *Myf5* (44). Each of these helps explain features of Waardenburg syndrome. Control of *MITF* by *PAX3* explains why the melanocyte features of WS1 and WS2 are so similar; *SOX10* is also involved in this control. *MET* is required for migration of muscle precursor cells from the neural crest into embryonic limb buds, and *MyoD* and/or *Myf5* is a master gene for muscle differentiation, thus explaining the muscle defects in WS3. People with loss of function mutations in *RET* often have Hirschsprung disease, but the precise role of the *PAX3-RET* relationship in WS-HSCR is not clear.

MITF and its mouse homolog *mi* appear to be master genes for melanocyte development. They encode transcription factors of the basic helix-loop-helix leucine zipper (bHLH-Zip) family. These bind their DNA target as dimers (homo- or heterodimers); the basic region affects the binding and the HLH and Zip regions govern dimerization. Known targets include several melanocyte-specific genes such as tyrosinase and *TRP2*. Transcription of *MITF* is under the control of *PAX3* and *SOX10*, and MITF protein is activated by phosphorylation downstream of the KIT receptor (explaining the similarities between WS2 and piebaldism, caused by *KIT* loss of function mutations) and probably also by GSK3β. MITF protein is also involved in eye development (homozygous mutant mice are microphthalmic) and must have other actions as well, because mice homozygous for certain *mi* mutations have skeletal and/or mast cell defects.

SOX10 is a member of the large SOX family of transcription factors, the best known member of which is *SRY*, the male-determining factor. SOX proteins contain an HMG box DNA-binding element, but in vitro this shows weak and very nonspecific binding. Specificity must be achieved by using different cofactors that presumably bind to adjacent sequences and then strengthen the DNA binding by protein-protein interaction (45). Exactly how *EDNRB/EDN3* mutations cause a WS-HSCR phenotype is not known, though studies of mice carrying manipulable transgenes that could be turned on or off at will have shown that EDN3/EDNRB function is needed only between days 10 and 12.5 to avoid the WS4 phenotype (46).

VII. THE MUTATIONAL SPECTRUM IN WAARDENBURG SYNDROME

PAX3 attracted interest as the first homeobox gene shown to be mutated in a heritable human disease. Many different mutations have been described in WS1 patients, including both truncating (nonsense and splice site) and missense mutations, as well as deletions of the whole gene. This spectrum demonstrates that the pathogenic mechanism is loss of function, and since WS1 is dominant, shows the importance of haploinsufficiency. A completely different condition is produced by a gain of function. Alveolar rhabdomyosarcoma, an aggressive childhood tumor, is commonly associated with a translocation t(2;13)(q35;14) that joins *PAX3* exons 1–7 on to sequence from the *FKHR* forkhead-related transcription factor (47). This somatic gene fusion creates a chimeric gene encoding an overactive version of the PAX3 protein (48).

Within WS1 patients there is no significant genotype-phenotype correlation, although careful analysis of a large series (49) showed a higher chance of pigmentary anomaly among patients with premature termination codons upstream of the homeodomain, compared to those with point mutations causing amino acid substitutions in the homeodomain. Unfortunately for genetic counselors, no predictor of hearing loss was found. Nonsense-mediated mRNA decay (50) makes it likely that alleles with premature termination codons produce no PAX3 protein.

Missense mutations are concentrated in sequences encoding two crucial DNA-binding regions, the N-terminal part of the paired domain and the third (recognition) helix of the homeodomain. X-ray crystallography of related proteins has shown that the amino acids involved form crucial DNA contacts (51). Truncating mutations are more widely spread through the gene, as expected. Most are seen only in single families, showing that recurrent mutation is the main mechanism responsible for the persistence of

Waardenburg syndrome. A few recurrent mutations are known. 873insG inserts an extra guanine nucleotide in a run of 6 G's, and has been seen in several independent families; homopolymeric runs are known to be mutation hotspots because of replication slippage.

Surprisingly, mutations of any sort have almost never been reported from the large region downstream of the homeobox, despite careful analysis of these regions in many patients. This is in contrast to *PAX6,* where truncating mutations are scattered across the entire coding sequence. The reason for this difference is hard to discern. This serine-threonine-rich downstream region of the PAX3 protein is presumed to constitute an activation domain. It seems unlikely that mutations in this region should cause no phenotype, or a phenotype so different from Waardenburg syndrome that the relevant patients have never been tested.

In a single family the *PAX3* missense mutation N47K is associated with a phenotype rather different from WS1, craniofacial-deafness-hand syndrome (MIM 122880) (52). It seems likely that amino acid 47 has some special functional significance in the PAX3 protein, because another substitution, N47H, is the cause of the only convincing example of familial WS3 (53).

For *MITF,* again the spectrum of mutations suggests loss of function and haploinsufficiency as the pathogenic mechanism. Since B-HLH-Zip family proteins act as dimers, there is the possibility of dominant negative effects, and it seems plausible that such effects explain two families in which *MITF* mutations cause Tietz syndrome (54,55). In both cases the basic region is mutated while the HLH and Zip domains remain intact, allowing the mutant protein to form dimers that might well be nonfunctional. The more severe and uniform phenotype of Tietz syndrome contrasts with the great variability of features in WS2-MITF families, the latter being typical of haploinsufficiency. However, we failed to find *MITF* mutations in several other families with Tietz syndrome (our unpublished data).

SOX10 mutations are rare, but the patients in which they have been found are surprisingly diverse. As well as a few with WS4, there are several with severe neurological features (56) and one described as having a form of the Yemenite deaf-blind-hypopigmentation syndrome (which does not include HSCR) (57). Much remains to be learned about the molecular pathology of *SOX10* mutants.

VIII. SUMMARY

The various forms of Waardenburg syndrome give us a window into aspects of neural crest and melanocyte differentiation. Detailed mechanistic explanations must await better definition of the natural targets of the various transcription factors involved.

REFERENCES

1. Waardenburg PJ. A new syndrome combining developmental anomalies of the eyelids, eyebrows and nose root with pigmentary defects of the iris and head hair and with congenital deafness. Am J Hum Genet 1951; 3:195–253.
2. Steel KP, Barkway C. Another role for melanocytes: their importance for normal stria vascularis development in the mammalian inner ear. Development 1989; 107:453–463.
3. Arias S. Genetic heterogeneity in the Waardenburg syndrome. Birth Defects Orig Art Series 1971; 7:87–101.
4. Shah KN, Dalal SJ, Sheth PN, Joshi NC, Ambani LM. White forelock, pigmentary disorder of the irides and long segment Hirschsprung disease: possible variant of Waardenburg syndrome. J Pediatr 1981; 99:432–435.
5. Gorlin RJ, Toriello HV, Cohen MM. Hereditary Hearing Loss and Its Syndromes. Oxford: OUP, 1995.
6. Farrer LA, Grundfast KM, Amos J, Arnos KS, Asher JH, Beighton P, Diehl SR, Fex J, Foy C, Frriedman TB, Greenberg J, Hoth C, Marazita M, Milunsky A, Morell R, Nance W, Newton V, Ramesar R, San Agustin TB, Skare J, Stevens CA, Wagner RG, Wilcox ER, Winship I, Read AP. Waardenburg syndrome (WS) type 1 is caused by defects at multiple loci, one of which is near ALPP on chromosome 2: first report of the WS Consortium. Am J Hum Genet 1992; 50:902–913.
7. Farrer LA, Arnos KS, Asher JH, Baldwin CT, Diehl SR, Friedman TB, Greenberg J, Grundfast KM, Hoth C, Lalwani AK, Landa B, Leverton K, Milunsky A, Morell R, Nance WE, Newton V, Ramesar R, Rao VS, Reynolds JE, San Agustin TB, Wilcox ER, Winship I, Read AP. Locus heterogeneity for Waardenburg syndrome is predictive of clinical subtypes. Am J Hum Genet 1994; 55:728–737.
8. Liu XZ, Newton VE, Read AP. Waardenburg syndrome Type 2: phenotypic findings and diagnostic criteria. Am J Med Genet 1995; 55:95–110.
9. Newton VE. Hearing loss and Waardenburg syndrome: implications for genetic counselling. J Laryngol Otol 1990; 104:97–103.
10. Merchant SN, McKenna MJ, Baldwin CT, Milunsky A, Nadol JB. Otopathology in a case of Type I Waardenburg's syndrome. Ann Otol Rhinol Laryngol 2001; 110:875–882.
11. da-Silva EO. Waardenburg I syndrome: a clinical and genetic study of two large Brazilian kindreds, and literature review. Am J Med Genet 1991; 40:65–74.
12. Bottani A, Antonarakis SE, Blouin JL. PAX3 missense mutations (G99S and R270C) in the original patient described with Klein-Waardenburg syndrome [abstr]. Am J Hum Genet 1999; 65(suppl):A143.

13. Zlotogora J, Lerer I, Bar-David S, Ergaz Z, Abielovich D. Homozygosity for Waardenburg syndrome. Am J Hum Genet 1995; 56:1173–1178.

14. Aymé S, Philip N. Possible homozygous Waardenburg syndrome in a fetus with exencephaly. Am J Med Genet 1995; 59:263–265.

15. Foy C, Newton VE, Wellesley D, Harris R, Read AP. Assignment of WS1 locus to human 2q37 and possible homology between Waardenburg syndrome and the Splotch mouse. Am J Hum Genet 1990; 46:1017–1023.

16. Morell R, Friedman TB, Moeljopawiro S, Hartono, Soewito, Asher JH. A frameshift mutation in the HuP2 paired domain of the probable human homolog of murine Pax-3 is responsible for Waardenburg syndrome type 1 in an Indonesian family. Hum Mol Genet 1992; 1:243–247.

17. Moase CE, Trasler DG. Splotch locus mouse mutants: model for neural tube defects and Waardenburg syndrome type I in humans. J Med Genet 1992; 29: 145–151.

18. Conway SJ, Henderson DJ, Kirby ML, Anderson RH, Copp AJ. Development of a lethal congenital heart defect in the splotch (Pax3) mutant mouse. Cardiovasc Res 1997; 36:163–173.

19. Steel KP, Smith RJH. Normal hearing in Splotch (Sp/+), the mouse homologue of Waardenburg syndrome Type 1. Nat Genet 1992; 2:75–79.

20. Steel KP. Inherited hearing defects in mice. Annu Rev Genet 1995; 29:675–701.

21. Burri M, Tromvoukis Y, Bopp D, Frigerio G, Noll M. Conservation of the paired domain in metazoans and its structure in three isolated human genes. EMBO J 1989; 8:1183–1190.

22. Epstein DJ, Vekemans M, Gros P. Splotch (Sp2^H), a mutation affecting development of the mouse neural tube, shows a deletion within the paired homeodomain of Pax-3. Cell 1991; 67:767–774.

23. Tassabehji M, Read AP, Newton VE, Harris R, Balling R, Gruss P, Strachan T. Waardenburg syndrome patients have mutations in the human homologue of the Pax-3 paired box gene. Nature 1992; 355:635–636.

24. Baldwin CT, Hoth CF, Amos JA, da-Silva EO, Milunsky A. An exonic mutation in the HuP2 paired domain gene causes Waardenburg's syndrome. Nature 1992; 355:637–638.

25. Asher JH, Friedman TB. Mouse and hamster mutants as models for Waardenburg syndrome in humans. J Med Genet 1990; 27:618–626.

26. Hughes A, Newton VE, Liu XZ, Read AP. A gene for Waardenburg syndrome type 2 maps close to the human homologue of the microphthalmia gene at chromosome 3p12-p14.1. Nat Genet 1994; 7:509–512.

27. Tachibana M, Perez-Jurado LA, Nakayama A, Hodgkinson CA, Li X, Schneider M, Miki T, Fex J, Francke U, Arnheiter H. Cloning of MITF, the human homolog of the mouse microphthalmia gene and assignment to chromosome 3p14.1-p12.3. Hum Mol Genet 1994; 3:553–557.

28. Tassabehji M, Newton VE, Read AP. MITF gene mutations causing Type 2 Waardenburg syndrome. Nat Genet 1994; 8:251–255.

29. Hosoda K, Hammer RE, Richardson JA, Baynash AG, Cheung JC, Giaid A, Yanagisawa M. Targeted and natural (piebald-lethal) mutations of endothelin-

B receptor gene produce megacolon associated with spotted coat color in mice. Cell 1994; 79:1267–1276.

30. Van Camp G, Van Thienen MN, Handig I, Van Roy B, Rao VS, Milunsky A, Read AP, Baldwin CT, Farrer LA, Bonduelle M, Standaert L, Meire F, Willems PJ. Chromosome 13q deletion with Waardenburg syndrome: further evidence for a gene involved in neural crest function on 13q. J Med Genet 1995; 32:531–536.

31. Puffenberger EG, Hosoda K, Washington SS, Nakao K, deWit D, Yanagisawa M, Chakravarti A. A missense mutation of the endothelin-B receptor gene in multigenic Hirschsprung's disease. Cell 1994; 79:1257–1266.

32. Attié T, Till M, Pelet A, Amiel J, Edery P, Boutrand L, Munnich A, Lyonnet S. Mutation of the endothelin-receptor B gene in Waardenburg-Hirschsprung disease. Hum Mol Genet 1995; 4:2407–2409.

33. Hofstra RM, Osinga J, Tan-Sindhunata G, Wu Y, Kamsteeg EJ, Stulp RP, van Ravenswaaij-Arts C, Majoor-Krakauer D, Angrist M, Chakravarti A, Meijers C, Buys CH. A homozygous mutation in the endothelin-3 gene associated with a combined Waardenburg type 2 and Hirschsprung phenotype (Shah-Waardenburg syndrome). Nat Genet 1996; 12:445–447.

34. Edery P, Attié T, Amiel J, Pelet A, Eng C, Hofstra RM, Martelli H, Bidaud C, Munnich A, Lyonnet S. Mutation of the endothelin-3 gene in the Waardenburg-Hirschsprung disease (Shah-Waardenburg syndrome). Nat Genet 1996; 12:442–444.

35. Southard-Smith EM, Kos L, Pavan WJ. *Sox10* mutation disrupts neural crest development in *Dom* Hirschsprung mouse model. Nat Genet 1998; 18:60–64.

36. Herbarth B, Pingault N, Bondurand N, Kuhlbrodt K, Hermans-Borgmeyer I, Puliti A, Lemort N. Herbarth B, Pingault V, Bondurand N, Kuhlbrodt K, Hermans-Borgmeyer I, Puliti A, Lemort N, Goossens M, Wegner M, et al. Mutation of the Sry-related *Sox10* gene in *Dominant megacolon*, a mouse model for human Hirschsprung disease. Proc Natl Acad Sci USA 1998; 95:5161–5165.

37. Pingault V, Bondurand N, Kuhlbrodt K, Goerich DE, Prehu MO, Puliti A, Herbarth B, Hermans-Borgmeyer I, Legius E, Matthijs G, Amiel J, Lyonnet S, Ceccherini I, Romeo G, Smith JC, Read AP, Wegner M, Goossens M. *SOX10* mutations in patients with Waardenburg-Hirschsprung disease. Nat Genet 1998; 18:171–173.

38. Bopp D, Burri M, Baumgartner S, Frigiero G, Noll M. Conservation of a large protein domain in the segmentation gene paired and in functionally related genes of *Drosophila*. Cell 1986; 47:1033–1040.

39. Vogan KJ, Underhill DA, Gros P. An alternative splicing event in the *Pax-3* paired domain identifies the linker region as a key determinant of paired domain DNA-binding activity. Mol Cell Biol 1996; 16:6677–6686.

40. Barber TD, Barber MC, Tomescu O, Barr FG, Ruben S, Friedman TB. Identification of target genes regulated by *PAX3* and *PAX3-FKHR*. Genomics 2002; 79:278–284.

41. Watanebe A, Takeda K, Ploplis B, Tachibana M. Epistatic relationship between Waardenburg syndrome genes *MITF* and *PAX3*. Nat Genet 1998; 18:283–286.

42. Epstein JA, Shapiro DN, Cheng J, Lam PYP, Maas RL. *Pax3* modulates expression of the c-Met receptor during limb muscle development. Proc Natl Acad Sci USA 1996; 93:4213–4218.

43. Lang D, Chen F, Milewski R, Li J, Lu MM, Epstein JA. *Pax3* is required for enteric ganglia formation and functions with *Sox10* to modulate expression of *c-ret*. J Clin Invest 2000; 106:963–971.

44. Tajbakhsh S, Rocancourt D, Cossu G, Buckingham M. Redefining the genetic hierarchies controlling skeletal myogenesis: *Pax-3* and *Myf-5* act upstream of MyoD. Cell 1997; 89:27–138.

45. Kamachi Y, Uchikawa M, Kondoh H. Pairing SOX off with partners in the regulation of embryonic development. Trends Genet 2000; 16:182–187.

46. Shin MK, Levorese JM, Ingram RS, Tilghman SM. The temporal requirement for endothelin receptor-B signalling during neural crest development. Nature 1999; 402:496–501.

47. Galili N, Davis RJ, Fredericks WJ, Mukhopadhyay S, Rauscher FJ, Emanuel BS, Rovera G, Barr FG. Fusion of a fork head domain gene to *PAX3* in the solid tumour alveolar rhabdomyosarcoma. Nat Genet 1993; 5:230–235.

48. Hollenbach AD, Sublett JE, McPherson CJ, Grosveld G. The Pax3-FKHR oncoprotein is unresponsive to the *Pax3*-associated repressor hDaxx. EMBO J 1999; 18:3702–3711.

49. DeStefano AL, Cupples LA, Arnos KS, Asher JH Jr, Baldwin CT, Blanton S, Carey ML, da Silva EO, Friedman TB, Greenberg J, Lalwani AK, Milunsky A, Nance WE, Pandya A, Ramesar RS, Read AP, Tassabejhi M, Wilcox ER, Farrer LA. Correlation between Waardenburg syndrome phenotype and genotype in a population of individuals with identified *PAX3* mutations. Hum Genet 1998; 102:499–506.

50. Frischmeyer PA, Dietz HC. Nonsense-mediated mRNA decay in health and disease. Hum Mol Genet 1999; 8:893–900.

51. Xu W, Rould MA, Jun S, Desplan C, Pabo CO. Crystal structure of a paired domain-DNA complex at 2.5A resolution reveals structural basis for Pax developmental mutations. Cell 1995; 80:639–650.

52. Asher JH Jr, Sommer A, Morrell R, Friedman TB. Missense mutation in the paired domain of *PAX3* causes craniofacial-deafness-hand syndrome. Hum Mutat 1996; 7:30–35.

53. Hoth CF, Milunsky A, Lipsky N, Sheffer R, Clarren SK, Baldwin CT. Mutations in the paired domain of the human *PAX3* gene cause Klein-Waardenburg syndrome (WS-III) as well as Waardenburg syndrome Type 1 (WS-1). Am J Hum Genet 1993; 52:455–462.

54. Amiel J, Watkin PM, Tassabehji M, Read AP, Winter RM. Mutation of the *MITF* gene in albinism-deafness syndrome (Tietz syndrome). Clin Dysmorphol 1998; 7:17–20.

55. Smith SD, Kenyon JB, Kelley PM, Hoover D, Comer B. Tietz syndrome (hypopigmentation/deafness) caused by mutation of MITF [abstr]. Am J Hum Genet 1997; 61(suppl):A347.

56. Touraine RL, Attie-Bitach T, Manceau E, Korsch E, Sarda P, Pingault V,

Encha-Razavi F, Pelet A, Auge J, Nivelon-Chevallier A, Holschneider AM, Munnes M, Doerfler W, Goossens M, Munnich A, Vekemans M, Lyonnet S. Neurological phenotype in Waardenburg syndrome type 4 correlates with novel *SOX10* truncating mutations and expression in developing brain. Am J Hum Genet 2000; 66:1496–1503.

57. Bondurand N, Kuhlbrodt K, Pingault V, Enderich J, Sajus M, Tommerup N, Warburg M, Hennekam RCM, Read AP, Wegner M, Goossens M. The Yemenite deaf-blind syndrome revisited: *SOX10* dysfunction causes different neurocristopathies. Hum Mol Genet 1999; 8:1785–1789.

7

Jervell and Lange-Nielsen Syndrome

Lisbeth Tranebjærg
*Wilhelm Johannsen Centre of Functional Genomics, Bispebjerg Hospital,
and University of Copenhagen, Copenhagen, Denmark*

I. INTRODUCTION

The scope of the chapter is the surdo-cardiac or Jervell and Lange-Nielsen syndrome (JLNS, MIM 220400). There will be some overlap with Romano-Ward or long-QT syndrome (RWS; LQTS) and sudden infant death syndrome (SIDS) because of the shared clinical, electrophysiological, and molecular genetic features involved.

II. BACKGROUND

The name of the cardiac-auditory disease, Jervell and Lange syndrome, was coined in 1957 after the description by Anton Jervell and Fred Lange-Nielsen, who discovered the rare combination of syncopes, congenital deaf-mutism, and elongated Q-T interval in the electrocardiogram (ECG) in one large Norwegian sibship (1). A description of fatal syncopal attacks, possibly the first report of JLNS, was given by Meissner in 1856: "The Patient was a deaf-mute girl in the Leipzig Institute for the deaf, who collapsed and died when she was being publicly admonished by the director for a misdemeanor. When the parents were informed, they evinced no surprise. It transpired then that one of their children had died suddenly after a terrible fright, and another after a violent fit of rage" (2,3). The condition is inherited in an autosomal recessive fashion, involves congenital profound hearing impairment associated with prolongation of the Q-T interval in the ECG, and predisposes to lethal cardiac arrhythmia, especially

117

under sympathic stimulation under stress such as swimming, scolding, and high sounds.

The clinically overlapping autosomal dominant RWS, named after the initial reports in 1963 and 1964 by Romano and Ward (4,5), and the delineation of the genetic predisposing factors behind the two conditions with apparently different modes of inheritance, have since become the focus of much scientific attention. Another early observation by Levine and Wordsworth in 1949 was not reported until 1958 because they waited for others to make the same observation of the rare association of profound hearing impairment and syncopal attacks (6). It was implied that the availability of electrocardiography in the 1950s paved the way for proper documentation of the cardiac abnormality in the syndrome (1). Fraser predicted in 1964 that the similarity between ECGs in the apparently different clinical entities might reflect a genetic relationship in causation (7). He specifically suggested the possibility that JLNS and isolated cardiac arrhythmia were due to either homozygosity or heterozygosity of mutations in the same gene(s).

This prediction has indeed been supported by several reports of autosomal dominant LQTS and autosomal recessive JLNS due to different mutations in the genes: *KCNQ1* and *KCNE1*. In addition, isolated autosomal recessive LQTS has been described in cases of mutations in *KCNQ1* without audiological affection, whereas no instances of isolated hearing impairment due to heterozygosity for a *KCNQ1* or *KCNE1* mutation have been identified so far. The mechanisms at the tissue level to explain this are still largely unknown.

The focus in reviews has often been on LQTS because of its higher frequency (8–10).

III. PREVALENCE ESTIMATES

The estimates of prevalence rely on reports with and without molecular confirmation, which makes it hard to estimate true figures.

Fraser et al. estimated prevalence rates of 1.6–6 per million (minimum and maximum estimates in 4–15-year-olds in England, Wales, and Ireland) inhabitants in England, Wales, and Ireland (7). Other studies lacking molecular investigation gave frequencies of 0.3% (2/154), 3.8% (5/132), and 6% (6/196) in Japan, Turkey, and the United States, respectively (11–14). The JLNS cases were identified either through the demonstration of elongated Q-T interval in populations of deaf children (11–13) or as congenital deafness associated with LQTS (14), and no molecular investigations

Table 1 *KCNQ1* Mutations Associated with JLNS

Nucleotide change	Mutation	Coding effect	Region	No. of families	Ethnic background	Phenotype	Ref.
IVS1+5G>A		Splice	S2	1	Fr	JLNS	28
451delCT		Frameshift	S2	1	Amish	JLNS	25
567insG		Frameshift	S2-S3	1	Sc	JLNS	18
623C>G	Y171X	Stop	S2	1	Fin	JLNS	21
572-576del		Frameshift	S2-S3	7	Nor	JLNS	15,16,17
728G>A	R243H	Missense	S4-S5	2	Fr, UK	JLNS	17,27
783G>C	E261D	Missense	S4-S5	1	Nor	JLNS	15,17
815G>A	G272D	Missense	S5	1	UK	JLNS	17
914G>C	W305S	Missense	Pore	2	Fr	JLNS	40
1008delC			S6	1	UK	JLNS	17
1188delC			S6	1	Haitian	JLNS	23
1552C>T	R518X	Stop	S6	9	Sw, Nor, USA	JLNS/LQTS	9,15,23,42
1588C>T	Q530X	Stop	S6	5	Nor, USA	JLNS/LQTS	9,15,17
1630,-7+8			S6	2	Fr	JLNS	19,43
1686-1G>A			S6	1	UK	JLNS	17
1760C>T	T587M	Missense	S6	2	USA	JLNS/LQTS	9,26,44
1781G>A	R594Q	Missense	S6	4	UK, USA	JLNS/LQTS	9,17
1876G>A	G589D	Missense	S6	34	Fin	JLNS/LQTS	21
1892del20		Frameshift	S6	1	Fr	JLNS	26
KCNE1 mutations associated with JLNS							
20C>T, 226G>A	T71, D76N	Missense		1	Lebanese	JLNS	22
139G>T	V47F,L51H	Missense		1	?	JLNS	46
172A>C, 176T>C, 177G>T	T59P, L60P	Missense		1	UK	JLNS	16,45
226G>A	D76N	Missense		2	?	JLNS/LQTS	37,46,47

were presented. Slightly variable diagnostic criteria were applied. The Turkish reports pinpointed the influence of consanguinity on the frequency (12,13). No molecular screening of populations of the deaf have been published. Estimates from Norway based on nationwide identification of all JLNS cases over several years may indicate a frequency of 1:200.000 (24/4.3 million) in the general population. Regional variation was found due to a founder mutation (15).

The syndome has been reported from Norway (1,15–17), England (7,16–18), Turkey (12,13,19,20), Sweden (Tranebjærg, unpublished data), Finland (21), Lebanon (22), Morocco (19), Kabylia (19), Haiti (23), "Caucasian American family" (23), Saudi-Arabia (24), the Amish (25), and France (26–28). See also Table 1.

IV. DIAGNOSTIC CRITERIA

In the ECG, the P wave represents atrial repolarization, the QRS complex represents ventricular depolarisation, and the T wave represents ventricular repolarization. A normal QTc is ~400 ms. QTc prolongation results from abnormal cardiac repolarization The diagnostic criteria for LQTS were described by Schwartz et al. (29) and modified by Priori et al. (30). LQTS is characterized by a QTc >440 ms in males and >460 ms in females associated with at least one of the following abnormalities: stress-related episodes of syncope, documented *torsades de pointes*, and a family history of early (under age 35) sudden cardiac death. Minor criteria include congenital deafness, episodes of T-wave alternans, low heart rate (in children), and abnormal ventricular repolarization. Diagnostic criteria for JLNS are congenital profound hearing impairment combined with a long Q-T. Syncopal attacks are most often associated with exercise, exertion or motion ("fear, flight, or fright") (29,30).

The hearing impairment in JLNS has without exception been congenital, profound, and stable. There has been no evidence for hearing impairment in heterozygous carriers of *KCNE1* or *KCNQ1* mutations (15; Kontula, personal communication).

V. OTHER CLINICAL ASPECTS

Older reports indicated an association with iron-deficient anemia in several instances (3,31), but we could not confirm this association to be an invariable part of the JLNS in our recent study (15). A likely explanation is anemia due to insufficient dietary iron intake.

A report from Turkish JLNS patients did not identify associated neurological abnormalities (20). Seizures in severely hearing-impaired individuals must always be considered to represent syncopal attacks due to unrecognized cardiac abnormalities as in JLNS, but otherwise no increased occurrence of epilepsy has been found (20). Numerous instances of misdiagnosed epilepsy and subsequent medical treatment are known (15).

Because of several reports of sudden unexpected childhood deaths in JLNS cases, it has been suggested that LQTS and JLNS might explain a recognizable fraction of sudden infant death syndrome (SIDS). Schwartz et al. provided clinical and electrocardiographic evidence for the possibility of unrecognized sudden infant death syndrome to be among cases with prolonged Q-T interval (32). A subsequent report confirmed a known LQTS-related *KCNQ1* mutation, C350T, in a SIDS patient (33).

In one Finnish family, a case of SIDS, identified by a questionnaire survey, was examined molecularly and identified to be a heterozygous carrier of the *KCNQ1* R589D mutation (21). In the published and well-characterized Norwegian JLNS families we found no cases of SIDS among relatives (15). The well-characterized spectrum of four identified *KCNQ1* mutations underlying JLNS in Norway makes this an excellent country to systematically screen a large number of SIDS cases for unrecognized JLNS mutations. An ongoing study has, so far, not identified any positive cases (Torleiv Rognum, 2002, personal communication). In summary, there is no evidence that a major fraction of SIDS cases are due to undiagnosed LQTS/JLNS.

VI. MOLECULAR GENETICS

All the genes identified so far in congenital LQTS encode ion channels responsible for the proper electrical activity of the cardiac cells. Among the estimated more than 70 human potassium genes, four out of five *KCNQ* genes have been associated with some channelopathy: cardiac arrhythmias, deafness, or epilepsy (34). Since 1995, six genes associated with cardiac arrhythmia susceptibility have been discovered: *KCNQ1* (formerly *KvLQT1*), *KCNH2* (formerly *HERG*), *SCN5A*, *KCNE1* (formerly *MinK*), *KCNE2* (formerly *MiRP1*), and *RyR2* (10). A seventh locus, LQT4, has been located to chromosome 4q25-27, but the gene awaits identification (35). Further genetic heterogeneity is predicted, since some LQTS families do not fit with linkage to either of the known loci or genes (10). Mutations in the sodium channel gene, *SCN5A*, and the ryanodine receptor gene, *RyR2*, also cause Brugada syndrome (right-bundle-branch block, ST segment elevation in leads V1–V3, and sudden death) and ventricular tachycardia (10).

The *KCNQ1* gene, found to be mutated in LQT cases, encodes for the (pore-forming) α-subunit of the voltage-gated K^+ channel protein that interacts with the (regulatory) β-subunit encoded by the *KCNE1* gene, and this gene immediately became an attractive candidate gene for mutation search in cases of normal *KCNQ1* sequence and LQT. Exclusion of the *KCNQ1* gene in some JLNS families was provided independently by two groups, reporting unrelated families with evidence against linkage to the *KCNQ1* locus on chromosome 11p15.5 (22,36), and soon after mutations were identified in the *KCNE1* gene (22). Individuals with JLNS have two mutations in either *KCNQ1* or *KCNE1* and therefore have no functional I_{Ks} channels. The hearing impairment segregates in a recessive fashion and the prolonged Q-T interval and cardiac arrhythmia in a semidominant way. So far, other loci or genes have not been implied as involved in JLNS although there are reports of clinically ascertained JLNS patients with one or no mutations detected (15,23,37).

KCNQ1 and KCNE1 interact to form the slow-activating delayed rectifying potassium channel (I_{Ks}) current and KCNH2 interact with KCNE2 to form the rapid delayed rectifying potassium current (I_{Kr}). This potassium channel repolarizes cardiac action potentials, and provides a pathway for the transepithelial potassium secretion in the inner ear (19,38) and is involved in keeping the potassium concentration high in the endolymph, which surrounds the organ of Corti. Mutations in the *KCNQ1* or *KCNE1* gene results in delayed repolarization and the inadequate endolymph production leads to degeneration of the organ of Corti (38). The molecular basis of the delayed rectifier current I_{Ks} in the heart was recently extensively reviewed (39).

Mutation in another KCNQ potassium channel gene, *KCNQ4*, is associated with autosomal dominant hearing impairment, but no cardiac abnormality (40). So far, no cases have been reported with impaired hearing associated with heterozygosity for mutations in *KCNQ1*, *KCNH1*, *KCNE1*, *KCNE2*, or *SCN5A*.

VII. SPECTRUM OF MUTATIONS

A compilation of the correct total number of patients and of all disease-causing mutations in *KCNQ1* and *KCNE1* genes is complicated by the fact that there are several cases with only one or no mutations reported in clinically diagnosed cases (13,23,37,48), and several examples of duplicate reports of identical patients. With that reservation, a total of at least 19 different *KCNQ1* mutations have been reported in JLNS patients (Table 1). They include seven missense and 12 frameshift/stop/splice mutations. At least seven other *KCNQ1* mutations are associated with autosomal recessive LQTS of "forme fruste" (49,50), which migh also cause JLNS. Table 1 summarizes all published JLNS mutations in the *KCNQ1* and the *KCNE1* genes. From Finland, two different mutations were identified and one of them, G589D, was found in heterozygosity in LQTS patients 'and in compound heterozygosity in a JLNS family. This mutation accounted for 30% of all LQTS mutations in Finland (21).

VIII.　GENETIC EPIDEMIOLOGY—THE SCANDINAVIAN PANORAMA

Our review from 1999 showed that 46% (11/24) of all disease alleles in diagnosed case of JLNS in Norway shared a new 5-bp *KCNQ1* mutation, and that the seven families all originated from mid-Norway (15). Three other mutations were also described. No other country but Norway has been implied to have a frequency of the condition as high as our estimate of 1:200,000 (24/4.3 million) nationwide (15).

Interestingly, the Finnish founder mutation, G589D, was associated with LQTS in the heterozygous state and with JLNS in the homozygous state (21). Only about one quarter of identified carriers of the mutation were symptomatic (LQTS).

A *KCNQ1* missense mutation, R518X, occurred in 5/24 disease alleles (four families) in Norway and has been identified in various countries in both LQTS and JLNS families (9,15–17,42). The mutation may be associated with autosomal dominant LQTS in heterozygosity and recessive LQTS or JLNS in homozygosity/compound heterozygosity form, making clinical prediction extremely difficult on the basis of heterozygosity for this mutation. Except for these examples no predominant mutations have been found.

IX.　HISTOPATHOLOGICAL AND FUNCTIONAL ASPECTS

To gain a deeper understanding of the pathogenesis of JLNS, it is of interest to compare older histological temporal bone investigations with more recent expression studies of the responsible genes. In three unrelated patients (11-year-old girl, 3-year-old boy, 12-year-old girl) (7,31,51,52) temporal bones demonstrated abnormal deposits of PAS-positive material in stria vascularis, as well as degeneration of the organ of Corti (52), whereas initial indications of spiral ganglion neuronal cell death (51) could not be confirmed later (52).

Despite a widespread expression of KCNQ1 in human kidney, placenta, lung, and placenta (53), the strongest expression was found in heart tissue and the pattern of expression as determined by in situ hybridation was restricted to the marginal cells of stria vascularis in mouse cochlea (19). Immunohistochemical and electrophysiological studies show that the I_{sk} protein localizes to the endolymphatic surface of stria vascularis in rat (54) and guinea pig (55), in perfect agreement with the histopathological findings in JLNS subjects (54,55).

Immunocytochemical and ultrastructural studies of wild-type and kcne $-/-$ (knockout) mice demonstrated colocalization of the KCNE1 and KCNQ1 proteins at the apical surface of vestibular dark cells already from gestational day 17 (56). The vestibular cells are normal at birth in kcne1 $-/-$ mice, but degenerative changes of the epithelial cells develop postnatally (56). Interestingly, the mice did not develop cardiac arrhythmia.

X. CLINICAL IMPLICATIONS OF *KCNQ1* AND *KCNE1* MUTATIONS

The clinical presentation as either LQTS or JLNS in carriers of *KCNQ1* or *KCNE1* mutation(s) depends on the nature of the underlying mutation(s) and the consequent functional impairment of the potassium channel (57). The term "lack of function" applies to a situation where a mutated gene does not lead to the synthesis of a full-length protein, either because of a deletion of parts of or the entire gene, or a frameshift mutation secondarily leading to a truncated peptide. This is thought to be the mechanism in those mutations presenting as recessive, in the sense that heterozygous carriers have no affection and homozygosity for the same of two different mutations leads to clinically JLNS. The majority of mutations in *KCNQ1* reported in JLNS patients belong to this type of disruption of the encoding gene. A few examples of splice site mutations also have been shown (Table 1). The term "dominant negative effect" refers to a situation where the normal protein functions in a structure consisting of several subunits, a multimere, and where the presence of a full-length, yet abnormally changed, peptide unit interfere with the assembly between the individual subunits. This is the usual mechanism for the large majority of missense mutations reported in instances of autosomal dominant LQTS, without hearing impairment associated. Yet, identical mutations in *KCNQ1* have been implicated in both JLNS and LQTS (9,15), indicating the complexity in trying to establish any genotype-phenotype correlation.

Recent electrophysiological studies of *KCNE1* and *KCNQ1* mutations involved in JLNS showed a spectrum of effects from simple loss of function to prominent dominant negative behavior (28,44). Why some individuals with such mutations, like E261D and R518X, in *KCNQ1* do not develop cardiac arrhythmia may rely on some myocardial depolarization reserve, and on genetically variable susceptibility in different individuals (44). This explanation would also be consistent with the reduced penetrance of clinical affection in some LQTS mutation carriers.

From the present compiled experience of a very low risk of cardiac affection in obligate mutation carriers of *KCNQ1* (15) or *KCNE1* mutations in JLNS cases, it seems that a certain reduction in the current of I_{Ks} is tolerated without adverse clinical manifestation. Apparently, there must be a complete absence of K^+ influx into the endolymph for hearing loss to be present (8,44).

The observations of families with autosomal recessive LQTS or "forme fruste" of LQTS (9,50) support the notion that C-terminal mutations in *KCNQ1* affect the function of the protein to a much lesser degree and further compromised function (by the presence of yet another mutation on the homolog chromosome) is necessary to develop overt LQTS.

The overall picture of missense mutations having a dominant negative effect and being associated with autosomal dominant LQTS and stop/frameshift mutations leading to lack of function and being associated with autosomal recessive JLNS is disturbed by several exceptions illustrating that it is not straightforward to predict a phenotype from a given genotype. Two *KCNQ1* mutations, R518X and R594Q, illustrate this complexity well. The R518X mutation was found in autosomal recessive LQTS and some heterozygous carriers had elongated Q-T interval but without fulfilling the criteria for overt LQTS. It was found in compound heterozygosity with another missense mutation, A525T (42). The same mutation was detected in four Norwegian JLNS families with either homozygosity or compound heterozygosity for this mutation. None of the carrier relatives were clinically affected (15,16).

The R518X mutation was present in compound heterozygosity with another missense mutation in a Scottish JLNS patient (15,17), and LQTS patients without further details about the inheritance pattern or affection status of relative given (9). Huang et al. found 1/45 carriers of the R518X clinically affected (45). An American JLNS patient had R518X in heterozygous form and a presumed (but not identified) second mutation (23).

Heterozygosity was associated with elongated Q-T interval, but no overt LQTS or impaired hearing (17,42). The mutation is in the C-terminal end of KCNQ1, and the mutation induced a weak dominant negative effect electrophysiologically when coinjected in a 3:1 ratio with wild-type cRNA (three times more mutant than wt cRNA), but not when injected in a 1:1 ratio (45). The *KCNQ1* mutation R594Q was also found in both LQTS and

JLNS patients, and with similar variable electrophysiological effects under different experimental conditions (9,17,45). The mutations Q530X and G589D show similar behavior (Table 1).

Seemingly, there are no instances of heterozygosity for *KCNE1* or *KCNQ1* mutations associated with isolated hearing impairment, and an invariable co-occurrence of hearing impairment and LQTS in patients with two *KCNQ1* mutations, except for R518X. Splawski et al. (9) do not specify if LQTS in patients with the mutations Q530X and R594Q was autosomal recessive or dominant. There were no instances of autosomal recessive inheritance in the Finnish group with the G589D mutation (Kontula, personal communication).

It could be expected about some of the *KCNQ1* mutations associated with "forme fruste"/recessive LQTS that hearing impairment might develop in some patients. Genetic counseling in such cases must be aware of the possible risk of hearing impairment.

XI. CLINICAL MANAGEMENT AND GENETIC COUNSELING

All severely hearing impaired children should have ECG taken to diagnose the elongated Q-T interval in JLNS. The recommended medical treatment of the cardiac component of JLNS follows the same guidelines as for LQTS. The current recommendations have changed over time and were recently comprehensively summarized by Chiang and Roden (58). Basically, beta-blockers are the first-choice drug, then cardiac pacemaker, left cardiac sympathetic denervation, and implantable cardioverter-defibrillator, if the combination of beta-blockers, denervation, and/or pacemaker fails to prevent the cardiac syncopes (58). It is still intensively discussed if asymptomatic carriers of a mutation should receive medical treatment.

After the clinical diagnosis of JLNS has been made, efforts should be made to identify the mutations in *KCNQ1*or *KCNE1*. In Norway, which has a high prevalence of JLNS and a limited spectrum of mutations in *KCNQ1*, all hearing-impaired persons who are referred for genetic evaluation and all instances of newly diagnosed LQTS patients are routinely investigated for the *KCNQ1* mutations: 572del5, R518X, Q530X, and E261D, and new families have been identified since our survey in 1999 (15; Tranebjærg, unpublished data). Our limited experience (15) strongly encouraged us to offer all identified carriers of LQTS mutations genetic counseling, cardiological examination, and written information about medication to be avoided, as well as being considered for prophylactic beta-blocker treatment.

The accumulated experience published so far indicates quite variable risk between different mutations in the *KCNQ1* gene. The individual JLNS families are often small and experience about the cardiac risk associated with being a carrier has been collected across the nuclear families sharing the same mutations. Only one obligate carrier out of 45 with *KCNQ1* R518X mutation had symptoms (45). Among 26 individuals identified to be carriers of the KCNQ1 572-576del mutation and deriving from seven different families, only one person had clinically symptomatic LQTS (15). In the Finnish study of *KCNQ1* G589D mutation carriers, 34 probands were identified and 316 heterozygous carriers were identified among 705 relatives, of whom only 83 (26%) were symptomatic. There was a slight overrepresentation of females among those with clinical affection. In the close relatives of the three JLNS probands, no symptomatic cases were found. This study is particularly interesting because of the demonstration of a founder background of this Finnish mutation, and the opportunity to compare the genotype and subsequent phenotype in such a large series of subjects on a fairly homogeneous population background (21).

The existing experience about most *KCNQ1* mutations associated with autosomal recessive LQTS is usually based on quite a few patients and the mutations demonstrated might be at risk for causing JLNS, similar to the existing experience with R518X. Genetic counseling should therefore include such aspects as well as all existing information about each mutation, including in vitro electrophysiological effects. The anxiety aroused in the extended family of a JLNS case must be taken into account by offering genetic counseling to relatives before a molecular carrier diagnosis is initiated. Clinical evaluation by means of ECG is not sufficiently sensitive nor specific to make a risk-stratification-based approach. We therefore recommend specific mutation analysis to assess the carrier status and risk of cardiac arrhythmia, and institute proper medical treatment.

Recently, a compilation of experience with a large number of JLNS patients showed a disappointing low efficacy of beta-blockers with a 51% rate of syncopal events and a 24% risk of lethal outcome despite treatment. In this abstract, no details of identified mutations nor assumed compliance were given (59). The overall message was that JLNS remains a malignant form of LQTS with a high risk of lethal outcome despite medical treatment. The main triggers were emotions and exercise (59).

The rapidly increasing use of cochlea implant as a treatment of severely hearing-impaired infants accentuates the recommendation of establishing a diagnosis of cardiac arrhythmia, to avoid lethal complications during surgery. So far, only one such case was published and the outcome was advantageous (48). Special precautions were taken before and during the surgery, with close cardiac monitoring and beta-blocker treatment, and after 11 months of follow-up, the situation was stable. One event of cardiac syncope led to the placement of an automatic pacemaker and defibrillator.

Special attention toward monitoring the cochlea implant is well justified considering the auditory stimuli eliciting severe syncopal attacks in many reports.

The increasing implementation of universal neonatal hearing screening in many countries also facilitates early diagnosis of JLNS, and timely institution of medical prophylaxis. Especially in a country like Norway with the described genetic epidemiology, molecular screening for the existing *KCNQ1* mutations could easily be incorporated as part of the panel of genetic tests offered to all newly diagnosed infants with severely impaired hearing capacity.

ACKNOWLEDGMENTS

The author wants to thank the Oticon Foundation for financial support and Prof. Torleiv Rognum and Prof. Kontula Kimmo for sharing unpublished findings.

REFERENCES

1. Jervell A, Lange-Neilsen F. Congenital deaf-mutism, functional heart disease with prolonged of the QT interval, and sudden death. Am Heart J 1957; 54: 103–106.
2. Meissner FL.Taubstummheit and taubstummentbildung. 1856; 119–120. Leipzig and Heidelberg: C.F. Winter'sche Verhandlung, 1856:119–120.
3. Jervell A. Surdocardiac and related syndromes in children. Adv Intern Med 1973; 17:425–438.
4. Romano C, Gemme G, Pongiglione R. Artimie cardiach rare dell'eta pediatrica II Accessi sincopali per fibrilliazione ventricolare parossitica. Clin Pediatr 1963; 45:656–683.
5. Ward O. A new familial cardiac syndrome in children. J Ir Med Assoc 1964; 54:103–106.
6. Levine SA, Woodworth CR. Congenital deafmutism, prolonged Q-T interval, syncopal attacks and sudden death. N Engl J Med 1958; 259:412.
7. Fraser GR, Froggatt P, Murphy T. Genetical aspects of the cardio-auditory syndrome of Jervell and Lange-Nielsen (congenital deafness and electrocardiographic abnormalities. Ann Hum Genet 1964; 28:133–151.
8. Roden DM, Lazzara R, Rosen M, Schwartz PJ, Towbin J, Vincent M. Multiple mechanisms in the long-QT syndrome: current knowledge, gaps and future directions. Circulation 1996; 94:1996–2012.
9. Splawski I, Shen J, Timothy KW, Lehmann MH, Priori S, Robinson JL, Moss AJ, Schwartz PJ, Towbin JA, Vincent M, Keating MT. Spectrum of mutations

in long-QT syndrome genes *KVLQT1*, *HERG*, *SCN5A*, *KCNE1*, and *KCNE2*. Circulation 2000; 102:1178–1185.

10. Keating MT, Sanguinetti MC. Molecular and cellular mechanisms of cardiac arrhythmias. Cell 2001; 104:569–580.

11. Hashiba K. Hereditary QT prolongation syndrome in Japan: genetic analysis and pathological findings of the conducting system. Jpn Circ J 1978; 42:1133–1139.

12. Komsuoglu B, Göldeli Ö, Kulan K, Budak F, Gedik Y, Tuncer C, Komsuoglu SS. The Jervell and Lange-Nielsen syndrome. Int J Cardiol 1994; 47:189–192.

13. Tuncer C, Cokkeser Y, Komsuoglu B, Özdemir R, Güven A, Pekdemir H, Sezgin AT, Ilhan A. Assessment of ventricular repolarization in deaf-mute children. Pediatr Cardiol 2000; 21:135–140.

14. Moss AJ, Schwartz PJ, Crampton RS, Locati E, Carleen E. The long QT syndrome: a prospective international study. Circulation 1985; 71(1):17–21.

15. Tranebjærg L, Bathen J, Tyson J, Bitner-Glindzicz. Jervell and Lange-Nielsen syndrome: a Norwegian perspective. Am J Med Genet 1999; 89:137–146.

16. Tyson J, Tranebjaerg L, Bellman S, Wren C, Taylor JFN, Bathen J, Aslaksen B, Sørland SJ, Lund O, Malcolm S, Pembrey M, Bhattacharya S, Bitner-Glindzicz M. IsK and KvLQT1: mutation in either of the two subunits of the slow component of the delayed rectifier potassium channel can cause Jervell and Lange-Nielsen syndrome. Hum Mol Genet 1997; 6(12):2179–2185.

17. Tyson J, Tranebjærg L, McEntagart M, Larsen LA, Christiansen M, Whiteford ML, Bathen J, Aslaksen B, Sørland SJ, Lund O, Pembrey M, Malcolm S, Bitner-Glindzicz M. Mutational spectrum in the cardioauditory syndrome of Jervell and Lange-Nielsen syndrome. Hum Genet 2000; 107:499–503. [Erratum in Hum Genet 2001; 108:75]

18. Splawski I, Timothy KW, Vincent GM, Atkinson DL, Keating MT. Molecular baisi of the long-QT syndrome associated with deafness. N Engl J Med 1997; 336(22):1562–1567.

19. Neyroud N, Tesson F, denjoy I, Leibovici M, Donger C, Barhanin J, Faure S, Gary F, Coumel P, Petit C, Schwartz K, Guicheney P. A novel mutation in the potassium channel gene KVLQT1 causes the Jervell and Lange-Nielsen cardioauditory syndrome. Nat Genet 1997; 15:186–189.

20. Ilhan A, Tuncer C, Komsuoglu SS, Kali S. Jervell and Lange-Nielsen syndrome: neurologic and cardiologic evaluation. Pediatr Neurol 1999; 21:809–813.

21. Piippo K, Swan H, Pasternak M, Chapman H, Paavonen K, Viitsalo M, Toivonen L, Kontula K. A founder mutation of the potassium channel KCNQ1 in long QT syndrome. Implications for estimation of disease prevalence and molecular diagnostics. J Am Coll Cardiol 2001; 37:562–568.

22. Schulze-Bahr E, Wang Q, Wedekind H, Haverkamp W, Chen Q, Sun Y, Rubie C, Hördt M, Towbin JA, Borggrefe M, Assmann G, Qu X, Somberg JC, Breithardt G, Oberti C, Funke H. *KCNE1* mutations cause Jervell and Lange-Nielsen syndrome. Nature Genet 1997; 17:267–268.

23. Wei J, Fish FA, Myerburg RJ, Roden DM, George AL. Novel KCNQ1 mutations associated with recessive and dominant congenital long QT syndromes:

evidence for variable hearing phenotype associated with R518X. Mutation 2000; Online Brief 317:1–5.

24. Rakaf M Al, Zakzouk SM, Shahwan SA Al. Jervell and Lange-Nielsen QT syndrome: a case report from Saudi Arabia. Int J Pediatr Otorhinol 1997; 39: 163–168.

25. Chen Q, Zhang D, Gingell RL, Moss AJ, Napolitano C, Priori SG, Schwartz PJ, Kehoe E, Robinson JL, Schulze-Bahr E, wang Q, Towbin JA. Homozygous deletion in KVLQT1 associated with Jervell and Lange-Nielsen syndrome. Circulation 1999; 99:1344–1347.

26. Neyroud N, Richard P, Vignier N, Donger C, Denjoy I, Demay L, Shkolnikova M, Pesce R, Chevalier P, Hainque B, Courmel P, Schwartz K, Guicheney P. Genomic organization of the KCNQ1 K+ channel gene and identification of C-terminal mutations in the long-QT syndrome. Circulation 1999; 84:290–297.

27. Mohammad-Panah R, Demolombe S, Neyroud N, Guicheney P, Kyndt F, van den Hoff M, Baro I, Escande D. Mutations in a dominant-negative isoform correlate with phenotype in inherited cardiac arrhythmias. Am J Hum Genet 1999; 64:1015–1023.

28. Chouabe C, Neyroud N, Richard P, Denjoy I, Hainque B, Romey G, Drici M-D, Guicheney P, Barhanin J. Novel mutations in KvLQT1 that affects I_{ks} activation through interactions with Isk. Cardiovasc Res 2000; 45:971–980.

29. Schwartz PJ, Moss AJ, Vincent GM, Crampton RS. Diagnostic criteria for the long QT syndrome: an update. Circulation 1993; 88(2):782–784.

30. Priori SG, Napolitano C, Schwartz PJ. Low penetrance in the long-QT syndrome: clinical impact. Circulation 1999; 99:186–189.

31. Fraser GR, Froggatt P, James TN. Congenital deafness associated with electrocardiographic abnormalities, fainting attacks and sudden death: a recessive syndrome. Q J Med 1964; 131:361–385.

32. Schwartz PJ, Stramba-Badiale M, Segantini A, Austoni P, Bosi G, Giorgetti R, Grancini F, Marni ED, Perticone F, Rosti D, Salice P. Prolongation of the QT interval and the sudden infant death syndrome. N Engl J Med 1998; 338(24): 1709–1714.

33. Schwartz PJ, Priori SG, Bloise R, Napolitano C, Ronchetti E, Piccini A, Goj C, Breithartd G, Schulze-Bahr E, Wedekind H, Nastoli J. Molecular diagnosis in a child with sudden infant death syndrome. Lancet 2001; 358:1342–1343.

34. Jentsch TF. Neuronal KCNQ potassium channels: physiology and role in disease. Nat Rev Neurosci 2000; 1:21–30.

35. Schott J, Charpentier F, Peltier S, Foley P, Drouin E, Bouhour J, Donnelly P, Vergnaud G, Bachner L, Moisan J-P, Le Marec H, Pascal O. Mapping of a gene for long QT syndrome to chromosome 4q25-27. Am J Hum Genet 1995; 57:1114–1122.

36. Bitner-Glindzicz M, Tyson J, Jameson R. Molecular basis of the long-QT syndrome. N Engl J Med 1997; 337:1011–1012.

37. Duggal P, Vesely MR, Wattanasirichaigoon D, Villafane J, Kaushik V, Beggs AH. Mutation of the gene for IsK associated with both Jervell and Lange-Nielsen and Romano-Ward forms of long-QT syndrome. Circulation 1998; 97:142–146.

38. Vetter DE, Mann JR, Wangemann P, Liu J, McLaughlin KJ, Lesage F, Marcus DC, Lazdunski M, Heinemann SF, Barhanin J. Inner ear defects induced by null mutations of the *isk* gene. Neuron 1996; 17:1251–1264.

39. Kurokawa J, Abriel H, Kass RS. Molecular basis of the delayed rectifier current I_{Ks} in the heart. J Mol Cell Cardiol 2001; 33:873–882.

40. Kubisch C, Schroeder BC, Friedreich T, Lütjohann B, El-Amraoui A, Marlin S, Petit C, Jentsch TJ. KCNQ4, a novel potassium channel expressed in sensory outer hair cells, is mutated in dominant deafness. Cell 1999; 96:437–446.

41. Neyroud N, Denjoy I, Donger C, Gary F, Villain E, Leenhardt A, Benali K, Schwartz K, Coumel P, Guicheney P. Heterozygous mutation in the pore of potassium channel gene KvLQT1 causes an apparently normal phenotype in long QT syndrome. Eur J Hum Genet 1998; 6(2):129–133.

42. Larsen LA, Fosdal I, Andersen PS, Kanters JK, Vuust J, Wetrell G, Christiansen M. Recessive Romano-Ward syndrome associated with compound heterozygosity for two mutations in the *KVLQT1* gene. Eur J Hum Genet 1999; 7:724–728.

43. Schmitt N, Schwarz M, Peretz A, Abitbol I, Attali B, Pongs O. A recessive C-terminal Jervell and Lange-Nielsen mutation of the KCNQ1 channel impairs subunit assembly. EMBO J 2000; 19(3):332–340.

44. Itoh T, Tanaka T, Nagai R, Kikuchi K, Ogawa S, Okada S, Yamagata S, Yano K, Yazaki Y, Nakamura Y. Genomic organization and mutational analysis of KVLQT1, a gene responsible for familial long QT syndrome. Hum Genet 1998; 103(3):290–294.

45. Huang L, Bitner-Glindzicz M, Tranebjærg L, Tinker A. A spectrum of functional effect for disease causing mutations in the Jervell and Lange-Nielsen syndrome. Cardiovasc Res 2001; 51:670–680.

46. Bianchi L, Shen Z, Dennis AT, Priori SG, Napolitano C, Ronchetti E, Bryskin R, Schwartz PJ, Brown AM. Cellular dysfunction of LQT5-minK mutants: abnormalities of IKs, IKr and trafficking in long QT syndrome. Hum Mol Genet 1999; 8(8):1499–1507.

47. Splawski I, Tristani-Firouzi M, Lehmann MH, Sanguinetti MC, Keating MT. Mutations in the hminK gene cause long QT syndrome and suppress I_{Ks} function. Nat Genet 1997; 17:338–340.

48. Green JD, Schuh MJ, Maddern BR, Haymond J, Helffrich RA. Cochlear implantation in Jervell and Lange-Nielsen syndrome. Ann Otol Rhinol Laryngol Suppl 2000; 185:27–28.

49. LQTS database http://www.ssi.dk/en/forskning/lqtsdb/ (last updated November 2000).

50. Donger C, Denjoy I, Berthet M, Neyroud, Cruaud C, Bennaceur M, Chivoret G, Schwartz K, Courmal P, Guicheney P. *KVLQT1* C-terminal missense mutation causes a forme fruste long-QT syndrome. Circulation 1997; 96:2778–2781.

51. Friedmann I, Fraser GR, Froggatt P. Pathology of the ear in the cardio-auditory syndrome of Jervell and Lange-Nielsen (Recessive deafness with electrocardiographic abnormalities). J Laryngol Otol 1966; 80:451–470.

52. Friedmann I, Fraser GR, Froggatt P. Pathology of the ear in the cardio-

auditory syndrome of Jervell and Lange-Nielsen. Report of a third case with an appendix on possible linkage with the Rh blood group locus. J Laryngol Otol 1968; 883–896.

53. Wang Q, Curran ME, Splawski I, Burn TC, Milholland JM, Van-ray TJ, Shen J, Timothy KW, Vincent GM, de Jager T, Schwartz PJ, Towbin JA, Moss AJ, Atkinson DL, Landes GM, Connors TD, Keating MT. Positional cloning of a novel potassium channel gene: KVLQT1 mutations cause cardiac arrythmias. Nat Genet 1996; 12:17–23.

54. Sakagami M, Fukazawa K, Matsunaga T, Fujita H, Mori N, Takumi T, Ohkubo H, Nakanishi S. Cellular localization of rat Isk protein in the stria vascularis by immunohistochemical observation. Hearing Res 1991; 56:168–172.

55. Mori N, Sakagami M, Fukazawa K, Matsunaga T. An immunohistochemical and electrophysiological study on I_{sk} protein in the stria vascularis of the guinea pig. Eur Arch Otorhinolaryngol 1993; 250:186–189.

56. Nicolas M-T, Dememes D, Martin A, Kuperschmidt S, Barhanin J. KCNQ1/KCNE1 potassium channels in mammalian vestibular dark cells. Hearing Res 2001; 153:132–145.

57. Bitner-Glindnizicz, Tranebjærg L. The Jervell and Lange-Nielsen syndrome. In: Kitamura K, Steele KP, eds. Genetics in Otorhinolaryngology. Adv Otorhinolaryngol 2000; 53:45–52. BaselKarger

58. Chiang C-E, Roden DM. The long QT syndromes: genetic basis and clinical implications. J Am Coll Cardiol 2000; 36:1–12.

59. Cerrone M, Schwartz PJ, Priori SG, Spazollini C, Denjoy I, Guicheney P, Schulze-Bahr E, Moss AJ, Zareba W, Hashiba K, Tanabe T, Tanaka T, Bathen J, Amlie JP, Bitner-Glindnicz M, Tyson J, Timothy KW, Vincent GMM, George AL, Naploitani C. Natural history and genetic aspects of the Jervell and Lange-Nielsen syndrome (abstract 2849). Circulation 2001; 104(suppl 17):602.

8
HDR Syndrome

Hilde Van Esch and Koenraad Devriendt
University of Leuven, Leuven, Belgium

I. INTRODUCTION

The combination of hypoparathyroidism, sensorineural deafness, and renal anomalies was described for the first time by Bilous et al. in 1992 (1) in a family with autosomal dominant hypoparathyroidism, sensorineural deafness, and renal dysplasia, and termed the HDR syndrome. This autosomal dominant malformation syndrome represents a new clinical entity and since the original publication, other patients with HDR have been published (2–4).

Recently, a member of the GATA-binding family of transcription factors was shown to be involved in this syndrome (5). All six members (GATA1–GATA6) of this family show a distinct tissue-specific expression (6), and play an essential role during vertebrate development (7–10). The identification of *GATA3* as the HDR gene occurred as part of a detailed studied of individuals with the DiGeorge syndrome (MIM 188400). These patients present abnormalities in organs derived from the third and fourth branchial arches, including the parathyroid glands, thymus, and outflow tract of the heart. In the majority of DiGeorge patients a microdeletion in chromosome 22q11 is present; however, in a small group of patients there is evidence of deletion or aberration in chromosome 10p (11). Molecular deletion analyses of these patients have resulted in the delineation of two nonoverlapping regions on chromosome 10p that contribute to this phenotype. Terminal 10p deletions (10p14–10pter) are associated with hypoparathyroidism, renal anomalies, and sensorineural deafness, whereas interstitial deletions (10p13–14) are associated with heart malformations and immune deficiency (12–14). Using deletion mapping studies, a critical HDR-region on chromosome 10p14–15 was delineated, which contained

133

Table 1 Clinical Data of All the Investigated HDR Patients

Patient	Parathyroid function	Sensorineural deafness	Renal anomalies	Other	GATA3 mutations
P-3/99	Primary hypoparathyroidism Age at diagnosis: 33 years Calcium deposits in basal ganglia.	Bil. -60 dB, more pronounced at the higher frequencies	Smaller left kidney with shrunken calyces Normal function.	Accessory left nipple Infertility, oligospermia	946–957 deletion in exon 5
P-4/99	Primary hypoparathyroidism Presenting with seizures	Bil. -50 dB	Single dysplastic left kidney and VUR	Uterus bicornis MR	Deletion of one GATA3 allele
P-5/99	Primary hypoparathyroidism	Bil. -85 dB	Agenesis left kidney	MR Exostoses	Deletion of one GATA3 allele
F-12/99	Primary hypoparathyroidism	Bilateral	No abnormalities detected on ultrasound	Biliary atresia	C828T in exon 4
P-16/99	Primary hypoparathyroidism Presenting with seizures at age of 5 years	Bil. flat audiograms	Agenesis right kidney		No mutations found
F-26/99	Primary hypoparathyroidism Age at diagnosis: 14 months	Bil. -70 dB, more pronounced at the higher frequencies	Right: multicystic kidney Left: renal dysplasia and VUR III		465–513 deletion in exon 3
P-BW	Primary hypoparathyroidism Presenting with seizures at age of 4 weeks	Bil. -70 dB, more pronounced at the higher frequencies	Agenesis right kidney Left kidney: VUR	Hypoplasia of vagina + internal genitalia	No mutations found
F-A	Transient hypocalcemia	Bil. -105 dB	Pelvicalyceal deformity		Deletion of one GATA3 allele
F-B	Primary hypoparathyroidism	Bil. -90 dB	VUR		Deletion of one GATA3 allele
F-C	Hypocalcemia	Bil. -90 dB	Aplasia of right kidney and VUR II	VSD	Deletion of one GATA3 allele
F-D	Primary hypoparathyroidism	Bil. -50 dB	Pelvicalyceal deformity		Deletion of one GATA3 allele
F-E	Primary hypoparathyroidism	Bil. -70 dB -70 dB right -110 dB left	Hypoplastic left kidney		T823A in exon 4
F-F	Primary hypoparathyroidism		Aplasia right kidney	Cerebral infarctions	C901AACCCT in exon 4
F-G	Primary hypoparathyroidism	Not examined	Proteinuria + hematuria		C1099T in exon 6
F-H	Primary hypoparathyroidism	Bil. -40 dB	Aplasia right kidney		No mutations found
F-I	Primary hypoparathyroidism	Bil. -105 dB	Chronic renal failure	Retinitis pigmentosa	No mutations found

Patients 4/99 and 5/99 were reported by Van Esch et al. (14), patients 3/99, 12/99, 16/99, and 26/99 were reported by Van Esch et al. (5), and families A–I were reported by Muroya et al. (15). P, patient; F, family; Bil, bilateral; VUR, vesicoureteric-reflux; dB, decibels; VSD, ventricular septum defect; MR, mental retardation.

the *GATA3* gene. Subsequent mutation analysis in HDR patients confirmed that haploinsufficiency for GATA3 is the underlying mechanism of the human HDR syndrome (5). Thus far, different mutations have been found including missense and nonsense mutations, intragenic deletions, insertions, and whole-gene deletions (5,15) (Table 1). These mutations result in a truncated protein that fails to bind the DNA, suggesting a loss of function.

II. CLINICAL CHARACTERISTICS

Clinically, the hypoparathyroidism is characterized by low serum calcium as a result of a deficient parathyroid hormone (PTH) secretion. PTH levels measured in serum of HDR patients range from low normal to undetectable. This leads to symptomatic or subclinical manifestations such as hypocalcemic seizures, calcium deposits, and bone demineralization. The renal anomalies observed in HDR patients belong to a spectrum of malformations including renal hypo- and dysplasia, vesicoureteral reflux, and agenesis of the kidney (16). The deafness found in HDR patients is of the sensorineural type, bilateral, and present at birth. The auditory loss is more pronounced at the higher frequencies and the severity ranges from moderate to severe, necessitating the use of hearing aids. Further deterioration of the hearing loss with advancing age is rarely the case. Phenotypic variability has been observed for the renal anomalies and the deafness. This might be due to variable penetrance of these anomalies; however, lack of appropriate investigations and possible phenotypic changes with age may account for the observed variability. Thus far, no mutations have been found in four families presenting with HDR syndrome, of which two also had additional features (5,15) (Table 1). It remains to be clarified whether a mutation in promotor or intron sequences remains undetected or whether the HDR syndrome is a heterogeneous disorder.

III. *GATA3* EXPRESSION

The HDR phenotype is consistent with the observed expression of *GATA3* in the developing kidney, inner ear, and parathyroids in human as well as in mouse embryos (17,18). *GATA3* expression can already be observed in the otic placode in the mouse at E8. From then on, *GATA3* is expressed in the main components of the developing auditory system, including the sensory epithelium, the afferent and efferent nerves, and the mesenchymal and ectodermal cells of the developing middle and outer ear (17,19). Based on its expression pattern, it has been suggested that *GATA3* is involved in the controlled suppression of hair cell differentiation in the mouse, to form the adult sensory cell pattern in the cochlea (20). Insufficient levels of *GATA3* and its regulated proteins could interfere with these strictly controlled processes and lead to a decreased auditory function. Besides expression in the cochlea, studies have shown that *GATA3* expression is downstream of *Hoxb1* expression during mouse hindbrain development (21). Lack of *GATA3* expression in rhombomere 4 inhibits the projection of contralateral vestibuloacoustic efferent neurons. This indicates that *GATA3* may play a role in the differentiation of the inner ear efferent neurons. However, clarification of these roles requires further studies, including identification of downstream target genes in these organs.

A homozygous *Gata3* knockout mouse has been reported by Pandolfi et al. (8) and displays multiple organ abnormalities, especially of the central nervous system together with a total block of T-cell differentiation and massive internal bleeding, lethal at midgestation. In contrast to human *GATA3* haploinsufficiency, heterozygous *Gata3* knockout mice were reported to be normal. However, careful reexamination of these animals showed the presence of sensorineural deafness in the heterozygous mutants (F. Grosveld, personal communication). This finding was already suspected from detailed *GATA3* expression studies during ear morphogenesis in normal and mutant mice (22).

REFERENCES

1. Bilous RW, Murty G, Parkinson DB, Thakker RV, Coulthard MG, Burn J, Mathias D, Kendall-Taylor P. Brief report: autosomal dominant familial hypoparathyroidism, sensorineural deafness, and renal dysplasia. N Engl J Med 1992; 327:1069–1074.
2. Beetz R, Zorowka P, Schonberger W, Kruse K, Wilichowski E, Zabel B, Mannhardt W, Schumacher R. Hypoparathyreoidismus und Innenohrschwerhorigkeit. Monatsschr Kinderheilkd 1997; 145:347–352.
3. Watanabe T, Mochizuki H, Kohda N, Minamitani K, Minagawa M, Yasuda T, Niimi H. Autosomal dominant familial hypoparathyroidism and sensorineural deafness without renal dysplasia. Eur J Endocrinol 1998; 139:631–634.
4. Hasegawa T, Hasegawa Y, Aso T, Koto S, Nagai T, Tsuchiya Y, Kim KC, Ohashi H, Wakui K, Fukushima Y. HDR syndrome (hypoparathyroidism, sensorineural deafness, renal dysplasia) associated with del(10)(p13). Am J Med Genet 1997; 73:416–418.
5. Van Esch H, Groenen P, Nesbit MA, Schuffenhauer S, Lichtner P,

Vanderlinden G, Harding B, Beetz R, Bilous RW, Holdaway I, Shaw NJ, Fryns JP, Van de Ven W, Thakker RV, Devriendt K. *GATA3* haploinsufficiency causes human HDR syndrome. Nature 2000; 406:419–422.

6. Simon MC. Gotta have GATA. Nat Genet 1995; 11:9.

7. Kuo CT, Morrisey EE, Anandappa R, Sigrist K, Lu MM, Parmacek MS, Soudais C, Leiden JM. *GATA4* transcription factor is required for ventral morphogenesis and heart tube formation. Genes Dev 1997; 11:1048–1060.

8. Pandolfi PP, Roth ME, Karis A, Leonard MW, Dzierzak E, Grosveld FG, Engel JD, Lindenbaum MH. Targeted disruption of the *GATA3* gene causes severe abnormalities in the nervous system and in fetal liver haematopoiesis. Nat Genet 1995; 11:40–44.

9. Pevny L, Simon MC, Robertson E, Klein WH, Tsai SF, D'Agati V, Orkin SH, Costantini F. Erythroid differentiation in chimaeric mice blocked by a targeted mutation in the gene for transcription factor *GATA-1*. Nature 1991; 349:257–260.

10. Tsai FY, Keller G, Kuo FC, Weiss M, Chen J, Rosenblatt M, Alt FW, Orkin SH. An early haematopoietic defect in mice lacking the transcription factor *GATA-2*. Nature 1994; 371:221–226.

11. Van Esch H, Groenen P, Fryns JP, Van de Ven W, Devriendt K. The phenotypic spectrum of the 10p deletion syndrome versus the classial DiGeorge syndrome. Genet Couns 1999; 10:59–65.

12. Lichtner P, R Kn, Hasegawa T, Van Esch H, Meitinger T, Schuffenhauer S. An HDR (hypoparathyroidism, deafness, renal dysplasia) syndrome locus maps distal to the DiGeorge syndrome region on 10p13/14. J Med Genet 2000; 37:33–37.

13. Fujimoto S, Yokochi K, Morikawa H, Nakano M, Shibata H, Togari H, Wada Y. Recurrent cerebral infarctions and del(10)(p14p15.1) de novo in HDR (hypoparathyroidism, sensorineural deafness, renal dysplasia) syndrome. Am J Med Genet 1999; 86:427–429.

14. Van Esch H, Groenen P, Daw S, Poffyn A, Holvoet M, Scambler P, Fryns JP, Van de Ven W, Devriendt K. Partial DiGeorge syndrome in two patients with a 10p rearrangement. Clin Genet 1999; 55:269–276.

15. Muroya K, Hasegawa T, Ito Y, Nagai T, Isotani H, Iwata Y, Yamamoto K, Fujimoto S, Seishu S, Fukushima Y, Hasegawa Y, Ogata T. *GATA3* abnormalities and the phenotypic spectrum of HDR syndrome. J Med Genet 2001; 38:374–380.

16. Van Esch H, Bilous RW. *GATA3* and kidney development: why case reports are still important. Nephrol Dial Transplant 2001; 16:2130–2132.

17. Debacker C, Catala M, Labastie MC. Embryonic expression of the human *GATA-3* gene. Mech Dev 1999; 85:183–187.

18. Labastie MC, Catala M, Gregoire JM, Peault B. The *GATA-3* gene is expressed during human kidney embryogenesis. Kidney Int 1995; 47:1597–1602.

19. Lawoko-Kerali G, Rivolta MN, Holley M. Expression of the transcription factors *GATA3* and *Pax2* during development of the mammalian inner ear. J Comp Neurol 2002; 442:378–391.

20. Rivolta MN, Holley MC. *GATA3* is downregulated during hair cell differentiation in the mouse cochlea. J Neurocytol 1998; 27:637–647.

21. Pata I, Studer M, van Doorninck JH, Briscoe J, Kuuse S, Engel JD, Grosveld F, Karis A. The transcription factor *GATA3* is a downstream effector of *Hoxb1* specification in rhombomere 4. Development 1999; 126:5523–5531.

22. Karis A, Pata I, van Doorninck JH, Grosveld F, de Zeeuw CI, de Caprona D, Fritzsch B. Transcription factor *GATA-3* alters pathway selection of olivocochlear neurons and affects morphogenesis of the ear. J Comp Neurol 2001; 429:615–630.

9
Branchio-oto-renal Syndrome

Shrawan Kumar
Boys Town National Research Hospital, Omaha, Nebraska, U.S.A.

I. INTRODUCTION

The occurrence of branchial anomalies was first recognized in the early nineteenth century (1) and thereafter additional reports were published about the association between ear anomalies and cervical fistula (2–5). However, the first report of a family with associated kidney problems did not appear until 1967 (6). Since then a great deal of progress has been made in clinical delineation and genetics of branchial anomalies (7–15). The hearing loss associated with branchial anomalies is variable; it can be progressive or stable or sensorineural or conductive; an illustrative example was a patient who had sensorineural hearing loss in one ear and conductive hearing loss in the other ear (16). Variable abnormalities associated with the external ear (malformed pinna, preauricular pits), middle ear (malformed ossicles), and inner ear (abnormal semicircular canal and cochlea) have also been reported (7,10,11,17–24). In each ear the hearing loss can vary from mild (20–40 dB loss) to moderate (40–60 dB) and to most severe (60–80 bB) or profound loss (> 80 dB). The cochlea is normally coiled in a spiral of 2–1/2 turns; however, patients with branchio-oto-renal (BOR) syndrome frequently have Mondini-type cochlear malformations, where cochlea is reduced to 1–1/2 turns (9). The penetrance of the disease gene appears to be 100% in persons carrying causative mutations. However, the clinical expression of BOR syndrome genes is extremely variable, and the phenotype can differ significantly within and between families. The major clinical features are hearing loss with pinnae deformities and preauricular pits, branchial arch anomalies, and renal defects (9,13,23,25,26). In most persons with BOR syndrome, auricular deformities, preauricular pits, ossicular malformations, and cervical sinuses/cysts/fistula occur together, reflecting the embryological origin of these structures from the first and second branchial arches.

The prevalence of BOR syndrome (MIM#113650; URL http://www. ncbi.nlm.nih.gov/Omim) is 1:40,000 and has been reported to be as high as 2% of the deaf population (27). However, the prevalence of BOR syndrome may be much higher than that reported earlier. In the general population, ear pits and ear tags are the most common ear malformations, which occur with a frequency of 5–6/1000 live births (28,29). It is not clear what proportion of those cases (ear anomalies, tags/pits) are later diagnosed as BOR. In the past, the families with single or only two major phenotypes were considered of different genetic origin than that of BOR (presence of three or more major clinical features). However, *EYA1* mutations (see below for details) have been detected in many familial and isolated cases with symptoms of preauricular sinuses and/or hearing as well as families with typical BOR loss (30–37). In the light of new findings reported in the last few years, such as identification of the *EYA1* gene and localization of the second BOR gene, more detailed studies are needed to determine the frequency of BOR syndrome.

II. CLINICAL ASPECTS OF BOR

Several studies have been conducted in the past to determine the frequency of different clinical phenotypes associated with BOR. Among all the anomalies reported, the hearing impairment was observed to be the most common feature (90%). Other symptoms associated with BOR were preauricular pits (77%), branchial cysts or fistulas usually found on the external lower third of the neck (63%), and renal anomalies (13%). In another study, renal anomalies were identified in 67% of individuals examined by ultrasound or excretory uregraphy (26). More recently, hypoplasia and dysplasia of the cochlea were described in several BOR patients by radiological techniques using temporal bones. An enlarged vestibular aqueduct, cochlear hypoplasia, and a widened vestibular sac were also reported (38–40). Other malformations included external (atretic, stenotic, or tortuous external canal) and middle ear anomalies (malformed enlarged or small) (26,38). Many other features, although not very common, such as abnormalities of the face, palate, ureters, and bladder, dysfunction of the lacrimal system, otitis media, palatoschisis, meatal atresia, malformation of facial nerve or paralysis, intracranial aneurysms, congenital cholesteatoma, and shoulder abnormalities, have also been associated with BOR (11,12,18,26,41–48). The

Table 1 The Overlapping Clinical Phenotypes Associated with Branchial Anomalies

Clinical features	BOR (43,44)	BO (43,44)	BR (10)	BOF (49–51)	BOU (52)	HMF (53,54)	OFC (6,55,56)
Branchial anomalies							
Facial asymmetry	+	+	+	+	−	+	+
Cleft sinus and fistula	+	+	+	−	−	−	+
Lacrimal duct stenosis	+	+	+	+	−	+	−
Nasal deformity	−	−	−	+	−	−	+
Skin tag	+	+	+	−	−	−	−
Commisural lip pits	−	+	−	−	−	−	−
Palate abnormality	+	+	+	+	−	−	+
Microtia	+	−	−	−	−	+	−
Micrognathia	+	+	+	−	+	+	−
Preauricular sinuses	+	+	+	−	+	+	+
Small and low-set ears	+	+	+	+	−	+	+
Pinnae malformation	+	+	+	−	+	+	+
Vestibular hypofunction	+	−	−	−	−	−	−
Facial paralysis	+	+	+	+	−	+	−
Upper lip deformity	−	−	−	+	−	−	−
Shoulder abnormality	−	+	−	−	−	−	+
Hearing disorder							
Sensorineural	+	+	+	+	+	+	+
Conductive	+	+	+	+	+	+	+
Mixed	+	+	+	+	+	+	+
Renal anomalies							
Uretral pelvic junction obstruction	+	−	−	−	−	−	−
Calceal cyst/diverticulum	+	−	−	−	−	−	−
Duplication of the ureters	−	−	+	−	+	−	−
Hydronephrosis	+	−	+	−	−	−	−
Bifid renal pelvis	+	−	+	−	−	−	−
Renal agenesis	+	−	+	−	−	−	−
Hypoplasia	+	−	+	−	−	−	−
Aplasia	+	−	+	−	−	−	−
Duplication of the collecting system	+	−	+	−	+	−	−

overlapping clinical features associated with branchial anomalies are presented in Table 1.

III. MOLECULAR GENETICS

BOR is inherited as an autosomal dominant disorder. Similar to other dominant developmental disorders, the phenotype is quite variable and not all the features of the syndrome are expressed in all carriers of BOR mutations. In the late seventies, many studies suggested that BO (branchio-oto), BOR, and BR (branchio-renal) are the result of mutations in a single gene. In 1992, the gene for BOR syndrome was localized to chromosome 8q (57,58). The *EYA1* gene was identified as the cause of BOR syndrome (59) and subsequently more than 30 mutations have been reported (30–37). Among many *EYA1* mutations reported in BOR cases, there are some mutations also identified in patients who had only eye defects (60), suggesting that the human *Eya1* gene is also involved in eye morphogenesis. *EYA1* is the human homolog of the *Drosophila* eye-absent (*Eya*) gene (61). More recent results indicate that families with branchial and hearing anomalies with no renal manifestation are not allelic to the BOR gene (62–64), suggesting the involvement of other gene(s). Recently, the second gene associated with branchial anomalies was localized to chromosome 1q (65).

The human *Eya1* cDNA is approximately 3.6 kb in length. The predicted protein of 539 amino acids is encoded by a 16-exon gene that spans approximately 156 kb of the genome and generates a 5.5-kb transcript (30). The human introns ranged in size from 0.1 to 27.5 kb in length. The transcript for *EYA1* and the encoded gene product have wide distribution in human tissues, including kidney, brain, lung, heart, and skeletal muscle (30).

Murine homologs of the *Drosophila eya* gene have also been identified (66). The new family of vertebrate genes designated *EYA1, EYA2, EYA3*, and *EYA4* share a high degree of sequence similarity with the *Drosophila Eya* gene. In mouse, Eya protein sequences reveal two distinct domains, a highly conserved 271-amino-acid carboxyl (C-) terminal region and a nonconserved amino (N-) terminal region. *Eya1* is widely expressed in cranial placodes, in the branchial arches and the CNS, and in complementary or overlapping patterns during organogenesis (67). The *EYA1* gene is a transcriptional coactivator and has been shown to interact with Six-family proteins (68) and possibly SIX, DACH, and/or G proteins are involved in the pathogenesis processes (69). The murine *EYA1* is coexpressed with *Six1* in early branchial and otic development and with *Six2* during early kidney development (70). These results suggest that despite enormous morphological differences, the conserved *Eya-Six* regulatory pathway is used during mammalian organogenesis.

A recent study has been conducted to inactivate the *EYA1* gene in mice to understand the developmental pathogenesis of organs affected in BOR syndromes (67,70,71). The knockout mice as well as a mouse strain with spontaneous mutation in the *EYA1* gene have cochlear and kidney anomalies (67,70,72). The phenotypic defects in mouse are strikingly similar to those of BOR syndrome. Using genetically well-defined mice with varying genetic background, linkage backcross mice bearing *EYA1* mutations will permit identification of genes that modify the phenotypic manifestation of the *EYA1* mutation. Also, they may provide insights into causes of the variable expressivity of human BOR syndrome. The mouse mutations also provide the means to study mutant *EYA1* gene expression during embryonic development and to examine the role of *EYA1* in molecular pathways leading to these common morphogenetic events.

Until recently, it was difficult to interpret whether syndromes with overlapping clinical phenotypes, such as BO, BOR, BOF (branchio-oculo-facial), BO, BOU (branchio-oto-uretral), or OFC (otofaciocervical), associated with branchial anomalies were caused by a single gene or more than one gene. After the localization of two loci associated with BOR syndrome and the identification of the *EYA1* gene, several reports were published on BOF (50,51) and BO indicating genetic heterogeneity (62,64). However, these reports should be interpreted with caution where the undetected *EYA1* mutation is not supported by genetic linkage studies. Recent reports indicate that BOF syndrome is not allelic to BO or BOR (50,51) and the OFC syndrome is a contiguous gene deletion syndrome involving the *EYA1* gene (56).

Many of our BOR families screened for *EYA1* do not show (approximately 60%) mutations in the *EYA1* gene (33). It is possible that most of the mutations lie in the noncoding regions of the gene or involve deletions and/or complex rearrangements. More than 30 mutations have now been reported in the *EYA1* gene (30–37). These mutations include nonsense, missense, frame shift, aberrant splicing, exon skipping, and large or small deletions. Most of the mutations are found in the highly conserved carboxy-terminal region of the gene, indicating that this region may play a predominant role in the structure and/or function of the *EYA1* gene.

IV. MUTATION IDENTIFICATION

Mutations in *EYA1* have been reported in approximately one-third of persons with phenotypic features of BOR syndromes. Only a few mutations, for example, the T→C change in exon 13 at base 1360, have been observed in more than one unrelated family (33). The data generated by our study and by others (30–37) add further support that no common *EYA1* mutation is associated with BOR syndrome. Interestingly, however, most of the mutations are clustered in the C-terminal region and within the *EYA1* homologous region or, exon 8 and exon 10 are commonly involved. While the effect of these mutations is not known, because the two nonsense mutations result in premature stop codons in exons 8 and 10 and mutations have been reported in the N-terminal region, it is possible that the phenotype reflects a dosage effect. The finding of splice site mutations (IVS 8-1 G→A) that alter correct *EYA1* splicing, resulting in exon skipping and premature truncation, supports this hypothesis.

About 65% of persons examined in our study did not have detectable mutations in the coding region of *EYA1*. To determine the prevalence of *EYA1* mutations in the syndrome, it is essential to screen for mutations in the UTRs, promoters, and intronic regions. It is unlikely that tightening diagnostic criteria for BOR syndrome will improve the correlation with *EYA1* mutations. A variety of *EYA1* mutations produce a continuum of disease, ranging from typical BOR to a mild clinical phenotype even within the same family. No obvious genotype-phenotype relationship could be discerned.

Further clinical studies of BOR syndrome should focus on detailed dysmorphology; genetic studies should be targeted to a more thorough mutation screen of *EYA1*. Families with undetected mutations should be verified for linkage to chromosome 8q and 1q to detect genetic heterogeneity. Our current results indicate the involvement of a third locus associated with branchial anomalies (73; Kumar et al., unpublished report). Also, two large families presenting with clinical features of branchio-otic type syndrome (62,64) have recently been reported that are unlinked to the BOR gene (8q region), indicating that mutations in other genes can produce phenotypes that overlap, at least some extent, with BOR syndrome. Thorough dysmorphological studies may reveal clinical features that permit unambiguous genotype-phenotype correlations, much as dystopin canthorm in Waardenburg syndrome, another heterogeneous developmental disorder with variable expressivity, implies mutations in *PAX3* and not MITF.

V. GENETIC TESTING AND GENOTYPE-PHENOTYPE CORRELATION

Recent mapping of new loci and identification of the *EYA1* gene have opened a door to the evaluation of possible correlations between specific mutations and the observed clinical variability. Unfortunately, to date, no distinct genotype-phenotype relationships have been demonstrated. This is due to the fact that a variety of *EYA1* mutations can produce a high degree of clinical variability among the patients with typical and atypical manifestations. In typical BOR, all three organs—branchial, auditory, and renal—are involved. However, atypical or variant and isolated cases are characterized by involvement limited to one or two organ systems, such as BO or BR. In our studies, no significant correlation between *EYA1* mutations of different types (33) and mild versus severe disease were found. However, correlations may be possible when a larger data series on genotype-phenotype and severity of the disease is available. With regard to genetic testing, several genetic diseases (e.g., polycystic kidney disease, cystic fibrosis, Usher syndrome type 2A, connexin 26 deafness, etc.) have common mutations, some of which are specific to particular ethnic groups. However, in BOR, several mutations have been described but no associations between specific mutations and particular ethnic populations have been reported. This makes genetic testing or counseling very difficult. It would be extremely helpful to determine whether there are such relationships. This would have important implications for genetic counseling and population screening to detect mutation carriers. We are now in the process of collecting BOR families from all over the world and a detailed study is underway in our laboratory to establish whether ethnic/racial-based differences exist in the mutations in the *EYA1* gene.

In summary, the major clinical features of a typical BOR syndrome are hearing loss (conductive, sensorineural, or mixed), branchial arch anomalies (preauricular pits, structural defects of the outer, middle, or inner ear, fistulas, cysts, or sinuses), and renal defects (hypoplasia or no kidney, renal agenesis). In several families in which the BOR phenotype segregates, mutations have been identified in the *EYA1* gene. However, in many affected families, mutation screening of *EYA1* has failed to document any allele variations. To determine the prevalence of mutations in the *EYA1*-coding region in persons with phenotypic features consistent with BOR syndrome, we screened 70 unrelated kindreds for *EYA1* allele variants. Several novel mutations were identified, and with the previously described mutations, suggest that *EYA1* allele variants in the coding region can be detected in 25–30% of persons with BOR syndrome. These findings imply either that the majority of BOR-causing mutations lie in intronic and/or 5'-3'-untranslated regions, involve chromosome rearrangement of the gene, or that the disease is genetically heterogeneous. Also, the absence of any common mutations associated with the *EYA1* gene somewhat reduces the likelihood of being able to offer testing using limited mutation panels in targeted populations, or the general population overall. However, mapping and cloning the other genes associated with branchiogenic disorders will have an important impact, leading to a more comprehensive understanding of the pathogenesis and etiology of this syndrome. How the BOR gene(s) influence both branchial/auditory and renal development is an interesting question. What is the common denominator in the development of both organs and what is the function of the gene associated with BOR? The delineation of gene(s) that exert control over branchial/auditory and/or renal development should shed considerable light on their underlying developmental processes and would define the spectrum of defects associated with this syndrome.

ACKNOWLEDGMENTS

I wish to thank all the family members for donating the blood samples and their participation in this research. I am also thankful to Dr. William J. Kimberling and Dr. Dana Orten for their valuable comments and suggestions. This work was supported by a grant from the National Institute of Dental and Craniofacial Research (NIDCR) 1 R01 DE14090-01.

REFERENCES

1. Ascherson FM. De Fistulis Colli Congenitis. 1832 Berolini.
2. Heusinger CF. Hals-Kiemen-Fisteln von noch nicht beobachteter Form. Virchows. Arch Pathol Anat Physiol 1864; 29:358–380.
3. Paget J. Cases of branchial fistulae in the external ears. Med Chir Trans 1878; 61:41–50.
4. Precechtel A. Pedigrees of anomalies in the first and second branchial cleft, inherited according to the laws of Mendel and a contribution to the technique of the extirpation of congenital lateral fistulae colli. Acta Otolaryngol (Stock) 1927; 11:23–30.
5. Fourman P, Fourman J. Hereditary deafness in a family with ear-pits (fistula auris congenital). Br Med J 1955; 2:1354–1356.
6. Fara M, Chlupackova V, Hrivnakova J. Dismorphia oto-facio-cervicalis familiaris. Acta Chir Plast (Prague) 1967; 9:255–268.
7. Fraser FC, Ling D, Clogg D, Nogrady B. Genetic aspects of the BOR syndrome-branchial fistulas, ear pits, hearing loss, and renal anomalies. Am J Med Genet 1978; 2:241–252.
8. Melnick M, Bixter D, Silk K, Yune H, Nance WE. Autosomal dominant branchio-oto-renal dysplasia. Birth Defects 1975; 11:121–128.
9. Melnick M, Bixler D, Nance WE, Silk K, Yune H. Familial branchio-oto-renal dysplasia: a new addition to the branchial arch syndromes. Clin Genet 1976; 9:25–34.
10. Melnick M, Hodes ME, Nance WE, Yune H, Sweeney A. Branchi-oto-renal

dysplasia and branchio-oto-dysplasia: two distinct autosomal dominant disorders. Clin Genet 1978; 13:425–442.

11. Cremers CWRJ, Fikkers-van Noord M. The earpits-deafness syndrome: clinical and genetic aspects. Int J Pediatr Otorhinolaryngol 1980; 2:309–322.

12. Cremers CWRJ, Thijssen HOM, Fischer AJEM, Marres EHMA. Otological aspects of the earpit-deafness syndrome. ORL 1981; 43:223–239.

13. Hunter AGW. Inheritance of branchial sinuses and preauricular fistulae. Teratology 1974; 9:225–228.

14. Martins AG. Lateral cervical and preauricular sinuses: their transmission as dominant characters. Br Med J 1961; 1:255–256.

15. Chitayat D, Hodgkinson KA, Chen MF, Haber GD, Nakishima S, Sando I. Branchio-oto-renal syndrome: further delineation of an underdiagnosed syndrome. Am J Med Genet 1992; 43:970–975.

16. Karmody CS, Feingold M. Autosomal dominant first and second branchial arch syndrome: a new inherited syndrome? Birth Defects Orig Artic Ser 1974; 10:31–40.

17. Ostri B, Johnsen T, Bergmann I. Temporal bone findings in a family with branchio-oto-renal syndrome (BOR). Clin Otolaryngol 1991; 16:163–167.

18. Fitch N, Srovolitz H. Severe renal dysgenesis produced by a dominant gene. Am J Dis Child 1976; 130:1356–1357.

19. Stoll C, Roth MP, Hessemann H, Paira M. Branchio-oto-renal dysplasia: a hereditary dominant autosomal syndrome with variable expression. Arch Fr Pediatr 1983; 40:763–766.

20. Gimsing S, Dyrmose J. Branchio-oto-renal dysplasia in three families. Ann Otol Rhinol Laryngol 1986; 95:421–426.

21. McLaurin JW, Kloepfer HW, Laguaite JK, Stallcup TA. Hereditary branchial anomalies and associated hearing impairment. Laryngoscope 1966; 76:1277–1288.

22. Rowley PT. Familial hearing loss associated with branchial fistulas. Pediatrics 1969; 44:978–985.

23. Bailleul JP, Libersa C, Laude M. Deafness and familial congenital auricular fistulas. Pediatrie 1972; 25:739–747.

24. Konig R, Fuchs S, Dukiet C. Branchio-oto-renal (BOR) syndrome: variable expressivity in a five-generation pedigree. Eur J Pediatr 1994; 153:446–450.

25. Cote A, O'Regan S. The branchio-oto-renal syndrome. Am J Nephrol 1982; 2:144–146.

26. Chen A, Francis M, Ni L, Cremers CW, Kimberling WJ, Sato Y, Phelps PD, Bellman SC, Wagner MJ, Pembrey M, et al. Phenotypic manifestations of branchio-oto-renal syndrome. Am J Med Genet 1995; 58:365–370.

27. Fraser FC, Sproule JR, Halal F. Frequency of the branchio-oto-renal (BOR) syndrome in children with profound hearing loss. Am J Med Genet 1980; 7: 341–349.

28. Kugelman A, Hadad B, Ben-David J, Podoshin L, Borochowitz Z, Bader D. Preauricular tags and pits in the newborn: the role of hearing tests. Acta Paediatr 1997; 86:170–172.

29. Kankkunen A, Thiringer K. Hearing impairment in connection with pre-auricular tags. Acta Paediatr Scand 1987; 76:143–146.

30. Abdelhak S, Kalatzis V, Heilig R, Compain S, Samson D, Vincent C, Levi-Acobas F, Cruaud C, Le Merrer M, Mathieu M, Konig R, Vigneron J, Weissenbach J, Petit C, Weil D. Clustering of mutations responsible for branchio-oto-renal (BOR) syndrome in the eyes absent homologous region (eyaHR) of *EYA1*. Hum Mol Genet 1997; 13:2247–2255.

31. Vincent C, Kalatzis V, Abdelhak S, Chaib H, Compain S, Helias J, Vaneecloo FM, Petit C. BOR and BO syndromes are allelic defects of *EYA1*. Eur J Hum Genet 1997; 5:242–246.

32. Kumar S, Kimberling WJ, Weston M, Schaefer BG, Anne Berg M, Marres HAM, Cremers CWRJ. Identification of three novel mutations in human EYA1 protein associated with branchio-oto-renal syndrome. Hum Mutat 1998; 11:443–449.

33. Kumar S, Deffenbacher K, Cremers CW, Van Camp G, Kimberling WJ. Branchio-oto-renal syndrome: identification of novel mutations, molecular characterization, mutation distribution, and prospects for genetic testing. Genet Test 1997–98; 1:243–251.

34. Fukuda S, Kuroda T, Chida E, Shimizu R, Usami S, Koda E, Abe S, Namba A, Kitamura K, Inuyama Y. A family affected by branchio-oto syndrome with *EYA1* mutations. Auris Nasus Larynx 2001; Suppl:S7–S11.

35. Rodriguez-Soriano J, Vallo A, Bilbao JR, Castano L. Branchio-oto-renal syndrome: identification of a novel mutation in the *EYA1* gene. Pediatr Nephrol 2001; 16:550–553.

36. Rickard S, Boxer M, Trompeter R, Bitner-Glindzicz M. Importance of clinical evaluation and molecular testing in the branchio-oto-renal (BOR) syndrome and overlapping phenotypes. J Med Genet 2000; 37:623–627.

37. Usami S, Abe S, Shinkawa H, Deffenbacher K, Kumar S, Kimberling WJ. *EYA1* nonsense mutation in a Japanese branchio-oto-renal syndrome family. J Hum Genet 1999; 44:261–265.

38. Ceruti S, Stinckens C, Creners CW, Casselman JW. Temporal bone anomalies in the branchio-oto-renal syndrome: detailed computed tomographic and magnetic resonance imaging findings. Otol Neurotol 2002; 23:200–207.

39. Stinckens C, Standaert L, Casselman JW, Huygen PL, Kumar S, Van de Wallen J, Cremers CW. The presence of a widened vestibular aqueduct and progressive sensorineural hearing loss in the branchio-oto-renal syndrome: family study. Int J Pediatr Otorhinolaryngol 2001; 59:163–172.

40. Kemperman MH, Stinckens C, Kumar S, Huygen PL, Joosten FB, Cremers CW. Progressive fluctuant hearing loss, enlarged vestibular aqueduct, and cochlear hypoplasia in branchio-oto-renal syndrome. Otol Neurotol 2001; 22:637–643.

41. Preisch JW, Bixler D, Ellis FD. Gustatory lacrimation in association with the branchio-oto-renal syndrome. Clin Genet 1985; 27:506–509.

42. Slack RWT, Phelps PD. Familial mixed deafness with branchial arch defects (earpits-deafness syndrome). Clin Otolaryngol 1985; 10:271–277.

43. Heimler A, Lieber E. Branchio-oto-renal syndrome: reduced penetrance and variable expressivity in four generations of a large kindred. Am J Med Genet 1986; 25:15–27.

44. Raspino M, Tarantino V, Moni L, Verrina E, Ciardi MR, Gusmano R. The branchio-oto-renal syndrome (report of two family groups). J Laryngol Otol 1988; 102:138–141.

45. Pennie BH, Marres HA. Shoulder abnormalities in association with branchio-oto-renal dysplasia in a patient who also has familial joint laxity. Int J Pediatr Otorhinolaryngol 1992; 23:269–273.

46. Cheong JH, Kim CH, Bak KH, Kim JM, Oh SJ. Multiple intracranial aneurysms associated with branchio-oto-dysplasia. J Korean Med Sci. 2001; 16:245–249.

47. Graham GE, Allanson JE. Congenital cholesteatoma and malformations of the facial nerve: rare manifestations of the BOR syndrome. AJMG 1999; 86:20–26.

48. Lipkin AF, Coker NJ, Jenkins HA. Hereditary congenital cholesteatoma: a variant of branchio-oto dysplasia. Arch Otolaryngol Head Neck Surg 1986; 112:1097–1100.

49. Fujimoto A. New autosomal dominant branchi-oculo-facial syndrome. Am J Med Genet 1987; 27:943–951.

50. Trummer T, Muller D, Schulze A, Vogel W, Just W. Branchio-oculo-facial syndrome and branchio-otic/branchio-oto-renal syndromes are distinct entities. J Med Genet 2002; 39:71–73.

51. Lin AE, Doherty R, Lea D. Branchio-oculo-facial and branchio-oto-renal syndromes are distinct entities. Clin Genet 1992; 41:221–223.

52. Fraser FC, Ayme S, Halal F, Sproule J. Autosomal dominant duplication of the renal collection system, hearing loss, and external ear anomalies: a new syndrome. Am J Med Genet 1983; 14:473–478.

53. Moeschler J, Clarren SK. Familial occurrence of hemifacial microsomia with radial limb defects. Am J Med Genet 1992; 12:371–375.

54. Rollnick BR, Kaye CI. Hemifacial microsomia and the branchio-oto-renal syndrome. J Craniofac Genet Dev Biol Suppl 1985; 1:287–295.

55. Dallapiccola B, Mingarelli R. Otofaciocervical syndrome: a sporadic patient supports splitting from the branchio-oto-renal syndrome. J Med Genet 1995; 32:816–818.

56. Rickard S, Parker M, van't Hoff W, Barnicoat A, Russell-Eggitt I, Winter RM, Bitner-Glindzicz M. Oto-facio-cervical (OFC) syndrome is a contiguous gene deletion syndrome involving *EYA1*: molecular analysis confirms allelism with BOR syndrome and further narrows the Duane syndrome critical region to 1 cM. Hum Genet 2001; 108:398–403.

57. Smith RJH, Coppage KB, Ankerstjerne JKB, Capper DT, Kumar S, Kenyon J, Kimberling WJ. Localization of the gene for branchiootorenal syndrome to chromosome 8q. Genomics 1992; 14:841–844.

58. Kumar S, Kimberling WJ, Kenyon JB, Smith RJH, Marres HAM, Cremers CWRJ. Autosomal dominant branchio-oto-renal syndrome—localization of a

disease gene to chromosome 8q by linkage in a Dutch family. Hum Mol Genet 1992; 7:491–495.

59. Abdelhak S, Kalatzis V, Heilig R, Compain S, Samson D, Vincent C, Weil D, Cruaud C, Sahly I, Leibovici M, Bitner-Glindzicz M, Francis M, Lacombe D, Vigneron J, Charachon R, Boven K, Bedbeder P, Van Regemorter N, Weissenbach J, Petit C. A human homologue of the *Drosophila* eyes absent gene underlies branchio-oto-renal (BOR) syndrome and identifies a novel gene family. Nat Genet 1997; 15:157–164.

60. Azuma N, Hirakiyama A, Inoue T, Asaka A, Yamada M. Mutations of a human homologue of the *Drosophila* eyes absent gene (*EYA1*) detected in patients with congenital cataracts and ocular anterior segment anomalies. Hum Mol Genet 2000; 9:363–366.

61. Bonini NM, Leiserson WM, Benzer S. The eyes absent gene: genetic control of cell survival and differentiation in the developing *Drosophila* eye. Cell 1993; 72:379–395.

62. Stratakis CA, Lin JP, Rennert OM. Description of a large kindred with autosomal dominant inheritance of branchial arch anomalies, hearing loss, and ear pits, and exclusion of the branchio-oto-renal (BOR) syndrome gene locus (chromosome 8q13.3). Am J Med Genet 1998; 79:209–214.

63. Kumar S, Kimberling WJ, Marres HA, Cremers CW. Genetic heterogeneity associated with branchio-oto-renal syndrome. Am J Med Genet 1999; 83:207–208.

64. Kumar S, Marres HAM, Cremeres CWRJ, Kimberling WJ. Autosomal dominant branchio-otic (BO) syndrome is not allelic to the branchio-oto-renal (BOR) gene at 8q13. Am J Med Genet 1998; 76:395–401.

65. Kumar S, Deffenbacher K, Marres HA, Cremers CW, Kimberling WJ. Genomewide search and genetic localization of a second gene associated with autosomal dominant branchio-oto-renal syndrome: clinical and genetic implications. Am J Hum Genet 2000; 66:1715–1720.

66. Xu P, Woo I, Her H, Beier DR, Maas RL. Mouse *Eya* homologues of the *Drosophila* eyes absent gene require *Pax6* for expression in lens and nasal placode. Development 1997; 124:219–231.

67. Xu PX, Cheng J, Epstein JA, Maas RL. Mouse *Eya* genes are expressed during limb tendon development and encode a transcriptional activation function. Proc Natl Acad Sci USA 1997; 94:11974–11979.

68. Ohto H, Kamada S, Tago K, Tominaga SI, Ozaki H, Sato S, Kawakami K. Cooperation of *six* and *eya* in activation of their target genes through nuclear translocation of *Eya*. Mol Cell Biol 1999; 19:6815–6824.

69. Ozaki H, Watanabe Y, Ikeda K, Kawakami K. Impaired interactions between mouse *Eya1* harboring mutations found in patients with branchio-oto-renal syndrome and *Six*, *Dach*, and G proteins. J Hum Genet 2002; 47:107–116.

70. Xu PX, Adams J, Peters H, Brown MC, Heaney S, Maas R. *Eya1*-deficient mice lack ears and kidneys and show abnormal apoptosis of organ primordia. Nat Genet 1999; 23:113–117.

71. Buller C, Xu X, Marquis V, Schwanke R, Xu PX. Molecular effects of *Eya1*

domain mutations causing organ defects in BOR syndrome. Hum Mol Genet 2001; 10:2775–2781.

72. Johnson KR, Cook SA, Erway LC, Matthews AN, Sanford LP, Paradies NE, Friedman RA. Inner ear and kidney anomalies caused by IAP insertion in an intron of the *Eya1* gene in a mouse model of BOR syndrome. Hum Mol Genet 1999; 8:645–653.

73. Koch SM, Kumar S, Cremers CW. A family with autosomal dominant inherited dysmorphic small auricles, lip pits, and congenital conductive hearing impairment. Arch Otolaryngol Head Neck Surg 2000; 126:639–644.

10

Treacher Collins Syndrome

Jill Dixon and Michael J. Dixon
University of Manchester, Manchester, England

I. INTRODUCTION

Although the condition was probably first described by Thompson in 1846 (1), Treacher Collins syndrome (TCS) is eponymously named after the ophthalmologist E. Treacher Collins, who described the essential components of the syndrome in 1900 (2). However, Franceschetti and Klein, who used the term mandibulofacial dysostosis to describe the facial appearance, detailed the first complete description of the condition (3).

II. CLINICAL FEATURES OF TREACHER COLLINS SYNDROME

TCS is an autosomal dominant disorder of facial development that affects approximately 1 in 50,000 live births (4,5). However, more than 60% of cases do not appear to have a previous family history and are thought to arise as the result of a spontaneous mutation (6). The major clinical features of TCS, with their frequencies in parentheses (7), include abnormalities of the external ears (77%) and atresia of external auditory canals (36%). Radiographic analysis of the middle ears of affected individuals has revealed malformation of the auditory ossicles with fusion between rudiments of the malleus and incus, partial absence of the stapes and oval window, or even complete absence of the middle ear and epitympanic space (8). As a result of these abnormalities, bilateral conductive hearing loss is common (50% of cases), whereas mixed or sensorineural hearing loss is rare (9). Lateral downward

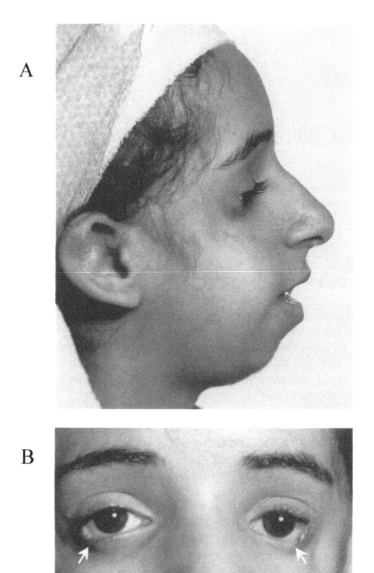

Figure 1 A patient with Treacher Collins syndrome. (A) A lateral view of the patient illustrates the mandibular hypoplasia and the abnormal external ear. (B) A frontal view of the same individual illustrates the colobomas (arrows) and paucity of eyelid lashes on the medial side of the abnormality. Immediately beneath the eyes, some "flattening" of the zygomatic complex is visible.

sloping of the palpebral fissures (89%), frequently with colobomas of the lower eyelids and a paucity of lashes medial to the defect (69%), are also frequently seen (Fig. 1). Hypoplasia of the facial bones, particularly affecting the mandible (78%) and zygomatic complex (81%), is also observed in TCS (Fig. 1). In severe cases, the zygomatic arch may be absent (10) and cleft palate (28%) may occur. These features are usually bilaterally symmetrical (Fig. 1) (11).

Although the genetic mutations underlying TCS are highly penetrant, the condition is characterized by marked inter- and intrafamilial phenotypic variability (7,12). Some individuals are so mildly affected that it can be extremely difficult to establish an unequivocal diagnosis and to provide accurate genetic counseling on clinical grounds alone. Indeed, some mildly affected TCS patients may only be diagnosed after the birth of a more severely affected child. At the other end of the phenotypic spectrum, severe cases of TCS have occasionally resulted in perinatal death due to a compromised airway (13).

III. DIFFERENTIAL DIAGNOSIS

In the differential diagnosis of TCS one should consider those conditions that form part of the oculoauriculovertebral (OAV) spectrum. This is a complex and heterogeneous set of conditions that includes hemifacial microsomia, a condition that primarily affects development of the ears, mouth, and mandible. Like TCS, hemifacial microsomia shows marked clinical variability but, unlike TCS, it usually affects one side of the face only. In cases where bilateral involvement has been described, there is generally marked asymmetry in the extent to which the different sides of the face are affected (14). Goldenhar syndrome is also considered to be part of the OAV spectrum but includes vertebral anomalies and epibulbar dermoids in addition to the facial involvement. In most cases, OAV spectrum occurs sporadically, and the condition therefore tends to be characterized by a low (empirical) recurrence risk. However, as 1–2% of cases have a previous family history with autosomal dominant and autosomal recessive inheritance being implicated in different cases, counseling should be provided on an individual family basis. Other conditions in which the facial gestalt may resemble TCS include Nager acrofacial dysostosis and Miller syndrome, but in both cases there are accompanying limb abnormalities. While OAV, Nager, and Miller syndrome are usually readily distinguished from TCS, caution should be exercised where individuals are affected minimally to ensure that these various conditions are not misdiagnosed.

IV. IDENTIFICATION OF THE GENE MUTATED IN TCS

The combined facts that TCS exhibits a well-defined mode of inheritance and the majority of cases can be diagnosed clinically ensured that the gene mutated in this condition could be isolated using a positional cloning strategy, i.e., on the basis of its position in the human genome alone (reviewed in Ref. 15). Using a series of clinically well-characterized families, the gene mutated in TCS, *TCOF1*, was initially mapped to a 9 cM region of human chromosome 5q31–q34 using restriction length fragment polymorphisms (16). Subsequent studies concentrated on the use of highly informative short tandem repeat polymorphisms to refine the location of the *TCOF1* critical region to a small genetic interval of chromosome 5q32–q33.1 (17–20). This region was then cloned using a combination of yeast artificial chromosome and cosmid clones (21–23), which were subsequently used in transcript mapping techniques to identify candidate genes that were screened for TCS-specific mutations. This strategy resulted in the identification of *TCOF1* (24).

V. CHARACTERISATION OF *TCOF1* AND TREACLE

TCOF1 encodes a low-complexity 1411-amino-acid protein, named Treacle, in which serine, alanine, lysine, proline, and glutamic acid account for over 60% of residues (25,26). Bioinformatics analyses have indicated that Treacle contains three domains: unique amino and carboxy termini, and a characteristic central repeat domain (25,26). The central repeat domain consists of 10 repeat units, each of which is encoded by an individual exon (exons 7–16). A single repeat consists of a cluster of acidic amino acid residues, containing numerous consensus sites for casein kinase II (CKII) phosphorylation, separated by basic amino acids comprising a majority of lysine, alanine, and proline residues. Further analysis of Treacle identified a number of potential monopartite nuclear localization signals (NLSs) of the consensus sequence K-K/R-X-R/K (27), embedded in the lysine-rich carboxy terminus of the protein.

Database searches revealed that Treacle does not exhibit strong homology to any previously identified genes or gene families. Such searches did, however, indicate that Treacle exhibits weak homology to rat nucleolar phosphoprotein Nopp140, with the greatest homology arising in the region of the repeated domain. These results have suggested that Treacle may also be a nucleolar protein (25,26). This hypothesis has been verified by subcellular localization studies using green fluorescent protein (GFP) reporters and anti-Treacle antibodies. These combined experiments demonstrated that the NLSs at the carboxy terminus of Treacle are functional and that Treacle localizes to the nucleolus (28,29). More recently, the subnucleolar localization of Treacle has been refined and the expression domain found to lie within that of nucleolin, precisely mirroring that of fibrillarin, suggesting localization to the dense fibrillar component of the nucleolus (30). However, unlike Nopp140, Treacle is absent from the coiled (Cajal) bodies.

Treacle has been further characterized using biochemical techniques. Western blotting indicated that anti-Treacle antibodies recognized a single protein band of approximately 220 kDa in cell lysates (30). However, as the predicted molecular weight of Treacle is 144 kDa, in vitro transcription and translation studies were used to confirm that this is the correct molecular weight of Treacle as determined by sodium dodecyl sulfate–polyacrylamide gel electrophoresis (SDS-PAGE) analyses. Isaac and co-workers noted that the discrepancy between the theoretical molecular weight of Treacle and its mobility on SDS-PAGE was reminiscent of that of Nopp140 (30). As most of the aberrant mobility of Nopp140 is due to phosphorylation in its central repeat domain, which shares homology with that of Treacle, in vitro trans-lated Treacle was treated with alkaline phosphatase in the presence or absence of phosphatase inhibitors. Treacle, like Nopp140, showed a ~40-kDa mobility shift upon phosphatase treatment and migrated at ~180 kDa, indicating a high degree of phosphorylation (30). Subsequently, it has also been determined that CKII and Treacle coimmunoprecipitate from HeLa cell lysates and that CKII is likely to be the kinase responsible for the posttransla-tional modification of Treacle (30). This is consistent with the results of Jones and colleagues, who showed that avian branchial arches contain a kinase activity that can phosphorylate Treacle peptides consistent with CKII site recognition (31).

Recently, another motif has been documented within the sequence of Treacle, a LIS1 homology (LisH) motif at amino acid positions 5–38 (32). The *LIS1* gene is mutated in patients with Miller-Dieker lissencepahly (33). In this bioinformatics-based study, over 100 eukaryotic intracellular proteins were found to contain a LisH motif and from their diverse functions the authors suggested that these motifs might contribute to the regulation of microtubule dynamics, either by mediating dimerization or by binding cy-toplasmic dynein heavy chain or microtubules directly. Currently, there have been no laboratory-based studies that support this hypothesis; however, it is interesting that Nopp140 also contains a LisH motif, reinforcing pre-vious observations that Treacle and Nopp140 share structural and func-tional similarities.

VI. MUTATION ANALYSIS OF *TCOF1*

To date, mutation analysis of *TCOF1* has resulted in the identification of over 120 mutations that are spread throughout the gene (24,26,34–36). While

the mutations include splicing mutations, insertions, and nonsense mutations, by far the majority (68%) are deletions, which range in size from one to
40 nucleotides. In any event, the result of these mutations is to introduce a
premature termination codon into Treacle, which suggests that the mechanism underlying TCS is haploinsufficiency. Although the majority of mutations tend to be family-specific, the recurrent mutation nt4135 del(GAAAA),
which occurs in exon 24 of *TCOF1*, accounts for 18.6% of mutations.

A small number of putative missense mutations have also been identified in *TCOF1* (34,36). Although one of these changes (K749K) initially
appeared to be silent, it resulted from a G > A transition in the last nucleotide
of exon 14. Unusually, the sequence of the associated splice donor site of
intron 14 was found to be gc rather than the more usual gt, a variation that is
present in the human, mouse, and dog *TCOF1* genes (25,26,37,38). In vitro
studies have shown that gc is the only substitution that will allow the 5′ splice
site to be accurately cleaved, although in such cases the surrounding sequence
is usually very closely matched to the consensus AG/gcaagt (39). In the case
of the mutation K749K, RT-PCR analysis indicated that the two variations
from the splice consensus sequence resulted in abnormal splicing with
readthrough into intron 14. As this mutation also results in the introduction
of a termination codon, the net effect is likely to be the same as the mutations
outlined above (34).

The remaining missense mutations I14F, A41V, W53C, and W53R
occur in the amino terminus of Treacle. Although their effect on protein
function remains unknown, it is noteworthy that this is the most highly conserved region of the protein (37,38,40). Moreover, although a high frequency
of single nucleotide polymorphisms (SNPs) has been observed in *TCOF1*, no
SNPs have been documented in that region of the gene encoding the amino
terminus of Treacle in over 100 normal individuals (24,26,34,36). Nevertheless, until the exact function of Treacle is determined, and, in particular,
the role that the unique amino and carboxy termini play in contributing to
that function, these missense changes should only be considered "putative"
mutations.

VII. MOLECULAR DIAGNOSIS OF TCS

Prior to the commencement of molecular studies on TCS, prenatal diagnosis
was only possible using fetoscopy or ultrasound imaging and both methods
have been used to make positive predictions (41–44). While the quality of
ultrasound imaging has improved markedly in recent years, allowing noninvasive prenatal diagnosis to be performed, it may still be difficult to make
a positive diagnosis, particularly where the fetus is mildly affected. Given

these circumstances the procedure is usually not diagnostic for apparently unaffected fetuses. Moreover, prenatal diagnosis using either fetoscopy or ultrasound imaging is not possible until the second trimester of pregnancy. Conversely, molecular diagnosis can be undertaken in the first trimester of pregnancy. Initially, this was achieved using linked polymorphic markers (13). More recently, in light of the identification of *TCOF1*, these predictions are now more reliable, since the presence or absence of a particular mutation can be assessed. However, genetic counseling of families with TCS is complicated by the fact that, in general, mutations between families are different (see above). Hence, the specific mutation must first be identified within a family before any counseling or prenatal diagnosis can be performed. Since this may require analysis of all 26 exons of *TCOF1*, it can be a time-consuming process. In addition, even if the fetus is found to carry the disease-causing mutation, no conclusions can be drawn about the severity with which the child will be affected. Therefore, parents may opt to delay any decision making until ultrasound can be used to provide further information on the extent of the abnormalities. However, for those cases in which the fetus does not carry the mutation, parents can be reassured that their child will be unaffected. The area in which molecular diagnosis is likely to find its greatest utility is in postnatal diagnosis of "at-risk" individuals. This will be particularly important in confirming the clinical diagnosis in mildly affected individuals and also in accurately counseling apparently unaffected parents of a child in which TCS has supposedly arisen as the result of a de novo mutation. Finally, it should be emphasized that the molecular diagnosis, although providing a useful adjunct to patient management in a subset of cases, is no substitute for careful patient examination leading to an accurate clinical diagnosis.

VIII. THE ROLE OF *TCOF1*/TREACLE IN CRANIOFACIAL DEVELOPMENT

To investigate the developmental mechanisms underlying TCS, research has largely focused on the mouse. Although the human and murine proteins display relatively low homology, 54.8% identity, and 71.6% similarity, their orthologous nature has been confirmed by genetic mapping (37,40). Expression analyses have further shown that, although the gene is widely expressed, the highest expression levels are observed in the neural folds immediately prior to fusion, and in the developing first pharyngeal arch (37). These observations are consistent with a role for the gene during craniofacial morphogenesis. These studies laid the foundations for the use of gene-targeting technology to study the function of the protein in vivo. To ensure

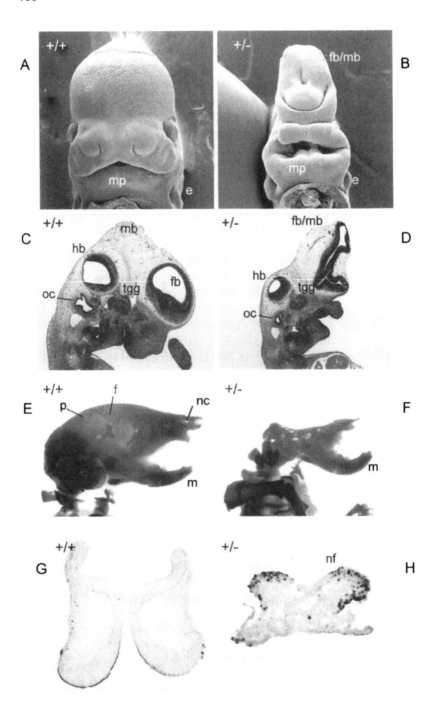

complete functional inactivation of *Tcof1*, Dixon and co-workers replaced exon 1, which contains the translation initiation codon, with a neomycin resistance cassette via homologous recombination in embryonic stem cells (45). The chimeric animals generated using these cells were intercrossed with C57BL/6 female mice. Confirmed *Tcof1* heterozygous (*Tcof1*$^{+/-}$) mice were found to die shortly after birth as a result of severe craniofacial anomalies that include agenesis of the nasal passages, abnormal development of the maxilla, acrania, exencephaly, and anophthalmia (45).

Developmental analysis showed that abnormalities were first detected in *Tcof1* heterozygous mice at embryonic day 8 (E8), after which they exhibited a generalized developmental delay. At E8.5, wild-type embryos displayed well-developed head folds and the first signs of optic development, whereas *Tcof1*$^{+/-}$ embryos exhibited smaller, more rounded neural folds and an absence of the optic evagination. While all wild-type embryos had completed the axial turning sequence and closed their rostral neuropore by E9, their *Tcof1*$^{+/-}$ littermates remained unturned with a patent rostral neuropore. By E10.5 the formation of the olfactory pit in wild-type mice divided the frontonasal mass into medial and lateral nasal processes. In contrast, *Tcof1*$^{+/-}$ embryos failed to develop either of these processes, and exhibited exencephaly with neuroepithelium protruding through the rostral neuropore (Fig. 2A–D). By E14.5, the lack of nasal passages and anophthalmia in *Tcof1*$^{+/-}$ mice were clearly apparent. Mutant mice also displayed mandibular hypoplasia, severe retrognathia of the middle third of the face, and low-

---

Figure 2 (A and B) Scanning electron microscope analysis of E12.5 wild-type and *Tcof1*$^{+/-}$ embryos, illustrating severe abnormalities of the developing facial complex, including underdevelopment of the brain, anophthalmia, and abnormal nasal passages. (C and D) Histological appearance of E12.5 wild-type and *Tcof1*$^{+/-}$ embryos. Parasagittal sections reveal underdevelopment of the entire otocyst as well as the lack of an endolymphatic appendage in the *Tcof1*$^{+/-}$ embryo. The trigeminal ganglion is severely hypoplastic in the *Tcof1* heterozygote. (E and F) Skeletal analysis of the skulls of postnatal wild-type and *Tcof1*$^{+/-}$ mice. The majority of the abnormalities are observed in the craniofacial region, including the lack of the frontal, parietal, and interparietal bones of the vault of the skull, as well as the abnormal nasal complex. (G and H) Whole-mount TUNEL analysis of wild-type and *Tcof1*$^{+/-}$ embryos at E8.5. A section through the neural folds of the wild-type embryo reveals infrequent apoptotic nuclei along the edges of the neural folds, whereas the *Tcof1* heterozygous embryo exhibits massively elevated levels of apoptotic nuclei throughout the entire neuroepithelium, particularly in the lateral regions. e, ear; f, frontal bone; fb, forebrain; mb, midbrain; hb, hindbrain; fb/mb, forebrain/midbrain mass; m, mandible; mp, mandibular process; nc, nasal complex; nf, neural fold; oc, otocyst; p, parietal bone; tgg, trigeminal ganglion.

set cup-shaped ears. Skeletal analysis of E18 $Tcof1^{+/-}$ mice revealed an absence of the frontal, parietal and interparietal bones of the vault of the skull. The nasal capsule and the maxilla were grossly malformed. The zygomatic arch, the tympanic ring, and the middle ear ossicles were also hypoplastic and misshapen in $Tcof1^{+/-}$ mice (Fig. 2E,F) (45).

As the phenotype suggested an abnormality of neural crest cell development, whole-mount TUNEL analysis, a technique that identifies cells undergoing apoptosis, was used by Dixon and co-workers (45). This technique revealed that the number of apoptotic cells was markedly elevated in the $Tcof1$ heterozygous embryos; in particular, the neuroepithelium of the cranial neural folds and the neural tube displayed a profusion of apoptotic cells (Fig. 2G,H). These abnormally high levels of apoptosis were observed in $Tcof1$ heterozygous mice throughout embryonic days 8 and 9, but thereafter they declined. The high levels of cell death in the neuroepithelium, together with the gross morphological phenotype, strongly suggested that a proportion of the premigratory neural crest cells were depleted. In addition, immunohistochemistry of embryonic day10.5 mice with an antineurofilament antibody indicated that the neural crest cell-derived cranial ganglia were severely hypoplastic, the ophthalmic branch of the trigeminal nerve and the glossopharyngeal ganglia/nerves were absent, and the dorsal root ganglia were markedly disorganized. These results suggest that the TCS phenotype results, at least in part, from a massive increase in apoptosis in the prefusion neural folds.

Subsequent studies in our own laboratory have investigated the contribution of different genetic backgrounds to the phenotype of the heterozygous mice. To date, the $Tcof1$ chimeras have been crossed with females from different inbred strains. Although these studies are currently ongoing, it is clear that the genetic background on which the $Tcof1$ mutation is placed is a key determinant in the severity of the resulting phenotype. Continued investigation of the contribution of the genetic background to phenotypic variation in mice may, in the long term, help us to understand the basis of the marked inter- and intrafamilial variation observed in TCS families.

REFERENCES

1. Thompson A. Notice of several cases of malformation of the external ear, together with experiments on the state of hearing in such persons. Monthly J Med Sci 1846; 7:420.
2. Treacher Collins E. Cases with symmetrical congenital notches in the outer part of each lid and defective development of the malar bones. Trans Ophthalmol Soc UK 1900; 20:190–192.

3. Franceschetti A, Klein D. Mandibulo-facial dysostosis: new hereditary syndrome. Acta Ophthalmol 1949; 27:143–224.

4. Rovin S, Dachi SF, Borenstein DB, Cotter WB. Mandibulofacial dysostosis, a familial study of five generations. J Pediatr 1964; 65:215–221.

5. Fazen LE, Elmore J, Nadler HL. Mandibulo-facial dysostosis (Treacher Collins syndrome). Am J Dis Child 1967; 113:406–410.

6. Jones KL, Smith DW, Harvey MA, Hall BD, Quan L. Older paternal age and fresh gene mutation: data on additional disorders. J Pediatr 1975; 86:84–88.

7. Marres HAM, Cremers CWRJ, Dixon MJ, Huygen PLM, Joosten FBM. The Treacher Collins syndrome: a clinical, radiological and genetic linkage study on two pedigrees. Arch Otol 1995; 121:509–514.

8. Stovin JJ, Lyon JA, Clemens RL. Mandibulofacial dysostosis. Radiology 1960; 74:225–231.

9. Phelps PD, Poswillo D, Lloyd GAS. The ear deformities in mandibulofacial dysostosis (Treacher Collins syndrome). Clin Otolaryngol 1981; 6:15–28.

10. Poswillo D. The pathogenesis of Treacher Collins syndrome (mandibulofacial dysostosis). Br J Oral Surg 1975; 13:1–26.

11. Kay ED, Kay CN. Dysmorphogenesis of the mandible, zygoma, and middle ear ossicles in hemifacial microsomia and mandibulofacial dysostosis. Am J Med Genet 1989; 32:27–31.

12. Dixon MJ, Marres HAM, Edwards SJ, Dixon J, Cremers CWRJ. Treacher Collins syndrome: correlation between clinical and genetic linkage studies. Clin Dysmorph 1994; 3:96–103.

13. Edwards SJ, Fowlie A, Cust MP, Liu DTY, Young ID, Dixon MJ. Prenatal diagnosis in Treacher Collins syndrome using combined linkage analysis and ultrasound imaging. J Med Genet 1996; 33:603–606.

14. Gorlin RJ, Cohen MM, Levin LS. Syndromes of the Head and Neck. Oxford: Oxford University Press, 1990.

15. Dixon MJ. Treacher Collins syndrome. Hum Mol Genet 1996; 5:1391–1397.

16. Dixon MJ, Read AP, Donnai D, Colley A, Dixon J, Williamson R. The gene for Treacher Collins syndrome maps to the long arm of chromosome 5. Am J Hum Genet 1991; 49:17–22.

17. Jabs EW, Li X, Coss CA, Taylor EW, Meyers DA, Weber JL. Mapping the Treacher Collins syndrome locus to 5q31.3–q33.3. Genomics 1991; 11:193–198.

18. Dixon MJ, Dixon J, Raskova D, Le Beau MM, Williamson R, Klinger K, Landes GM. Genetic and physical mapping of the Treacher Collins syndrome locus: refinement of the localisation to chromosome 5q32–q33.2. Hum Mol Genet 1992; 1:249–253.

19. Dixon MJ, Dixon J, Houseal T, Bhatt M, Ward DC, Klinger K, Landes GM. Narrowing the position of the Treacher Collins syndrome locus to a small interval between three new microsatellite markers at 5q32–q33.1. Am J Hum Genet 1993; 52:907–914.

20. Loftus SK, Edwards SJ, Scherpbier-Heddema T, Buetow KH, Wasmuth JJ, Dixon M. A combined genetic and radiation hybrid map surrounding the Treacher Collins syndrome locus on chromosome 5q. Hum Mol Genet 1993; 2:1785–1792.

21. Dixon J, Gladwin AJ, Loftus SK, Riley J, Perveen R, Wasmuth JJ, Anand R, Dixon MJ. A yeast artificial chromosome contig encompassing the Treacher Collins syndrome critical region at 5q31.3–q32. Am J Hum Genet 1994; 55:372–378.

22. Li X, Wise CA, Le Paslier D, Hawkins AL, Griffin CA, Pittler SJ, Lovett M, Jabs EW. A YAC contig of approximately 3 Mb from human chromosome 5q31–q33. Genomics 1994; 19:470–477.

23. Loftus SK, Dixon J, Koprivnikar K, Dixon MJ, Wasmuth JJ. Transcriptional map of the Treacher Collins candidate gene region. Genome Res 61996; 26–34.

24. The Treacher Collins Syndrome Collaborative Group. Positional cloning of a gene involved in the pathogenesis of Treacher Collins syndrome. Nat Genet 1996; 12:130–136.

25. Dixon J, Edwards SJ, Anderson I, Brass A, Scambler PJ, Dixon MJ. Identification of the complete coding sequence and genomic organisation of the Treacher Collins syndrome gene. Genome Res 1997; 7:223–234.

26. Wise CA, Chiang LC, Paznekas WA, Sharma M, Musy MM, Ashley JA, Lovett M, Jabs EW. *TCOF1* encodes a putative nucleolar phosphoprotein that exhibits mutations in Treacher Collins syndrome throughout its coding region. Proc Natl Acad Sci USA 1997; 94:3110–3115.

27. Chelsky D, Ralph R, Jonak G. Sequence requirements for synthetic peptide-mediated translocation to the nucleus. Mol Cell Biol 1989; 9:2487–2492.

28. Marsh KL, Dixon J, Dixon MJ. Mutations in the Treacher Collins syndrome gene lead to mislocalisation of the nucleolar protein treacle. Hum Mol Genet 1998; 11:1795–1800.

29. Winokur ST, Shiang R. The Treacher Collins syndrome (*TCOF1*) gene product, treacle, is targeted to the nucleolus by signals in its C-terminus. Hum Mol Genet 1998; 7:1947–1952.

30. Isaac C, Marsh KL, Dixon J, Paznekas W, Dixon MJ, Jabs EW, Meier UT. Characterization of the nucleolar gene product of Treacher Collins syndrome in patient and control cells. Mol Biol Cell. 2000; 11:3061–3071.

31. Jones NC, Farlie PG, Minichiello J, Newgreen DF. Detection of an appropriate kinase activity in branchial arches I and II that coincide with peak expression of the Treacher Collins sydrome gene product, treacle. Hum Mol Genet 1999; 8:2239–2245.

32. Emes RD, Ponting CP. A new sequence motif linking lissencephaly, Treacher Collins and oral-facial-digital type 1 syndromes, microtubule dynamics and cell migration. Hum Mol Genet 2001; 10:2813–2820.

33. Lo Nigro C, Chong CS, Smith AC, Dobyns WB, Carrozzo R, Ledbetter DH. Point mutations and an intragenic deletion in *LIS1*, the lissencephaly causative gene in isolated lissencephaly sequence and Miller-Dieker syndrome. Hum Mol Genet 1997; 6:157–164.

34. Gladwin AJ, Dixon J, Loftus SK, Edwards SJ, Wasmuth JJ, Hennekam RCM, Dixon MJ. Treacher Collins syndrome may result from insertions, deletions or splicing mutations, which introduce a termination codon into the gene. Hum Mol Genet 1996; 5:1533–1538.

35. Edwards SJ, Gladwin AJ, Dixon MJ. The mutational spectrum in Treacher Collins syndrome reveals a predominance of mutations that create a premature termination codon. Am J Hum Genet 1997; 60:515–524.

36. Splendore A, Silva EO, Alonso LG, Richieri-Costa A, Alonso N, Rosa A, Carakushanky G, Cavalcanti DP, Brunoni D, Passos-Bueno MR. High mutation detection rate in *TCOF1* among Treacher Collins syndrome patients reveals clustering of mutations and 16 novel pathogenic changes. Hum Mutat 2000; 16:315–322.

37. Dixon J, Hovanes K, Shiang R, Dixon MJ. Sequence analysis, identification of evolutionary conserved motifs and expression analysis of murine *TCOF1* provide further evidence for a potential function for the gene and its human homologue, *TCOF1*. Hum Mol Genet 1997; 6:727–737.

38. Haworth KE, Islam I, Breen M, Putt W, Makrinou E, Binns M, Hopkinson D, Edwards Y. Canine *TCOF1*: cloning, chromosome assignment and genetic analysis in dogs with different head types. Mamm Genome 2001; 12:622–629.

39. Aebi M, Hornig H, Weissmann C. 5′ cleavage site in eukaryotic pre-mRNA splicing is determined by the overall 5′ splice region, not by the conserved GU. Cell 1987; 50:237–246.

40. Paznekas WA, Zhang N, Gridley T, Jabs EW. Mouse *TCOF1* is expressed widely, has motifs conserved in nucleolar phosphoproteins, and maps to chromosome 18. Biochem Biophys Res Commun 1997; 238:1–6.

41. Nicolaides KH, Johansson D, Donnai D, Rodeck CH. Prenatal diagnosis of mandibulofacial dysostosis. Prenat Diagn 1984; 4:201–205.

42. Meizner I, Carmi R, Katz M. Prenatal ultrasonic diagnosis of mandibulofacial dysostosis [Treacher Collins syndrome]. J Clin Ultrasound 1991; 19:124–127.

43. Milligan DA, Harlass FE, Duff P, Kopelman JN. Recurrence of Treacher Collins syndrome with sonographic findings. Mil Med 1994; 159:250–252.

44. Cohen J, Ghezzi F, Goncalves L, Fuentes JD, Paulyson KJ, Sherer DM. Prenatal sonographic diagnosis of Treacher Collins syndrome: a case and review of the literature. Am J Perinatol 1995; 12:416–419.

45. Dixon J, Brakebusch C, Fässler R, Dixon MJ. Increased levels of apoptosis in the prefusion neural folds underlie the craniofacial disorder. Treacher Collins syndrome. Hum Mol Genet 2000; 10:1473–1480.

11
MYH9

Anil K. Lalwani and Anand N. Mhatre
New York University, New York, New York, U.S.A.

I. INTRODUCTION

In 1993, a five-generation family with hereditary hearing impairment associated with cochleosaccular degeneration was identified (Fig. 1) (1). Through linkage analysis, this family was mapped to chromosome 22q12.2–q13.3, spanning a 17–23-cM region, defining a new locus for nonsyndromic hereditary hearing impairment DFNA17 (2). Subsequently, a mutation in *MYH9*, responsible for the DFNA17 was identified (3). The mutation R705H, a consequence of G–A transition in the nucleotide sequence, is considered critical for the ATPase activity of the myosin motor domain. Simultaneously, mutations in MYH9 have also been identified in hereditary macrothrombocytopenia (4,5). Herein, the DFNA17 phenotype and genotype-phenotype correlations are discussed.

II. AUDIOLOGICAL FINDINGS

Of the 22 member of the family, eight had hearing impairment; six were males and two were females. In the affected members of the family, hearing loss began as a mild high-frequency deficit apparent by age 10–12 that progressed during adolescence (Fig. 2). By the third decade of life, the hearing loss was moderate to severe. Despite the similarity in the nature and progression of hearing loss, there was variation in the severity of hearing loss among the affected family members (Fig. 3). Because of the limited

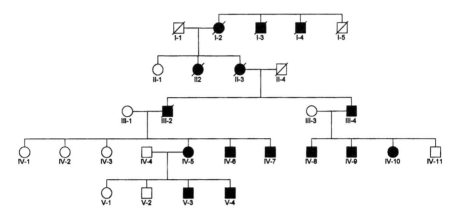

Figure 1 Pedigree of the DFNA17 family with progressive high-frequency hearing impairment associated with cochleosaccular degeneration.

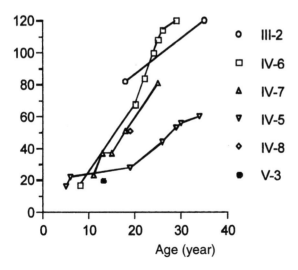

Figure 2 Pure tone thresholds for the right ear averaged for 500, 1000, 2000, and 3000 Hz. Test results show a mild hearing impairment in all subjects at age 13 with progression of the loss with aging.

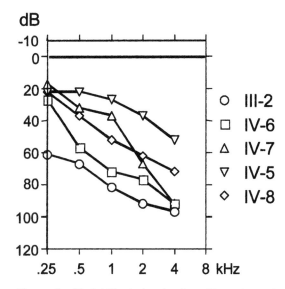

Figure 3 Variability in hearing loss. Shown is the hearing impairment observed for different affected individuals between the ages of 18 and 20 years. The proband, III-2, shows the most significant hearing impairment when compared with his three children and his nephew.

number of affected individuals, it was not possible to determine the rate of progression of hearing impairment. In some members of the family with significant hearing impairment, the word identification scores were good considering the degree of hearing loss. The preservation of clarity with a significant sensorineural hearing impairment is reminiscent of Schucknecht's strial presbyacusis.

Distortion product otoacoustic emissions (DPOAE) were also performed on the affected and unaffected members of the family. Presence or absence of otoacoustic emissions reflected the level of hearing loss of the individual being tested. OAE were present in individuals with mild hearing loss and absent in members with profound impairment. Therefore, OAE cannot be used for early identification of individuals harboring the mutated gene prior to the development of hearing impairment. Similar to OAE, auditory brainstem responses (ABR) reflected the severity of hearing impairment. ABR were normal in individuals with mild hearing impairment and absent in deaf individuals.

III. TEMPORAL BONE FINDINGS

The temporal bone of the proband, a 61-year-old profoundly deaf man, demonstrated classic findings associated with Scheibe, or cochleosaccular, degeneration: degeneration of the stria vascularis, the organ of Corti, and the saccular sensory epithelium. There was collapse of Reissner's membrane onto the spiral ligament and area of organ of Corti. Stria vascularis was either absent or replaced by basophilic granules. The population of spiral ganglion neurons was reduced to one third of normal levels. Consistent with cochleosaccular degeneration, the utricle and the ampullae of the semicircular canals appeared to be completely normal.

IV. MYH9, A CONVENTIONAL NONMUSCLE MYOSIN

The DFNA17 locus was mapped to a relatively large genetic region of 17–23 cM on chromosome 22q12.2–q13.3, typical for the size of the family studied (2). The low resolution of the linked region precluded use of the positional cloning approach to identify the disease gene. The candidate gene approach, default alternative to positional cloning, was thus pursued to identify the mutant gene within the DFNA17 locus. Analysis of the chromosome 22-gene map identified 163 candidate genes within the region spanning the DFNA17 locus (6). One of the candidate genes encoding the nonmuscle myosin heavy chain A (*MYH9*), was selected for further analysis. The selection of *MYH9*, a member of the class II or conventional myosin, was based upon identification of mutations in several other myosin heavy-chain genes that are pathogenically linked to HHI (7).

The class II myosins are broadly expressed in skeletal, cardiac, and smooth muscles as well as nonmuscle tissues and consist of a pair of heavy chains, a pair of light chains, and a pair of regulatory light chains (8). The N-terminal motor domain is the most highly conserved region of the myosin heavy chain and contains the ATP- and actin-binding sites. The apparent molecular weight of the class II myosin heavy chain is 200 kDa. The myosin that mediates skeletal muscle contraction, also known as the sarcomeric myosin, represents the most well-characterized representative of the class II myosin family. Cardiac and smooth muscle cells also express isoforms of class II myosin, distinct from the sarcomeric myosin that mediates contraction in these muscle cells.

Characterization of myosins in nonmuscle cells has identified two distinct isoforms of myosin II: nonmuscle myosin-IIA (MYH9) (9,10) and nonmuscle myosin-IIB (MYH10) (10). *MYH9* and *MYH10* have been mapped to 22q11.2 and 17q13, respectively, and exhibit 85% identity in their motor domains. Several skeletal-muscle heavy-chain genes have also been localized to the region containing *MYH10*. Most cells express relatively equal amounts of each of these myosins, with a few exceptions; platelets express MYH9 only (11,12) while neuronal tissues predominantly express MYH10. MYH9 and MYH10 demonstrate overlapping but distinct intracellular locations when coexpressed within the same cell type (13,14). In vitro motility studies of these two isoforms has shown that MYH9 is several-fold faster than MYH10 in its rate of ATP hydrolysis and movement of actin filaments (15). The differences in their localization and their in vitro characteristics suggest differing in vivo functions.

Sequence analysis of *MYH9* in the DFNA17 family identified a G–A transition at nucleotide 2114 that cosegregated with the inherited autosomal dominant hearing impairment (3). This missense mutation changes codon

Myosin Heavy Chain	aa #	peptide sequence
		linker region
DFNA17	690	DQLRCNGVLEGIRICHQGFPNRVVFQEFRQ
MYH9 (non-muscle A)	690	DQLRCNGVLEGIRICRQGFPNRVVFQEFRQ
MYH10 (non-muscle B)	697	DQLRCNGVLEGIRICRQGFPNRIVFQEFRQ
skeletal muscle a	697	HQLRCNGVLEGIRICRKGFPSRILYADFKQ
skeletal muscle b	695	HQLRCNGVLEGIRICRKGFPSRILYADFKQ
perinatal	694	HQLRCNGVLEGIRICRKGFPSRILYGDFKQ
featal	695	HQLRCNGVLEGIRICRKGFPSRILYGDFKQ
embryonic	692	HQLRCNGVLEGIRICRKGFPNRILYGDFKQ
extraocular	695	HQLRCNGVLEGIRICRKGFPSRILYADFKQ
cardiac muscle a	691	HQLRCNGVLEGIRICRKGFPNRILYGDFRQ
cardiac muscle b	691	HQLRCNGVLEGIRICRKGFPNRLLYGDFRQ
smooth muscle	583	EQLRCNGVLEGIRICRQGFPNRIVFQEFRQ
rat MYH9	690	DQLRCNGVLEGIRICRQGFPNRVVFQEFRQ
chicken MYH9	690	DQLRCNGVLEGIRICRQGFPNRVVFQEFRQ
chicken MYH10	697	DQLRCNGVLEGIRICRQGFPNRIVFQEFRQ
xenopus MYH9	690	DQLRCNGVLEGIRICRQGFPNRVVFQEFRQ
xenopus MYH10	713	DQLRCNGVLEGIRICRQGFPNRIVFQEFRQ
drosophila MYH9	741	DQLRCNGVLEGIRICRQGFPNRIPFQEFRQ
drosophila MYH10	696	DQLRCNGVLEGIRICRQGFPNRIPFQEFRQ
dictostylium	674	DQLRCNGVLEGIRITRKGFPNRIIYADFVK
acanthamoeba	695	DQLRCNGVLEGIRIARKGWPNRLKYDEFLK
C elegans	706	DQLRCNGVLEGIRICRQGFPTRLPFQEFRQ

SH2   SH1

Figure 4 DFNA17 mutation R705H resides in a highly conserved and functionally important myosin heavy-chain motor domain.

705 from an invariant arginine (R) to histidine (H), R705H. The identified mutation R705H within *MYH9* occurs in a highly conserved and functionally critical region within the carboxy-terminal half of the myosin heavy-chain motor domain that forms the globular head in the hexameric myosin molecule (Fig. 4). Within the motor domain, R705 resides in a highly conserved linker region spanning 16 amino acids that contains two free thiol groups, C704 (SH1) and C694 (SH2). Crystal structure of the globular head of the skeletal muscle myosin has shown that the two thiols are part of two short α-helices joined through a kink at the conserved G696 residue (16,17). The SH1 and SH2 helices are believed to play a key role in the conformational changes that occur in the myosin head during force generation coupled to ATP hydrolysis. X-ray crystallographic studies suggest that during the power stroke, the light-chain-binding domain (LCBD) swings relative to the catalytic/ATP-binding domain. The pivot point of this swinging motion is considered to be in the vicinity of the SH1-SH2 helix (18). Not surprisingly, in vitro and in vivo modifications of the SH1 helix including cross-linking of SH1-SH2 groups or alteration/substitution of SH1/SH2 have been shown to disrupt the mechanical function of the myosin motor domain (19,20). Thus, studies investigating myosin structure and function have demonstrated that the functional integrity of myosin is critically dependent upon its flexibility at the SH1–SH2 helix. The strict conservation of this linker region among myosin II subtypes within and between species further underscores its functional importance. The R705H mutation in the DFNA17 family may cause an altered conformation of the SH1 helix that affects its flexibility and movement, thus disrupting the mechanical function of the motor domain.

V. *MYH9* EXPRESSION IN THE MAMMALIAN COCHLEA

Localization of MYH9 expression in situ in the mammalian cochlea has particular importance for understanding and interpreting the histopathology associated with its dysfunction. Within the rat cochlea, MYH9 expression was localized in three distinct tissue types: the organ of Corti, the subcentral region of the spiral ligament, and Reissner's membrane (Fig. 5) (3). Within the organ of Corti, the MYH9 expression was identified throughout the outer hair cells including the cuticular plate. The CSD histopathology of the affected DFNA17 proband demonstrated a collapsed Reissner's membrane, a two-cell-layer-wide membranous barrier that forms the upper boundary of the cochlear duct. MYH9 dysfunction in the Reissner's membrane may contribute to its compromised cytoarchitecture, thus disturbing cochlear fluid homeostasis and affecting cochlear function. The cochlear tissue con-

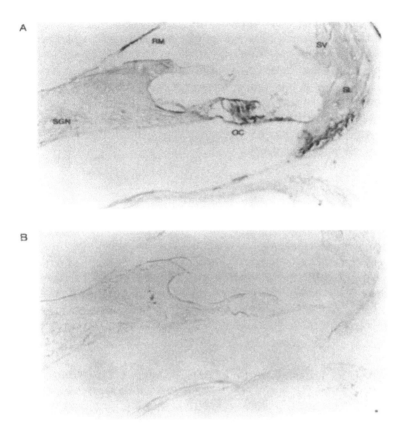

Figure 5 (A) Within the rat cochlea, MYH9 expression was localized in three distinct tissue types: the organ of Corti, the subcentral region of the spiral ligament, and Reissner's membrane. (B) Control cochlear section with competing peptide shows no staining.

spicuous by its absence of MYH9 expression is the stria vascularis, the lateral wall of the cochlear duct, and whose dysfunction is generally considered to be the cause of CSD. The absence of MYH9 expression is the stria vascularis suggests that this tissue type is not directly responsible for the underlying pathophysiology of CSD.

MYH9 is also expressed within the spiral ligament consisting of connective tissue made up of fibrocytes. These fibrocytes of the spiral ligament are classified according to the distinct isoforms of the Na^+, K^+-ATPase that they express as well as by their cytoskeletal components. The subcentric region of the spiral ligament, immnoreactive to the MYH9 antibody, is characterized by the presence of type III and type IV fibrocytes. The type III fibrocytes are rich in actin and other contractile/contraction-associated proteins (21,22). The postulated role for these cells includes providing anchorage for surrounding cells and/or developing or reacting to tension generated in the basilar membrane–spiral ligament complex. Maintenance of this tension is likely more crucial in the high-frequency-sensitive basal turn of the cochlea where the basilar membrane is wider relative to the apex. This may be the simple explanation for the observed high-frequency hearing impairment in DFNA17.

VI. HEREDITARY MACROTHROMBOCYTOPENIAS

Hereditary macrothrombocytopenias (MTCPs) are a family of related disorders inherited in an autosomal dominant manner, characterized by large platelets with or without leukocyte inclusion bodies, and a reduction in total number of platelets. These syndromes include May-Hegglin anomaly (MHA), Sebastian syndrome (SBS), Fechtner syndrome (FTNS), Epstein syndrome (EPS), and Alport syndrome with platelet defects (APSM) (Table 1). While sharing the presence of MTCP, each of these syndromes is distinguished from the others by the presence or absence of nephritis, cataracts, and deafness. Molecular genetic analysis has recently identified mutations in *MYH9* as the pathogenic cause of each of the five inherited MTCPs (Table 2) (4,5,23). Single base pair missense or nonsense mutations in both the motor and rod domain have been linked to MCTP and DFNA17. Mutations in the head domain are proposed to affect the motor function while the rod domain mutations are thought to affect the assembly of the

Table 1 Clinical Features Associated with the Autosomal Dominant MTCP

Disorder	MTCP	LI	HI	Nephritis	Cataracts
MHA	+	+	−	−	−
SBS[a]	+	+	−	−	−
Brodie	+	−	+	−	−
FTNS[a]	+	+	+	+	+
EPS	+	−	+	+	+
APSM	+	−	+	+	+

MHA, May-Hegglin anomaly; SBS, Sebastian syndrome; FTNS, Fechtner syndrome; APSM, Alport syndrome with platelet defect; EPS, Epstein syndrome; MTCP, macrothrombocytopenia; LI, leukocyte inclusions; HI, hearing impairment.
[a] In SBS and FTNS, the inclusion are smaller and less organized in comparison to MHA.

Table 2 Reported Amino Acid Changes in MYH9 and the Associated Phenotype

AA change	Nt change	Exon	Diagnosis
N93K	C279G	1	MHA
A95T	G283A	1	
S96L	C287T	1	Fe/Ep, Ep
K371N		10	MHA/SBS
R702C	C2104T	16	FTNS; EPS; APSM
R705H	G2111A	16	DFNA17
S1114P		25	APSM
T1155I		25	MHA
R1165C		26	MHA
R1165L	G3494T	26	
R1400W		30	
D1424H	G4270C	30	FTNS, MHA
D1424N	G4270A	30	FTNS, SBA, MHA
D1424Y	G4270T	30	MHA
E1841K		38	FTNS, MHA, MHA/SBS
R1933X	C5797T	40	MHA, MHA/SBS, FTNS
	5779delC	40	

AA, amino acid; Nt, nucleotide; MHA, May-Hegglin anomaly; SBS, Sebastian syndrome; FTNS, Fechtner syndrome; APSM, Alport syndrome with platelet defect; EPS, Epstein syndrome.

myosin complex. The clinical symptoms associated with *MYH9* mutations serve to identify the critical biological role of *MYH9* in the affected target organs. However, the precise mechanism of pathogenesis in the affected target organs remains to be determined. The finding of mutations at the same location causing different phenotypes suggests that the genetic background may be influential in determining the clinical severity associated with a particular MYH9 mutation.

VII. SUMMARY

Mutations in MYH9 are associated with syndromic and nonsyndromic deafness. The mechanism by which MYH9 dysfunction leads to hearing loss and the observed inner ear histopathology, cochleosaccular dysplasia (CSD), in the DFNA17 proband in some and hereditary MCTPs in others remains to be determined. Future development of animal models with loss of function of *Myh9* will facilitate a direct and effective means of understanding the role of MYH9 and its mutant allele in hearing and its dysfunction.

ACKNOWLEDGMENTS

This study was supported in part by grants from the National Institute on Deafness and Other Communication Disorders, National Institute of Health (K08 DC 00112 to AKL); American Hearing Research Foundation; National Organization for Hearing Research; Deafness Research Foundation; and Hearing Research, Inc.

REFERENCES

1. Lalwani AK, Linthicum FH, Wilcox ER, et al. A five-generation family with late-onset progressive hereditary hearing impairment due to cochleosaccular degeneration. Audiol Neuro-Otol 1997; 2:139–154.
2. Lalwani AK, Luxford WM, Mhatre AN, et al. A new locus for nonsyndromic hereditary hearing impairment, DFNA17, maps to chromosome 22 and represents a gene for cochleosaccular degeneration [letter]. Am J Hum Genet 1999; 64:318–323.
3. Lalwani AK, Goldstein JA, Kelly MJ, et al. Human Nonsyndromic Deafness DFNA17 is due to a mutation in nonmuscle myosin MYH9. Am J Hum Genet 2000; 67:1121–1128.
4. Kelley MJ, Jawien W, Ortel TL, Korczak JF. Mutation of MYH9, encoding non-muscle myosin heavy chain A, in May-Hegglin anomaly. Nat Genet 2000; 26:106–108.
5. Seri M, Cusano R, Gangarossa S, et al. Mutations in MYH9 result in the May-Hegglin anomaly, and Fechtner and Sebastian syndromes. The May-Hegglin/Fechtner Syndrome Consortium. Nat Genet 2000; 26:103–105.
6. Dunham I, Shimizu N, Roe BA, et al. The DNA sequence of human chromosome 22 [see comments] [published erratum appears in Nature 2000 Apr 20;404(6780):904]. Nature 1999; 402:489–495.
7. Friedman TB, Sellers JR, Avraham KB. Unconventional myosins and the genetics of hearing loss. Am J Med Genet 1999; 89:147–157.
8. Sellers JR. Myosins: a diverse superfamily. Biochim Biophys Acta 2000; 1496: 3–22.
9. Saez CG, Myers JC, Shows TB, Leinwand LA. Human nonmuscle myosin heavy chain mRNA: generation of diversity through alternative polyadenylation. Proc Natl Acad Sci USA 1990; 87:1164–1168.
10. Simons M, Wang M, McBride OW, et al. Human nonmuscle myosin heavy chains are encoded by two genes located on different chromosomes. Circ Res 1991; 69:530–539.

11. Maupin P, Phillips CL, Adelstein RS, Pollard TD. Differential localization of myosin-II isozymes in human cultured cells and blood cells. J Cell Sci 1994; 107:3077–3090.

12. Phillips CL, Yamakawa K, Adelstein RS. Cloning of the cDNA encoding human nonmuscle myosin heavy chain-B and analysis of human tissues with isoform-specific antibodies. J Muscle Res Cell Motil 1995; 16:379–389.

13. Kolega J. Cytoplasmic dynamics of myosin IIA and IIB: spatial "sorting" of isoforms in locomoting cells. J Cell Sci 1998; 111:2085–2095.

14. Kolega J. Fluorescent analogues of myosin II for tracking the behavior of different myosin isoforms in living cells. J Cell Biochem 1998; 68:389–401.

15. Kelley CA, Sellers JR, Gard DL, et al. *Xenopus* nonmuscle myosin heavy chain isoforms have different subcellular localizations and enzymatic activities [published erratum appears in J Cell Biol 1997 Jul 14;138(1):215]. J Cell Biol 1996; 134:675–687.

16. Gulick AM, Rayment I. Structural studies on myosin II: communication between distant protein domains. Bioessays 1997; 19:561–569.

17. Rayment I. The structural basis of the myosin ATPase activity [see comments]. J Biol Chem 1996; 271:15850–15853.

18. Houdusse A, Kalabokis VN, Himmel D, Szent-Gyorgyi AG, Cohen C. Atomic structure of scallop myosin subfragment S1 complexed with MgADP: a novel conformation of the myosin head. Cell 1999; 97:459–470.

19. Patterson B, Ruppel KM, Wu Y, Spudich JA. Cold-sensitive mutants G680V and G691C of *Dictyostelium* myosin II confer dramatically different biochemical defects. J Biol Chem 1997; 272:27612–27617.

20. Suzuki J, Aikawa M, Isobe M, et al. Altered expression of smooth muscle and nonmuscle myosin heavy chain isoforms in rejected hearts: a sensitive marker for acute rejection and graft coronary arteriosclerosis. Transplant Proc 1995; 27:578.

21. Henson MM, Henson OW Jr, Jenkins DB. The attachment of the spiral ligament to the cochlear wall: anchoring cells and the creation of tension. Hearing Res 1984; 16:231–242.

22. Henson MM, Burridge K, Fitzpatrick D, et al. Immunocytochemical localization of contractile and contraction associated proteins in the spiral ligament of the cochlea. Hearing Res 1985; 20:207–214.

23. Heath KE, Campos-Barros A, Toren A, et al. Nonmuscle myosin heavy chain IIA mutations define a spectrum of autosomal dominant macrothrombocytopenias: May-Hegglin anomaly and Fechtner, Sebastian, Epstein, and Alport-like syndromes. Am J Hum Genet 2001; 69:1033–1045.

12
Mitochondrial Hearing Loss

Nathan Fischel-Ghodsian
Cedars-Sinai Medical Center and David Geffen School of Medicine at UCLA, Los Angeles, California, U.S.A.

I. INTRODUCTION

The last decade has led to the identification of several mitochondrial DNA mutations associated with hearing loss. Since the only known function of the human mitochondrial chromosome is to participate in the production of chemical energy through oxidative phosphorylation, it was not unexpected that mitochondrial mutations interfering with energy production could cause systemic neuromuscular disorders, which have as one of their features hearing impairment. Surprisingly, however, inherited mitochondrial mutations have also been found to be a cause of nonsyndromic hearing loss, and predispose to aminoglycoside-induced hearing loss, while acquired mitochondrial mutations have been proposed as one of the causes of presbycusis. This chapter will first give a short background review of mitochondrial genetics, outline the different mitochondrial mutations associated with hearing loss, and discuss the clinical relevance of diagnosing these mutations. The latter part of the chapter will concentrate on the fact that the clinical expression of these mitochondrial mutations is dependent on environmental exposures and nuclear-encoded modifier genes. Preventive and therapeutic strategies will depend on identification and avoidance of the environmental exposures, and the identification of the nuclear-encoded modifier genes. Experimental approaches to identify these modifier genes will be presented.

II. NORMAL MITOCHONDRIAL GENETICS

There are hundreds of mitochondria in each cell, which help in the protection against reactive oxygen species, are intimately involved in the regulation of cell death, and serve a variety of metabolic functions, the most important being the synthesis of ATP by oxidative phosphorylation. Each mitochondrion contains in its matrix 2–10 mitochondrial chromosomes. Each of these mitochondrial DNA molecules in humans is 16,569 bp long, double-stranded, forms a closed circle, and replicates and is transcribed within the mitochondrion in ways reminiscent of its bacterial origin. The mitochondrial DNA molecule encodes 13 mRNA genes, as well as two rRNAs and 22 tRNAs, which are required for assembling a functional mitochondrial protein-synthesizing system. The 13 mRNAs are translated on mitochondrion-specific ribosomes, using a mitochondrion-specific genetic code, into 13 proteins. These proteins interact with approximately 60 nuclear encoded proteins to form the five enzyme complexes required for oxidative phosphorylation. These complexes are bound to the mitochondrial inner membrane, and are involved in electron transport and ATP synthesis (reviewed in Ref. 1).

Mitochondrial DNA is transmitted exclusively through mothers. This leads to the expectation that a defect in a mitochondrial gene should lead to disease equally in both sexes, but can only be transmitted through the maternal line. Normally, most healthy individuals appear to have only a single mitochondrial DNA genotype, i.e., are homoplasmic, but in many mitochondrial disease states the mitochondrial DNA population is mixed, i.e., heteroplasmic (2). The amount of heteroplasmy varies from tissue to tissue, and for cells within a tissue, and the severity of the symptoms does not always correlate well with the proportion of mutant mitochondrial chromosomes. While for most of the multisystemic mitochondrial syndromes the homoplasmic state would presumably be lethal, homoplasmy of mutant mitochondrial DNA is observed for two tissue-specific diseases, the ocular disorder Leber's hereditary optic neuroretinopathy (3) and maternally inherited hearing loss.

III. HEARING IMPAIRMENT DUE TO MITOCHONDRIAL MUTATIONS

Hearing loss can be due to both inherited and acquired, heteroplasmic and homoplasmic, mitochondrial mutations. These data have recently been reviewed (4), and are summarized with the inclusion of the most recent data in Table 1.

Table 1 Mitochondrial Mutations and Hearing Impairment

Hearing impairment	Mutations identified	Inherited	Acquired	Homoplasmy	Heteroplasmy
Syndromic					
Syst. neuromuscular	Deletions, A3243G, ...	Rare	Usually	No	Yes
Diabetes + deafness	A3243G-tRNAleu(UUR)	Yes	Possible	No	Yes
	Deletion/rearrangement	Yes	Not observed	No	Yes
	A8296G-tRNAlys	Yes	Not known	No	Yes
	T14709C in the tRNAglu	Yes	Not observed	No	Yes
PPK + deafness	A7445G—noncoding	Yes	Not observed	Yes	Minimal
Nonsyndromic[a]	A1555G-12S rRNA	Yes	Not observed	Yes	Minimal
	A7445G—noncoding	Yes	Not observed	Yes	Minimal
	Cins7472-tRNAser(UCN)	Yes	Not observed	Nearly	Yes
	T7511C-tRNAser(UCN)	Yes	Not observed	Nearly	Yes
Ototoxic	A1555G-12S rRNA	Yes	Not observed	Yes	No
	ΔT961Cn	Yes	Possible	Yes	"Multiple"
Presbycusis	"Random"	Not known	Yes	No	Yes

[a]A pathogenic role has been proposed, but not been established, for the T7510C and G7444A sequence changes (see text).

A. Mitochondrial Mutations and Syndromic Hearing Loss

Systemic neuromuscular syndromes such as Kearns-Sayre syndrome, mito-chondrialencephalomyopathy, lactic acidosis, and strokelike episodes (MELAS), and mitochondrial encephalomyopathy with ragged red fibers (MERRF), have hearing loss frequently as one of their clinical signs (5–7). In these cases the heteroplasmic mutation can be found generally at highest levels in nerves and muscle. Because of the higher energy requirements of muscle and nervous tissue, and the fact that small numbers of dysfunctional muscle and nerve cells can interrupt the function of many neighboring normal cells, mitochondrial DNA mutations in those tissues are thought to be particularly harmful. It is not unexpected that generalized neuronal dysfunction is also expressed in the auditory system.

In 1992 several families with diabetes mellitus and sensorineural hearing loss were described, and surprisingly were found to have inherited the heteroplasmic A3243G mutation in the gene for tRNAleu(UUR) the very same mutation associated with the systemic MELAS syndrome (8,9). In none of these cases were other neurological symptoms present. One family had instead of the 3243 mutation a heteroplasmic large deletion/insertion event (10), and more recently the heteroplasmic point mutations T14709C in the tRNAglu gene and A8296G in the tRNAlys gene were also found to be associated with maternally inherited diabetes and deafness (11,12). This association between diabetes mellitus, hearing loss, and mitochondrial mutations has been confirmed in population studies of diabetic patients (13–20). Kadowaki et al., for example, found the 3243 mutation in 2–6% of diabetic patients in Japan, and in three of five patients with diabetes and deafness. Twenty-seven of their 44 patients with diabetes and the 3243 mutation had hearing loss (15). The hearing loss is sensorineural and usually develops only after the onset of diabetes. In the non-Japanese populations examined, the 3243 mutation accounts for less than 1% of the diabetic patients (17–19). More recently, the phenotype of diabetes in those patients was shown to be of the nonobese type, with relatively young age of onset in most patients, a low frequency of diabetic proliferative retinopathy, and a high frequency of macular pattern dystrophy, diabetic nephropathy, and associated neuromuscular conditions (20–23). In most of these cases the heteroplasmic A3243G mutation was found (20,21), while in the other cases a heteroplasmic large deletion was identified (22,23). In addition, diabetes mellitus, diabetes insipidus, optic atrophy, and deafness have been well described as the Wolfram syndrome, a usually autosomal recessive condition (24), but which may also occur as a consequence of mitochondrial deletions (25,26).

Some of the mutations described below in the nonsyndromic section have been found associated occasionally with other symptoms. Most prominently, the A7445G in the tRNAser gene mutation was initially described as a nonsyndromic deafness mutation, but was subsequently found to be also associated with the skin condition palmoplantar keratoderma (PPK) in at least some of the cases (27–29). Another mutation in the tRNAser gene has also been found in one family to be associated with ataxia and myoclonus (30). The most common nonsyndromic mutation, the A1555G mutation in the 12S rRNA gene, has been described in one family with Parkinson's disease, in another with a constellation of spinal and pigmentary disturbances, and in one case of a woman with a restrictive cardiomyopathy (31–33). It remains, however, not unlikely that these associations occurred by chance and are not causally related. Similarly, the homoplasmic mitochondrial sequence change A5568G in the tRNAtrp gene was proposed as pathogenic for a family with hearing loss and hypopigmentation, but the evidence for pathogenicity is speculative at this time (34).

B. Mitochondrial Mutations and Nonsyndromic Hearing Loss

The first mutation associated with nonsyndromic deafness was identified in an Arab-Israeli pedigree, when the striking pattern of transmission only through mothers was noted (35,36). Most of the deaf family members had onset of severe to profound sensorineural hearing loss during infancy, but a minority of family members had onset during childhood or even adulthood (37). The homoplasmic A1555G mutation in the mitochondrial 12S ribosomal RNA gene was identified as the pathogenic mutation (36). Initially, in all additional pedigrees and individual patients with the same A1555G mutation the hearing loss occurred only after aminoglycoside exposure, as described below (37a,38–42). However, subsequently a significant number of pedigrees were described in Spain, with family members who went deaf with and without aminoglycosides (43,44). It is interesting that the age of onset of hearing loss in the Spanish families was rarely congenital, which is different from the Arab-Israeli pedigree. In particular the study by Estivill et al. is remarkable for two reasons, both of which indicate a higher than previously expected frequency of this mutation. First, it describes 19 families with the A1555G mutation out of a total of 70 families with sensorineural hearing loss collected. Even if the selection of families led to a bias toward families with multiple affected individuals, and even when only the individuals without aminoglycoside exposure are considered, this represents an unexpectedly high frequency of familial sensorineural hearing loss due to the A1555G mutation. Second, the fact that the mutation was identified on different haplotypes, a finding supported by the study of Torroni et al., indicates that it is likely that this mutation exists in other populations as well, and may not be rare (44,45). Similarly, in Mongolia the mutation appears to be common, although it is not clear to what extent this is a selection bias due to aminoglycoside exposure (46). However, unpublished results from screening of hearing-impaired populations in other parts of the world seem so far to indicate a very low frequency of the A1555G mutation. Despite that, most recently individual families with the A1555G and non-syndromic, nonototoxic hearing loss have been described in different places in the world (47–50).

Another close to homoplasmic inherited mutation leading to hearing loss is the A7445G mutation. It was first described in a family from Scotland, and confirmed and established in two unrelated pedigrees from New Zealand and Japan (27–29). In the New Zealand and Japanese pedigrees, a mild form of the skin condition palmoplantar keratoderma also segregates in the maternal line (29). Interestingly, the penetrance of this mutation for hearing loss in the Scottish pedigree is quite low, while in the New Zealand and Japanese pedigrees it is very high. Thus, in similarity to the Arab-Israeli pedigree, the mitochondrial mutation by itself does not appear to be sufficient to cause hearing loss, but requires additional genetic or environmental factors, which seem to be rare in the Scottish pedigree and common in the New Zealand and Japanese pedigrees. The difference in penetrance in this situation appears to be due to a difference in mitochondrial haplotype. In the New Zealand pedigree complete sequencing of the mitochondrial DNA revealed three additional sequence changes in complex I protein genes, two of which have also been labeled as secondary Leber's hereditary optic neuroretinopathy mutations (28). Since these or similar sequence changes are not present in the Scottish pedigree (51), mitochondrial haplotype appears to account for the differences in penetrance in this case.

A third mitochondrial mutation, a cytosine insertion at position 7472 in the tRNAser(UCN) gene, was identified in one large Dutch family (52). The same mutation had been previously described in a Sicilian family with hearing loss, some of the family members also having other neurological symptoms, such as ataxia and myoclonus (30). In the Dutch family, the hearing loss is sensorineural progressive with onset in early adulthood. Most of the individuals over 30 years of age were deaf, indicating that the penetrance in this family is high. The mutation is heteroplasmic, although most individuals have over 90% of abnormal mitochondrial chromosomes in the tissues examined.

More recently, a large African American pedigree with maternal inheritance and nonsyndromic hearing loss has been identified (53), and shown to have a close to homoplasmic T7511C mutation in the tRNAser(UCN) gene (54). The same mutation was subsequently found in a Japanese and two French families (49,55). Also, a British family with a T7510C mutation and nonsyndromic deafness was described, although the mitochondrial chromosome was not fully evaluated (56). Finally, the G7444A substitution has been described in deaf individuals with and without the A1555G mutation, but its pathogenicity has not been established (46).

C. Mitochondrial Mutations and Ototoxic Hearing Loss

Aminoglycoside ototoxicity is one of the most common causes of acquired deafness. Although vestibulocochlear damage is nearly universal when high drug levels are present for prolonged periods, at lower drug levels there appears to be a significant genetic component influencing susceptibility to aminoglycoside ototoxicity. The existence of families with multiple individuals with ototoxic deafness induced by aminoglycoside exposure was noticed early on. Konigsmark and Gorlin in 1976 summarized most existing descriptions of familial aminoglycoside ototoxicity and concluded that inheritance of the predisposition is probably autosomal dominant with incomplete penetrance. However, they also noted that no male-to-male transmission has been seen, and concluded that the inheritance could be multifactorial (57). In 1989 Higashi reviewed the literature, and concluded that the most likely explanation for the maternal inheritance observed is a mitochondrial DNA defect (58). In 1991, Hu et al. in China described another 36 families with maternally transmitted predisposition to aminoglycoside ototoxicity, and concluded also that a mitochondrial defect may be responsible for this predisposition (59). Additional evidence for a genetic basis for aminoglycoside susceptibility comes from animal studies. Macaque monkeys are resistant to dihydrostreptomycin, while patas monkeys are highly sensitive to that drug (60).

We analyzed three Chinese families in which several individuals developed deafness after the use of aminoglycosides, and identified the A1555G mutation in the 12S ribosomal RNA gene in all three of them, but not in hundreds of controls (36). In addition, a small proportion of "sporadic" Chinese patients, without a positive family history for aminoglycoside ototoxicity, exhibit this particular mutation (37a). These findings were confirmed in two Japanese families and additional Chinese sporadic cases (38). Subsequently, the same mutation was found in families and sporadic patients with aminoglycoside ototoxicity from Zaire the United States, Mongolia, Spain, South Africa, and Israel (39–44,61). Interestingly, in one streptomycin-induced deaf individual with a strong familial history of aminoglycoside-induced hearing loss and the mitochondrial 1555 mutation, detailed vestibular examination revealed severe hearing loss with completely normal vestibular function (37). This unexpected relative sparing of the vestibular system has recently been confirmed in Japanese patients (62).

Since the A1555G mutation in the mitochondrial 12S rRNA gene accounts only for 17–33% of patients with aminoglycoside ototoxicity, it is possible that other susceptibility mutations can be found in the same gene. DNA from 35 Chinese sporadic patients with aminoglycoside ototoxicity and without the A1555G mutation was analyzed for sequence variations in the 12S rRNA gene. Three sequence changes were found; only one of them, an absence of a thymidine at position 961 with varying numbers of cytosines inserted (ΔT961Cn), appeared likely to be a pathogenic mutation (63). Analysis of 34 similar U.S. patients of varying ethnic backgrounds did not reveal this mutation, but most recently we identified an Italian family with five maternally related members who all became deaf after aminoglycoside treatment, and were found to have the ΔT961Cn mutation (64). This sequence change was not found in 799 control individuals (63).

D. Mitochondrial Mutations and Presbycusis

Another condition associated with acquired heteroplasmic mutations and hearing loss is presbycusis. Presbycusis is the hearing loss that occurs with age in a significant proportion of individuals. Since mitochondrial DNA mutations, and the resulting loss of oxidative phosphorylation activity, seem to play an important role in the aging process (reviewed in Ref. 65), it is not unlikely that mitochondrial mutations in the auditory system can also lead to presbycusis. We recently examined the spiral ganglion and membranous labyrinth from archival temporal bones of five patients with presbycusis for mutations within the mitochondrially encoded cytochrome oxidase II gene

(66). When compared to controls, results indicated that at least a proportion of people with presbycusis have a significant load of mitochondrial DNA mutations in auditory tissue, and that there is great individual variability in both quantity and cellular location of these mutations. Similar data were obtained by Bai et al. when screening cochlear tissue from temporal bones for the presence of the 4977 bp deletion, although the ages of the presbycusis and control groups were not well matched (67). The greatest advantage of studying acquired mutations in the ear relates to the availability of temporal bone tissue banks, which have functional audiological data available, and thus allow correlation of measurable functional status, histology, immuno-histochemistry of oxidative phosphorylation complexes, and mitochondrial DNA analysis.

IV. CLINICAL RELEVANCE OF MITOCHONDRIAL MUTATIONS ASSOCIATED WITH HEARING IMPAIRMENT

The major clinical relevance of mitochondrial mutations to hearing loss remains the prevention of aminoglycoside-induced hearing loss. In countries where aminoglycosides are used commonly, aminoglycoside-induced oto-toxicity is a major cause of hearing loss. For example, in a study that reviewed all deaf-mutes in a district of Shanghai, 21.9% had aminoglyco-side-induced hearing loss, representing 167 individuals from a population of nearly half a million (59). The 1555 mutation accounted for at least 30% of these. In the United States the 1555 mutation accounts for about 15% of all aminoglycoside-induced deafness cases (40). The difference in frequency may reflect use of aminoglycosides in the United States more commonly for severe in-hospital infection. These patients receive significantly higher levels for more prolonged periods, and are more likely to have other medical conditions that exacerbate or cause the hearing loss. The frequency of the 961 predisposing mutation is unknown, but appears from our samples to be significantly lower. The frequency of these mutations in the general pop-ulation has not been established, but at least outside of Spain is probably in the less than 0.2% range.

Whatever the precise frequency, prevention of a major cause of ami-noglycoside-induced ototoxicity is now possible. Physicians need to inquire about a family history of aminoglycoside-induced hearing loss prior to the administration of systemic aminoglycosides, as well as prior to the local administration of aminoglycosides into the cochlea as treatment for Men-iere's disease. In addition, every individual with aminoglycoside-induced hearing loss should probably be screened at least for the presence of the mitochondrial 1555 and 961 mutations, since presence of a mutation will allow counseling to all maternally related relatives to avoid aminoglycosides. Similarly, the description by Estivill et al. (44) indicates that it might not be unreasonable to screen every individual with nonsyndromic hearing loss for the mutation, unless maternal inheritance can clearly be excluded. Since the test is easily done, and since prevention of hearing loss in maternal relatives can easily be accomplished, this may be cost-effective medical practice. The avoidable hearing loss in at least 40 patients in the report by Estivill et al. is a case in point.

With the exception of aminoglycosides and mitochondrial mutations in the 12S rRNA gene, there are no proven preventive or therapeutic interventions for mitochondrially related hearing impairments. The diagnosis of such defects is, however, useful for genetic counseling and is indicated in all families with an inheritance pattern of hearing loss consistent with maternal transmission, and possibly in all patients who have both diabetes mellitus and adult-onset hearing loss.

V. PATHOPHYSIOLOGY OF MITOCHONDRIAL DEAFNESS MUTATIONS

For aminoglycoside ototoxicity due to the A1555G mutation, it is interesting that this mutation lies exactly in the region of the gene for which the resistance mutations in yeast and *Tetrahymena* have been described, and in which aminoglycoside binding has been documented in bacteria (68–70). In addition, the mutation makes the mitochondrial RNA gene in this region more similar to the bacterial ribosomal RNA gene (36). Since aminoglycosides are concentrated within cochlear cells, and remain there for prolonged periods (71), we proposed that susceptible individuals with the 1555 mutation have increased binding to aminoglycosides leading to altered protein synthesis in the mitochondria (36), the tissue specificity being due to the concentration of the drug in those cells. Subsequent binding experiments have proven that increased binding to the mitochondrial 12S ribosomal RNA occurs (72). However, when examining lymphoblastoid cell lines of individuals with the 1555 mutation, exposure of the cell lines to high concentrations of neomycin or paromomycin led to a decreased rate of growth in glucose medium, but no mutant proteins were detected (73). Similar results of decreased protein synthesis but no mutant proteins were obtained in Japan using mitochondrial transfer from human skin fibroblast line with the 1555 mutation ρ0 HeLa cells exposed to very high levels of streptomycin (74). This may indicate that the effect of aminoglycosides in these cell lines could be nonspecific and be different than in the cochlea, perhaps because of different transport of the antibiotic into the mitochondria.

For nonsyndromic hearing loss, at first glance it is possible to speculate that mitochondrial mutations interfere with energy production, that the cochlea is highly dependent on sufficient energy production, and that insufficient energy production leads to degeneration of cochlear cells. However, the cochlea is not the most energy-dependent tissue in the body, and in the systemic neuromuscular disorders listed in Sec. III.A, the extraocular muscles appear to be the most energy-sensitive cells, and hearing loss is certainly not the most prominent clinical sign. Thus, to understand the pathophysiological pathways leading from the mitochondrial mutations to hearing loss, two major biological questions need to be answered: Why does the same mutation cause severe hearing loss in some family members but not in others, and why is the ear the only organ affected?

Study of the mitochondrial mutations leading to hearing loss has led to three possible precipitating factors modulating phenotypic expression, and it is likely that a combination of them play also a significant role in the phenotypic expression of acquired mitochondrial disorders. The first such factor involves environmental agents, and aminoglycosides are the prime example as a triggering event in the case of the 1555 mutation. It is not unlikely that other, as-yet-unrecognized, environmental factors could play similar, but perhaps less dramatic, roles. Diet and drugs affecting oxygen radical formation and breakdown come to mind. The second factor involves the mitochondrial haplotype, and, as noted above, the 7445 mutation provides a dramatic example of that effect. The third factor involves nuclear genes. The Arab-Israeli pedigree and some of the Spanish and Italian pedigrees are good examples of the role of nuclear genes. For example, the entire Arab-Israeli family lives in the similar environmental surroundings of a small Arab village in Israel, and all maternal relatives share the same mitochondrial haplotype.

Biochemical differences between lymphoblastoid cell lines of hearing and deaf family members with the identical mitochondrial chromosomes provide direct support for the role of nuclear factors (73). An extensive genome-wide search has led to the conclusion that this nuclear effect is unlikely to be due to the effect of a single nuclear locus but involves a number of modifier genes (75,76). The chromosomal location of one of these modifer genes has been identified, and linkage equilibrium has been obtained in families from varied ethnic backgrounds (76,77). Thus, the model that emerges for explaining penetrance is a threshold model, where a combination of environmental, mitochondrial, and nuclear factors can push a cell over a threshold, with dramatic clinical differences on either side of this threshold.

The second major biological question relates to tissue specificity: If a homoplasmic mutation affects oxidative phosphorylation (the only known function of the human mitochondrial chromosome and an essential process in every nucleated cell of the human body), it is unclear how the clinical defect remains confined to the cochlea, rather than affecting every tissue. We propose that cochlea-specific isoforms or splice variants involved in mitochondrial RNA processing or translation interact abnormally with the mutated rRNA, tRNA, or polycistronic mRNA, and lead to qualitative or quantitative changes in the protein products. Different processing of mitochondrial RNA and protein, leading to tissue-specific defects or functions, has been described: Several examples of tissue specificity in oxidative phosphorylation and of tissue-specific secondary functions of mitochondrial RNAs exist. Tissue-specific subunits for oxidative phosphorylation have been described (78). Even more relevant is the case report of a 22-year-old patient who died from respiratory failure due to a mitochondrial myopathy. It was shown that the causative mutation in the mitochondrial tRNA-Leu(UUR) gene caused a RNA-processing defect in skeletal muscle but not in the patient's fibroblasts (79), raising the possibility of a skeletal-muscle-specific mitochondrial RNA-processing gene. Examples of secondary function include the mitochondrial large ribosomal RNA gene in *Drosophila melanogaster*, which, in addition to being involved in mitochondrial translation, can in a few cells also be processed for export into the cytoplasm where it induces pole cell formation in embryos, a key event in the determination of the germ line (80). Similarly, in the mouse the ND1 protein can be processed in two different ways, part of it being presented on the cell membrane with a minor histocompatibility protein (81).

VI. EXPERIMENTAL APPROACHES TO ELUCIDATE THE PATHOPHYSIOLOGY OF MITOCHONDRIAL DEAFNESS MUTATIONS

The pathophysiological pathways of the mitochondrial deafness mutations in the inner ear, with the possible exception of aminoglycoside-induced ototoxicity, are not understood at this time. However, it can be hoped that the identification of the nuclear modifier genes will shed light on these pathways, and provide targets for prevention and therapy of the hearing impairment. Three complementary approaches have been taken to identify these modifier genes:

(1) The genetic approach: Taking advantage of families with maternally inherited hearing impairment, the goal will be to use positional cloning to initially identify the chromosomal locations of the modifier genes, and then identify the genes themselves. While a priori it was not clear whether

enough families have been identified to attempt such efforts for a complex genetic disease, the recent finding of linkage and linkage disequilibrium to a chromosomal region on chromosome 8 is very encouraging (76,77). Analysis of candidate genes in that region, and additional linkage analyses using the chromosome 8 locus as a stratification parameter, will eventually lead to the identification of the chromosome 8 modifier gene and the identification of additional chromosomal loci.

(2)   The candidate gene approach: The most likely candidates for being modifiers of the mitochondrial mutated gene are identified and screened for linkage disequilibrium in families and then for mutations. Two initial candidates, the ribosomal protein S12, which physically interacts with the 12S ribosomal RNA, and connexin 26, because of a suggestive linkage result, were screened in this manner and excluded as potential modifier genes (82). More recently we have started a concerted effort to identify all genes involved in mitochondrial RNA processing and translation. The reasons have been summarized (83), but in short are as follows: (a) all the mitochondrial mutations associated with nonsyndromic hearing loss involve ribosomal or transfer RNA (see Table 1); (b) biochemical analysis of the effect of these mutations demonstrates a RNA-processing defect or a decrease in translational efficiency (73,84–86); and (c) different processing of mitochondrial RNA and protein, leading to tissue-specific defects or functions, has been described (78–81). We have thus proposed that cochlea-specific subunits of mitochondrial ribosomes or RNA-processing proteins interact abnormally with the mitochondrial defect, leading to insufficient oxidative phosphorylation or loss of a secondary function in the cochlea. Similarly, allelic variations in some of these proteins may also be responsible for the penetrance differences observed between patients.

(3)   The mouse model approach: Recently the first mouse model of a naturally occurring pathogenic mitochondrial DNA mutation has been identified (87). In that model a mitochondrial DNA mutation in the *tRNA-Arg* gene worsens hearing impairment when combined with the nuclear-encoded *Ahl* gene locus on mouse chromosome 10, which has been described as a major gene for age-related hearing loss in mice (87,88). This mouse model provides a ready experimental model to dissect the complex genetic factors and interactions. It is likely that the pathways in mice and human are similar, and thus the human homologs of all nuclear genes and/or pathways identified in mice will become candidates for testing in humans.

VII.   SUMMARY

In conclusion, mitochondrial-related hearing loss can be caused by a variety of mutations, and can present in a variety of clinical forms with different degrees of severity. These mutations are not uncommon and, because of the susceptibility of individuals with the 1555 and 961 mutations and their maternal relatives to aminoglycosides, are important to diagnose. Despite the fact that these mostly homoplasmic mitochondrial mutations represent the simplest model of a mitochondrial DNA disease, it remains unclear how mitochondrial mutations lead to the clinically crucial features of penetrance and tissue specificity: Within the same family some individuals with the mutation can have profound hearing loss while others have completely normal hearing, and only the hearing is affected although all tissues have the mutation and are dependent on mitochondrial ATP production. Experimental approaches using genetic linkage studies in human families, candidate gene analysis, and spontaneous mouse models of mitochondrial hearing impairment may help in elucidating the pathophysiology between mitochondrial mutations and hearing loss, and eventually provide approaches to prevention and therapies.

ACKNOWLEDGMENTS

The author is supported by NIH/NIDCD grants RO1DC01402 and RO1DC04092.

REFERENCES

1. Attardi G, Schatz G. Biogenesis of mitochondria. Annu Rev Cell Biol 1988; 4:289–333.
2. Wallace DC. Diseases of the mitochondrial DNA. Annu Rev Biochem 1992; 61:1175–1212.
3. Howell N. Mitochondrial gene mutations and human diseases: a prolegomenon. Am J Hum Genet 1994; 55:219–224.
4. Fischel-Ghodsian N. Mitochondrial deafness mutations reviewed. Hum Mutat 1999; 13:261–270.
5. Schon EA, Bonilla E, DiMauro S. Mitochondrial DNA mutations and pathogenesis. J Bioenerg Biomembr 1997; 29:131–149.
6. Chomyn A. The myoclonic epilepsy and ragged-red fiber mutation provides new insights into human mitochondrial function and genetics. Am J Hum Genet 1998; 62:745–751.
7. Sue CM, Lipsett LJ, Crimmins DS, Tsang CS, Boyages SC, Presgrave CM, Gibson WP, Byrne E, Morris JG. Cochlear origin of hearing loss in MELAS syndrome. Ann Neurol 1998; 43:350–359.
8. Reardon W, Ross RJM, Sweeney MG, Luxon LM, Pembrey ME, Harding AE, Trembath RC. Diabetes mellitus associated with a pathogenic point mutation in mitochondrial DNA. Lancet 1992; 340:1376–1379.

9. van den Ouwel JMW, Lemkes HHPJ, Ruitenbeek W, Sandkuijil LA, De Vijlder MF, Struyvenberg PAA, van de Kamp JJP, Massen JA. Mutation in mitochondrial tRNALeu(UUR) gene in a large pedigree with maternally transmitted type II diabetes mellitus and deafness. Nat Genet 1992; 1:368–371.

10. Ballinger SW, Shoffner JM, Hedaya EV, Trounce I, Polak MA, Koontz DA, Wallace DC. Maternally transmitted diabetes and deafness associated with a 10.4 kb mitochondrial deletion. Nat Genet 1992; 1:11–15.

11. Vialettes BH, Paquis-Flucklinger V, Pelissier JF, Bendahan D, Narbonne H, Silvestre-Aillaud P, Montfort MF, Righini-Chossegros M, Pouget J, Cozzone PJ, Desnuelle C. Phenotypic expression of diabetes secondary to a T14709C mutation of mitochondrial DNA: comparison with MIDD syndrome (A3243G mutation): a case report. Diabetes Care 1997; 20:1731–1737.

12. Kameoka K, Isotani H, Tanaka K, Azukari K, Fujimura Y, Shiota Y, Sasaki E, Majima M, Furukawa K, Haginomori S, Kitaoka H, Ohsawa N. Novel mitochondrial DNA mutation in tRNA(Lys) (8296A– > G) associated with diabetes. Biochem Biophys Res Commun 1998; 245:523–527.

13. Oka Y, Katagiri H, Yazaki Y, Murase T, Kobayashi T. Mitochondrial gene mutation in islet-cell-antibody-positive patients who were initially non-insulin-dependent diabetics. Lancet 1993; 342:527–528.

14. Alcolado JC, Majid A, Brockington M, Sweeney MG, Morgan R, Rees, Harding AE, Barnett AH. Mitochondrial gene defects in patients with NIDDM. Diabetologia 1994; 37:372–376.

15. Kadowaki T, Kadowaki H, Mori Y, Tobe K, Sakuta R, Suzuki Y, Tanabe Y, Sakura H, Awata T, Goto Y-I, Hayakawa T, Matsuota K, Kawamori R, Kamada T, Horai S, Nonaka I, Hagura R, Akanuma Y, Yazaki Y. A subtype of diabetes mellitus associated with a mutation of mitochondrial DNA. N Engl J Med 1994; 330:962–968.

16. Katagiri H, Asano T, Ishihara H, Inukai K, Anai M, Yamanouchi T, Tsukuda K, Kikuchi M, Kitaoka H, Ohsawa N, Yazaki Y, Oka Y. Mitochondrial diabetes mellitus: prevalence and clinical characterization of diabetes due to mitochondrial tRNA[Leu(UUR)] gene mutation in Japanese patients. Diabetologia 1994; 37:504–510.

17. Sepehrnia B, Prezant TR, Rotter JI, Pettitt DJ, Knowler WC, Fischel-Ghodsian N. Screening for mtDNA diabetes mutations in Pima Indians with NIDDM. Am J Med Genet 1995; 56:198–202.

18. Newkirk JE, Taylor RW, Howell N, Bindoff LA, Chinnery PF, Alberti KG, Turnbull DM, Walker M. Maternally inherited diabetes and deafness: prevalence in a hospital diabetic population. Diabetes Med 1997; 14:457–460.

19. Rigoli L, Di Benedetto A, Romano G, Corica F, Cucinotta D. Mitochondrial DNA [tRNA(Leu)(UUR)] in a southern Italian diabetic population [letter]. Diabetes Care 1997; 20:674–675.

20. Guillausseau PJ, Massin P, Dubois-LaForgue D, Timsit J, Virally M, Gin H, et al. Maternally inherited diabetes and deafness: a multicenter study. Ann Intern Med 2001; 134:721–728.

21. Harrison TJ, Boles RG, Johnson DR, LeBlond C, Wong LJ. Macular pattern

retinal dystrophy, adult-onset diabetes, and deafness: a family study of A3243G mutation mitochondrial heteroplasmy. Am J Ophthalmol 1997; 124: 217–221.

22. Nicolino M, Ferlin T, Forest M, Godinot C, Carrier H, David M, Chatelain P, Mousson B. Identification of a large scale mitochondrial DNA deletion in endocrinopathies and deafness: report of two unrelated cases with diabetes mellitus and adrenal insufficiency, respectively. J Clin Endocrinol Metab 1997; 82:3063–3067.

23. Souied EH, Sales MJ, Soubrane G, Coscas G, Bigorie B, Kaplan J, Munnich A, Rotig A. Macular dystrophy, diabetes, and deafness associated with a large mitochondrial DNA deletion. Am J Opthalmol 1998; 125:100–103.

24. Cremers CWRJ, Wijdeveld PGAB, Pinckers AJLG. Juvenile diabetes mellitus, optic atrophy, hearing loss, diabetes insipidus, atonia of the urinary tract and bladder and other abnormalities (Wolfram syndrome): a review of 88 cases from the literature with personal observations on 3 new patients. Acta Paediatr Scand 1977; 264(suppl):1–16.

25. Rotig A, Cormier V, Chatelain P. Deletion of mitochondrial DNA in a case of early-onset diabetes mellitus, optic atrophy, and deafness (Wolfram syndrome, MIM 222300). J Clin Invest 1993; 91:1095–1098.

26. Bu X, Rotter JI. Wolfram syndrome: a mitochondrial-mediated disorder? Lancet 1993; 342:598–600.

27. Reid FM, Vernham GA, Jacobs HT. A novel mitochondrial point mutation in a maternal pedigree with sensorineural deafness. Hum Mutat 1994; 3:243–247.

28. Fischel-Ghodsian N, Prezant TR, Fournier P, Stewart IA, Maw M. Mitochondrial tRNA mutation associated with non-syndromic deafness. Am J Otolaryngol 1995; 16:403–408.

29. Sevior KB, Hatamochi A, Stewart IA, Bykhovskaya Y, Allen-Powell DR, Fischel-Ghodsian N, Maw M. Mitochondrial A7445G mutation in two pedigrees with palmoplantar keratoderma and deafness. Am J Med Genet 1998; 75:179–185.

30. Tiranti V, Chariot P, Carella F, Toscano A, Soliveri P, Girlanda P, Carrara F, Fratta GM, Reid FM, Mariotti C, Zeviani M. Maternally inherited hearing loss, ataxia and myoclonus associated with a novel point mutation in mitochondrial tRNASer(UCN) gene. Hum Mol Genet 1995; 4:1421–1427.

31. Shoffner JM. Oxidative phosphorylation disease diagnosis. Semin Neurol 1999; 19:341–351.

32. Nye JS, Hayes EA, Amendola M, Vaughn D, Charrow J, McLone DG, Speer MC, Nance WE, Pandya A. Myelocystocele-cloacal exstrophy in a pedigree with a mitochondrial 12S rRNA mutation, aminoglycoside-induced deafness, pigmentary disturbances, and spinal anomalies. Teratology 2000; 61:165–171.

33. Santorelli FM, Tanji K, Manta P, Casali C, Krishna S, Hays AP, Mancini DM, DiMauro S, Hirano M. Maternally inherited cardiomyopathy: an atypical presentation of the mtDNA 12S rRNA gene A1555G mutation. Am J Hum Genet 1999; 64:295–300.

34. Hutchin TP, Thompson KR, Read AP, Mueller RF. Identification of a novel

mtDNA mutation in the tRNAthr gene in a family with hearing impairment and cutaneous hypopigmentation with an albinoid appearance. The Molecular Biology of Hearing and Deafness. Bethesda, MD, Oct. 4–7, 2001.

35. Jaber L, Shohat M, Bu X, Fischel-Ghodsian N, Yang HY, Wang SJ, Rotter JI. Sensorineural deafness inherited as a tissue specific mitochondrial disorder. J Med Genet 1992; 29:86–90.

36. Prezant TR, Agapian JV, Bohlman MC, Bu X, Oztas S, Qiu WQ, Arnos KS, Cortopassi GA, Jaber L, Rotter JI, Shohat M, Fischel-Ghodsian N. Mitochondrial ribosomal RNA mutation associated with both antibiotic-induced and non-syndromic deafness. Nat Genet 1993; 4:289–294.

37. Braverman I, Jaber L, Levi H, Adelman C, Arnos KS, Fischel-Ghodsian N, Shohat M, Elidan J. Audio-vestibular findings in patients with deafness caused by a mitochondrial susceptibility mutation and precipitated by an inherited nuclear mutation or aminoglycosides. Arch Otolaryngol Head Neck Surg 1996; 122:1001–1004.

37a. Fischel-Ghodsian N, Prezant TR, Bu X, Öztas S. Mitochondrial ribosomal RNA gene mutation associated with aminoglycoside ototoxicity. Am J Otolaryngol 1993; 14:399–403.

38. Hutchin T, Haworth I, Higashi K, Fischel-Ghodsian N, Stoneking M, Saha N, Arnos C, Cortopassi G. A molecular basis for human hypersensitivity to aminoglycoside antibiotics. Nucleic Acids Res 1993; 21:4174–4179.

39. Matthijs G, Claes S, Longo-Mbenza B, Cassiman J-J. Non-syndromic deafness associated with a mutation and a polymorphism in the mitochondrial 12S ribosomal RNA gene in a large Zairean pedigree. Eur J Hum Genet 1996; 4: 46–51.

40. Fischel-Ghodsian N, Prezant TR, Chaltraw W, Wendt KA, Nelson RA, Arnos KS, Falk RE. Mitochondrial gene mutations: a common predisposing factor in aminoglycoside ototoxicity. Am J Otolaryngol 1997; 18:173–178.

41. Pandya A, Xia X, Radnaabazar J, Batsuuri J, Dangaansuren B, Odgerel D, Fischel-Ghodsian N, Nance WE. Mutation in the mitochondrial 12S rRNA gene in two families from Mongolia with matrilineal aminoglycoside ototoxicity. J Med Genet 1997; 34:169–172.

42. Gardner JC, Goliath R, Viljoen D, Sellars S, Cortopassi G, Hutchin T, Greenberg J, Beighton P. Familial streptomycin ototoxicity in a South African family: a mitochondrial disorder. J Med Genet 1997; 34:904–906.

43. El-Schahawi M, deMunain L, Sarrazin AM, Shanske AL, Basirico M, Shanske S, DiMauro S. Two large Spanish pedigrees with non-syndromic sensorineural deafness and the mtDNA mutation at nt 1555 in the 12SrRNA gene: evidence of heteroplasmy. Neurology 1997; 48:453–456.

44. Estivill X, Govea N, Barcelo A, Perello E, Badenas C, Romero E, Moral L, Scozzari R, D'Urbano L, Zeviani M, Torroni A. Familial progressive sensorineural deafness is mainly due to the mtDNA A1555G mutation and is enhanced by treatment with aminoglycosides. Am J Hum Genet 1998; 62: 27–35.

45. Torroni A, Cruciani F, Sellitto D, Lopez-Bigas N, Rabionet R, Govea N, Loped De Munain A, Sarduy M, Romero L, et al. The A1555G mutation in the 12S rRNA gene of human mtDNA: recurrent origins and founder events in

families affected by sensorineural deafness. Am J Hum Genet 1999; 65:1349–1358.

46. Pandya A, Erdenetungalag R, Xia X, Welch KO, Radnaabazar J, Dangaa-suren B, Arnos KS, Nance WE. The role and frequency of mitochondrial mutations in two distinct populations: the USA and Mongolia. The Molecular Biology of Hearing and Deafness. Bethesda, MD, Oct. 4–7, 2001.

47. Usami S, Kasai AS, Shinkawa H, Moeller B, Kenyon JB, Kimberling WJ. Genetic and clinical features of sensorineural hearing loss associated with the 1555 mitochondrial mutation. Laryngoscope 1997; 107:483–490.

48. Casano RAMS, Bykhovskaya Y, Johnson DF, Torricelli F, Bigozzi M, Fischel-Ghodsian N. Hearing loss due to the mitochondrial A1555G mutation in Italian families. Am J Med Genet 1998; 79:388–391.

49. Feldmann D, Marlin S, Chapiro E, Denoyelle F, Sternberg D, Weil D, Petit C, Garabedian EN, Couderc R. Prevalence of mitochondrial mutations in familial sensorineural hearing impairment: importance of A1555G and T7511C. Am J Hum Genet 2001; 69(suppl):A2122.

50. Mingroni-Netto RC, Abreu-Silva RS, Braga MCC, Lezirovitz K, Della-Rosa VA, Pirana S, Spinelli M, Otto PA. Mitochondrial mutation A1555G (12SrRNA) and connexin 26 35delG mutation are frequent causes of deafness in Brazil. Am J Hum Genet 2001; 69(suppl):A2124.

51. Reid FM, Vernham GA, Jacobs HT. Complete mtDNA sequence of a patient in a maternal pedigree with sensorineural deafness. Hum Mol Genet 1994b; 3:1435–1436.

52. Verhoeven K, Ensink RJH, Tiranti V, Huygen P, Johnson DF, Schatteman I, Van Laer L, Verstreken M, Van de Heyning P, Fischel-Ghodsian N, Zeviani M, Cremers CWRJ, Willems PJ, Van Camp G. Different penetrance of neurological symptoms associated with a mutation in the mitochondrial tRNASer (UCN) gene. Eur J Hum Genet 1999; 7:45–51.

53. Friedman RA, Bykhovskaya Y, Bradley R, Fallis-Cunningham R, Paradies N, Smith RJ, Grodin J, Pensak ML, Fischel-Ghodsian N. Maternal in-herited deafness due to a novel genetic defect. Am J Med Genet 1999; 84:369–372.

54. Sue CM, Tanji K, Hadjigeorgiou G, Andreu AL, Nishino I, Krishna S, Bruno C, Hirano M, Shanske S, Bonilla E, Fischel-Ghodsian N, DiMauro S, Friedman R. Maternally inherited hearing loss in a large kindred with a novel T7511C mutation in the mitochondrial DNA tRNASer(UCN) gene. Neurol-ogy 1999; 52:1905–1908.

55. Ishikawa K, Tamagawa Y, Takahashi K, Kimura H, Saito K, Ichimura K. Hereditary hearing loss in a Japanese family with a T7511C mutation in the mitochondrial tRNAser(UCN) gene. The Molecular Biology of Hearing and Deafness. Bethesda, MD, Oct. 4–7, 2001.

56. Hutchin TP, Parker MJ, Young ID, Davis A, Mueller RF. Mitochondrial DNA mutations in the tRNASer(UCN) gene causing maternally inherited hearing impairment. J Med Genet 2000; 37:692–694.

57. Konigsmark BW, Gorlin RJ. Genetic and Metabolic Deafness. Philadelphia: W.B. Saunders Co, 1976:364–365.

58. Higashi K. Unique inheritance of streptomycin-induced deafness. Clin Genet 1989; 35:433–436.
59. Hu D-N, Qui W-Q, Wu B-T, Fang L-Z, Gu Y-P, Zhang Q-H, Yan J-H, Dingm Y-Q, Wong H. Genetic aspects of antibiotic induced deafness: mitochondrial inheritance. J Med Genet 1991; 28:79–83.
60. Stebbins WC, McGinn CS, Feitosa AG. Animal models in the study of ototoxic hearing loss. In: Lerner SA, Matz GL, Hawkins JE, eds: Aminoglycoside Ototoxicity. Boston: Little, Brown & Co., 1981:5–25.
61. Shohat M, Fischel-Ghodsian N, Legum C, Halpern GJ. Aminoglycoside induced deafness in an Israeli Jewish family with a mitochondrial ribosomal RNA gene mutation. Am J Otolaryngol 1999; 20:64–67.
62. Tono T, Kiyomizu K, Matsuda K, Komune S, Usami S, Abe S, Shinkawa H. Different clinical characteristics of aminoglycoside-induced profound deafness with and without the 1555 A→G mitochondrial mutation. J Oto-Rhino-Laryngol Related Spec 2001; 63:25–30.
63. Bacino CM, Prezant TR, Bu X, Fournier P, Fischel-Ghodsian N. Susceptibility mutations in the mitochondrial small ribosomal RNA gene in aminoglycoside induced deafness. Pharmacogenetics 1995; 5:165–172.
64. Casano RAMS, Johnson DF, Hamon M, Bykhovskaya Y, Torricelli F, Bigozzi M, Fischel-Ghodsian N. Inherited susceptibility to aminoglycoside ototoxicity: genetic heterogeneity and clinical implications. Am J Otolaryngol 1999; 20:151–156.
65. Nagley P, Zhang C, Martinus RD, Vaillant F, Linnane AW. Mitochondrial DNA mutations and human aging: molecular biology, bioenergetics, and redox therapy. In: DiMauro S, Wallace DC, eds. Mitochondrial DNA in Human Pathology. New York: Raven Press, 1993.
66. Fischel-Ghodsian N, Bykhovskaya Y, Taylor K, Kahen T, Cantor R, Ehrenman K, Smith R, Keithley E. Temporal bone analysis of patients with presbycusis reveals high frequency of mitochondrial mutations. Hearing Res 1997; 110:147–154.
67. Bai U, Seidman MD, Hinojosa R, Quirk WS. Mitochondrial DNA deletions associated with aging and possibly presbycusis: a human archival temporal bone study. Am J Otol 1997; 18:449–453.
68. Li M, Tzagaloff A, Underbrink-Lyon K, Martin NC. Identification of the paramomycin-resistance mutation in the 15S rRNA gene of yeast mitochondria. J Biol Chem 1982; 257:5921–5928.
69. Spangler EA, Blackburn EH. The nucleotide sequence of the 17S ribosomal RNA gene of *Tetrahymena thermophila* and the identification of point mutations resulting in resistance to the antibiotics paromomycin and hygromycin. J Biol Chem 1985; 260:6334–6340.
70. Gravel M, Melancon P, Brakier-Gingras L. Cross-linking of streptomycin to the 16S ribosomal RNA of *Escherichia coli*. Biochemistry 1987; 26:6227–6232.
71. Henley CM, Schacht J. Pharmacokinetics of aminoglycoside antibiotics in blood, inner-ear fluids and tissues and their relationship to ototoxicity. Audiology 1988; 27:137–146.

72. Hamasaki K, Rando RR. Specific binding of aminoglycosides to a human rRNA construct based on a DNA polymorphism which causes aminoglycoside-induced deafness. Biochemistry 1997; 36:12323–12328.

73. Guan M, Fischel-Ghodsian N, Attardi G. Biochemical evidence for nuclear gene involvement in phenotype of non-syndromic deafness associated with mitochondrial 12S rRNA mutation. Hum Mol Genet 1996; 5:963–972.

74. Inoue K, Takai D, Soejima A, Isobe K, Yamasoba T, Oka Y, Goto Y, Hayashi J. Mutant mtDNA at 1555 A to G in the 12S rRNA gene and hypersusceptibility of mitochondrial translation to streptomycin can be co-transferred to ρ^0 HeLa cells. Biochem Biophys Res Commun 1996; 223:496–501.

75. Bykhovskaya Y, Shohat M, Ehrenman K, Johnson DF, Hamon M, Cantor R, Aouizerat B, Bu X, Rotter JI, Jaber L, Fischel-Ghodsian N. Evidence for complex nuclear inheritance in a pedigree with non-syndromic deafness due to a homoplasmic mitochondrial mutation. Am J Med Genet 1998; 77: 421–426.

76. Bykhovskaya Y, Estivill X, Taylor K, Hang T, Hamon M, Casano RAMS, Yang H, Rotter JI, Shohat M, Fischel-Ghodsian N. Candidate locus for a nuclear modifier gene for maternally inherited deafness. Am J Hum Genet 2000; 66:1905–1910.

77. Bykhovskaya Y, Yang H, Taylor K, Hang T, Tun RYM, Estivill X, Casano RAMS, Majamaa K, Shohat M, Fischel-Ghodsian N. Modifier locus for mitochondrial DNA disease: linkage and linkage disequilibrium mapping of a nuclear modifier gene for maternally inherited deafness. Genet Med 2001; 3: 177–180.

78. Arnaudo E, Hirano M, Seelan RS, Milatovich A, Hsieh C, Fabriscke GM, Grossman LI, Francke U, Schon EA. Tissue-specific expression and chromosome assignment of genes specifying two isoforms of subunit VIIa of human cytochrome c oxidase. Gene 1992; 119:299–305.

79. Bindoff LA, Howell N, Poulton J, McCullough DA, Morten KI, Lightowlers RN, Turnbull DM, Weber K. Abnormal RNA processing associated with a novel tRNA mutation in mitochondrial DNA. J Biol Chem 1993; 268:19559–19564.

80. Kobayashi S, Amikura R, Okada M. Presence of mitochondrial large ribosomal RNA outside mitochondria in germ plasm of *Drosophila melanogaster*. Science 1993; 260:1521–1524.

81. Wang CR, Loveland BE, Fischer-Lindahl K. H-2M3 encodes the MHC class I molecule presenting the maternally transmitted antigen of the mouse. Cell 1991; 66:335–345.

82. Johnson DF, Hamon M, Fischel-Ghodsian N. Cloning and characterization of the human mitochondrial ribosomal S12 gene. Genomics 1998; 52:363–368.

83. Fischel-Ghodsian N. Mitochondrial RNA processing and translation—link between mitochondrial mutations and hearing loss? Mol Genet Metab 1998; 65:97–104.

84. Guan M, Enriquez JA, Fischel-Ghodsian N, Puranam RS, Lin C, Maw M, Attardi G. Deafness-associated mtDNA 7445 mutation has pleiotropic effects,

affecting tRNASer(UCN) precursor processing and expression of NADH dehydrogenase ND6 subunit gene. Mol Cell Biol 1998; 18:5868–5879.

85. Guan M-X, Attardi G, Fischel-Ghodsian N. A biochemical basis for the inherited susceptibility to aminoglycoside ototoxicity. Hum Mol Genet 2000; 9: 1787–1793.

86. Guan M-X, Fischel-Ghodsian N, Attardi G. Transmitochondrial cell lines carrying the deafness-associated mitochondrial 12S rRNA mutation reveal a determinant role of nuclear background in the biochemical phenotype. Hum Mol Genet 2001; 10:573–580.

87. Johnson KR, Zheng QY, Bykhovskaya Y, Spirina O, Fischel-Ghodsian N. A nuclear-mitochondrial DNA interaction affecting hearing impairment in mice. Nat Genet 2001; 27:191–194.

88. Johnson KR, Zheng QY, Erway LC. A major gene on chromosome 10 affecting age-related hearing loss is common to at least ten inbred strains of mice. Genomics 2000; 70:171–180.

13

Gene Localization and Isolation in Nonsyndromic Hearing Loss

Patrick J. Willems
GENDIA, Antwerp, Belgium

I. GENE LOCALIZATION AND ISOLATION

Until 1992 not a single nuclear locus for nonsyndromic hearing loss (HL) had been mapped on the human genome. It is remarkable how long the genetic dissection of a very common genetic disorder such as HL lagged behind that of other sensory handicaps such as blindness. There are several explanations for this. In the first place, scientists and clinicians have always been attracted to study organs with clinically visible and/or pathologically identifiable defects such as presented by the eye. Many eye disorders can be identified by simple inspection, and classified into a large spectrum of specific defects of specific parts of the eye caused by specific genetic diseases. The cochlea, however, is still not much more than a black box with only one phenotype, hearing loss. Furthermore, owing to the inaccessibility of the auditory system, pathological studies of human HL still are scarce, and insights into the pathogenic pathways leading to HL are still based for the major part upon studies of mouse models with HL. As key proteins involved in normal hearing and HL have only been identified in the last decade, the cloning of genes implicated in human HL by *functional genetics* has been precluded for a long time. Also the *positional cloning* of HL genes lagged behind that of other disease genes.

Until 10 years ago it was generally assumed that mapping genes through linkage analysis was hardly possible in the case of HL. This assumption was based on the fact that the genetic community initially focused on prelingual HL in Western countries, as this type of HL is congenital and severe, thereby leading to deaf-mutism and social isolation in many Western countries. As prelingual HL usually has an autosomal recessive mode of inheritance, most Western pedigrees contain only a limited number of affected family members. Furthermore, the linkage data from different families cannot be combined in view of the large genetic heterogeneity of nonsyndromic HL, with involvement of many genes. As the linkage power of such single one-generation pedigrees was too small to localize genes by conventional linkage analysis, hardly any recessive gene has been mapped in Western pedigrees. Another complicating factor in the localization of recessive HL loci in the Western world was the assortative mating in the deaf community, which often introduces different mutant genes into a single family, thereby hampering linkage analysis. However, ethnic isolates in developing countries turned out to be a reservoir of consanguineous multiplex families with autosomal recessive HL present in many family members owing to the frequent inbreeding in these countries. Another advantage of these ethnic isolates was the nearly absent assortative mating, together with the limited living area of these families with extended pedigrees living together in a small area, providing easy access to a large number of affected family members. Most autosomal recessive forms of HL have therefore been mapped in ethnic isolates.

Another assumption precluding linkage analysis in HL was the idea that most monogenetic HL constitutes prelingual HL, which in most cases shows autosomal recessive inheritance with the above-mentioned limitations for linkage analysis. Only in the 1990s was it recognized that many individuals with monogenic HL have a postlingual progressive type of HL, with in most cases autosomal dominant inheritance. Multiplex pedigrees with many affected family members with autosomal dominant HL turned out to be very frequent, providing enough linkage power for gene localization and isolation. This was instrumental in the localization of many forms of dominant HL. In 1992 the localization of the first autosomal dominant form of postlingual HL in an extended family from Costa Rica (1) marked the start of an impressive international effort to hunt down the genes implicated in nonsyndromic HL.

Within the last 10 years more than 60 loci and more than 25 genes have been implicated in nonsyndromic HL (2–9). This impressive catchup in the genetic dissection of nonsyndromic HL is unparalleled in genetics. Several factors have contributed to this success. First, the human genome process has paved the way for gene localization and isolation for any given disease. In the 1980s gene localization still was painstaking owing to the paucity of highly polymorphic markers with a known position on the human genome, and the technological constraints whereby each of the markers had to be labeled radioactively and analyzed separately. Consequently, gene localization by genome screening took many months, if successful at all. Today any disease for which sufficient linkage power is found, can be mapped on the genome in a few weeks owing to the availability of extended sets of highly informative microsatellite markers covering the whole genome, and improved technology using automated analysis of fluorescence-labeled marker sets. Other favoring factors were the development of cochlea-specific cDNA libraries that represent an excellent reservoir of candidate genes for HL (10), together with the availability of murine models for HL (11).

Finally, the setup of an international collaborative effort with many ear, nose, and throat specialists and clinical geneticists rendered impetus to the identification of genes implicated in nonsyndromic HL.

II. LOCI FOR NONSYNDROMIC HEARING LOSS

More than 65 nuclear loci for nonsyndromic HL have been mapped on the human genome. These loci have been classified as DFN (DeaFNess) followed by a number indicating the chronological order of identification

Table 1 Autosomal Dominant Loci and Genes for Nonsyndromic HL[a]

Locus	Location	Gene	Locus	Location	Gene
DFNA1	5q31	*DIAPH1*	DFNA19	10	
DFNA2	1p34	*KCNQ4*	DFNA20	17q25	
		GJB3			
DFNA3	13q12	*GJB2*	DFNA22	6q13	*MYO6*
		GJB6			
DFNA4	19q13		DFNA23	14q21-22	
DFNA5	7p15	*ICERE1*	DFNA24	4q	
DFNA6/14/38	4p16	*WFS1*	DFNA25	12q21-24	
DFNA7	1q21–23		DFNA26	17q25	
DFNA8/12	11q22–24	*TECTA*	DFNA27	4q12	
DFNA9	14q12–13	*COCH*	DFNA28	8q22	
DFNA10	6q22–23	*EYA4*	DFNA30	15q26	
DFNA11	11q12–21	*MYO7A*	DFNA32	11p15	
DFNA13	6p21	*COL11A2*	DFNA34	1q44	
DFNA15	5q31	*POU4F3*	DFNA36	9q13-21	*TMC1*
DFNA16	2q24		DFNA37	1p21	
DFNA17	22q	*MYH9*	DFNA41	12q24-ter	
DFNA18	3q22				

[a] Only loci and genes published until June 2002 are included. DFNA loci not listed here represent reserved or withdrawn loci, or loci shown to be involved in syndromic HL.

Table 2 Autosomal Recessive Loci and Genes for Nonsyndromic HL[a]

Locus	Location	Gene	Locus	Location	Gene
DFNB1	13q12	*GJB2*	DFNB18	11p14-15	*USH1C*
		GJB6			
DFNB2	11q13	*MYO7A*	DFNB19	18p11	
DFNB3	17p11	*MYO15*	DFNB20	11q25-ter	
DFNB4	7q31	*SLC26A4*	DFNB21	11q	*TECTA*
DFNB5	14q12		DFNB22	16p12	*OTOA*
DFNB6	3p14-21		DFNB23	10p11-q21	
DFNB7/11	9q13-21	*TMC1*	DFNB24	11q23	
DFNB8/10	21q22	*TMPRSS3*	DFNB25	4p15-q12	
DFNB9	2p22-23	*OTOF*	DFNB26	4q31	
DFNB12	10q21-22	*CDH23*	DFNB27	2q23-31	
DFNB13	7q34-36		DFNB28	22q13	
DFNB14	7q31		DFNB29	21q22	*CLDN14*
DFNB15	3q21-25		DFNB30	10p	*MYO3A*
	or 19p13				
DFNB16	15q21-22	*STRC*	DFNB31	9q32-34	
DFNB17	7q31		DFNB33	9q34	

[a] Only loci and genes published until June 2002 are included. DFNB loci not listed here represent reserved or withdrawn loci, or loci shown to be involved in syndromic HL.

of the locus. DFNA is used for autosomal dominant loci, DFNB for autosomal recessive loci, and DFN for X-linked loci. Up to June 2002, 31 DFNA loci (Table 1), 30 DFNB loci (Table 2), and four DFN loci (Table 3) had been published, with many more in press. The loci and genes are also cataloged on-line (9). All of these loci have been mapped by positional genetics using conventional linkage analysis.

Table 3 X-Linked Recessive Loci and Genes for Nonsyndromic HL[a]

Locus	Location	Gene
DFN2	Xq22	
DFN3	Xq21	*POU3F4*
DFN4	Xp21	
DFN6	Xp22	

[a] Only loci and genes published until June 2002 are included. DFN loci not listed here represent reserved or withdrawn loci, or loci shown to be involved in syndromic HL.

Table 4 Genes Involved in Nonsyndromic HL

Protein	Gene	Nonsyndromic HL	Additional phenotype
Cytoskeletal proteins			
Myosin VI	*MYO6*	DFNA22	
Myosin VIIA	*MYO7A*	DFNA11–DFNB2	Usher 1B
Myosin XV	*MYO15*	DFNB3	
Myosin heavy chain 9	*MYH 9*	DFNA17	Fechtner/May-Hegglin
Myosin IIIA	*MYO3A*	DFNB30	
Diaphanous	*DIAPH1*	DFNA1	
Structural proteins			
Alpha tectorin	*TECTA*	DFNA8/12–DFNB21	
Stereocilin	*STRC*	DFNAB16	
Collagen type 11	*COL11A2*	DFNA13	OSMED
Otoancorin	*OTOA*	DFNB22	
Transcription factors			
POU3F4	*POU3F4*	DFN3	
POU4F3	*POU4F3*	DFNA15	
EYA4	*EYA4*	DFNA10	
Ion transport proteins			
Connexin 26	*GJB2*	DFNA3–DFNB1	Vohlwinkel/PPD[a]
Connexin 30	*GJB6*	DFNA3	
Connexin 31	*GJB3*	DFNA2	Erythrokeratodermia
Connexin 43	*GJA1*		
Pendrin	*SLC26A4*	DFNB4	Pendred
KCNQ4	*KCNQ4*	DFNA2	
TMC1	*TMC1*	DFNA36–DFNB7/B11	
Claudin 14	*CLDN14*	DFNB29	
Unknown function			
Icere	*DFNA5*	DFNA5	
Cochlin	*COCH*	DFNA9	
Otoferlin	*OTOF*	DFNB9	
CDH23	*CDH23*	DFNB12	Usher 1D
TMPRSS3	*TMPRSS3*	DFNB8/B10	
Wolframin	*WFS1*	DFNA6/A14/A38	Wolfram
Harmonin	*USH1C*	DFNB18	Usher 1C

[a] PPD: palmoplantar keratodermia.

III. GENES FOR NONSYNDROMIC HEARING LOSS

The first nuclear gene involved in nonsyndromic HL was identified in 1995 as *POU3F4*. Two more genes, myosin 7A and connexin 26, were isolated in 1997. In the last 5 years an impressive list of 25 additional genes have been identified, bringing the total of nonsyndromic HL genes to 28 in June 2002.

The spectrum of genes (Table 4) includes cytoskeletal proteins, such as diaphanous and the myosins 3A, 6, 7A, 15 and myosin heavy chain 9; structural proteins of the organ of Corti, such as alpha tectorin, stereocilin, *COL11A2* en otoancorin; transcription factors, such as *POU3F4*, *POU4F3*, and *EYA4*; ion transport and channel proteins such as connexins 26, 30, 31, and 43, pendrin, *KCNQ4*, *TMC1*, and claudin 14; and proteins of unknown function such as icere, cochlin, otoferlin, wolframin, *CDH23*, *USH1C*, and *TMPRSS3*. The largest groups of homologous genes are the myosins and the connexins (each four genes). Apart from the nuclear genes, mutations in mitochondrial genes (*12S rRNA* and *tRNA-ser*) have also been found to be associated with nonsyndromic HL.

Some of the HL genes, including *MYO7A*, *MYH9*, *COL11A2*, *GJB2*, *GJB3*, *SLC26A4*, *WFS1*, *CDH23*, and *tRNA-ser*, are responsible for both nonsyndromic and syndromic HL. Most of these genes are involved in only a limited number of pedigrees up to now, with the exception of *GJA2* (connexin 26), *KCNQ4*, *SLC26A4*, *COCH*, *POU3F4*, and *12S rRNA*. Connexin 26 mutations are among the most frequent mutations in the human genome, being present in 1–4% of most Caucasian individuals, and representing almost half of all autosomal recessive deafness.

REFERENCES

1. Leon PE, Raventos H, Lynch E, Morrow J, King MC. The gene for an inherited form of deafness maps to chromosome 5q31. Proc Natl Acad Sci USA 1992; 89:5181–5184.
2. Tekin M, Arnos KS, Pandya A. Advances in hereditary deafness [Review]. Lancet 2001; 358:1082–1090.
3. Resendes BL, Williamson RE, Morton CC. At the speed of sound: gene discovery in the auditory system [Review]. Am J Hum Genet 2001; 69:923–935.
4. Steel KP, Kros CJ. A genetic approach to understanding auditory function [Review]. Nat Genet 2001; 27:143–149.
5. Willems PJ. Genetic causes of hearing loss. N Engl J Med 2000; 342:1101–1109.
6. Van Camp G, Willems PJ, Smith RJ. Nonsyndromic hearing impairment: unparalleled heterogeneity [Review]. Am J Hum Genet 1997; 60:758–764.
7. Kalatzis V, Petit C. The fundamental and medical impacts of recent progress in research on hereditary hearing loss [Review]. Hum Mol Genet 1998; 7:1589–1597.

8. Morton CC. Genetics, genomics and gene discovery in the auditory system. Hum Mol Genet 2002; 11:1229–1240.

9. www.uia.ac.be/dnalab/hhh/

10. Skvorak AB, Weng Z, Yee AJ, Robertson NG, Morton CC. Human cochlear expressed sequence tags provide insight into cochlear gene expression and identify candidate genes for deafness. Hum Mol Genet 1999; 8:439–452.

11. Steel KP. Inherited hearing defects in mice [Review]. Annu Rev Genet 1995; 29:675–701.

14
Connexins

Paolo Gasparini
Second University of Naples and Telethon Institute of Genetics and Medicine, Naples, Italy

I. INTRODUCTION

Connexins are a large family of proteins involved in formation of gap junctions that allow the direct transfer of small molecules and ions between neighboring cells (1). Transmission at gap junction synapses is very fast allowing the production of almost instantaneously acting potentials. Gap junctions are rare between mammalian neurons, but are common in nonneural cells, such as glia, epithelial cells, and smooth and cardiac muscle cells. Three groups of connexins exist, named alpha, beta, and non-alpha–non-beta, as shown in Figure 1. Each connexin is identified by a number directly related to its molecular weight. Connexins form hexameric hemichannels (termed "connexons") in the endoplasmic reticulum, which are then translocated into the plasma membrane. The connexon then "docks" with a connexon of an adjacent cell to form a functional channel termed a "gap junction." Connexons can form either homotypic, heterotypic, or heteromeric channels. Connexins are expressed in many different tissues, including skin and inner ear. In the epidermis, gap junctions appear to play a role in the coordination of keratinocyte growth and differentiation (2), whereas several arguments support the idea that gap junctions have an important role in auditory transduction. The auditory organ has gap junctions between the outer hair cells and supporting cells (including melanocytes), providing a morphological basis for the occurrence of intracellular responses to sound in supporting cells and for electric coupling of receptor cells. The endothelium of the scala media of the cochlea is involved in the production of a receptor response to the auditory stimulus and is separated

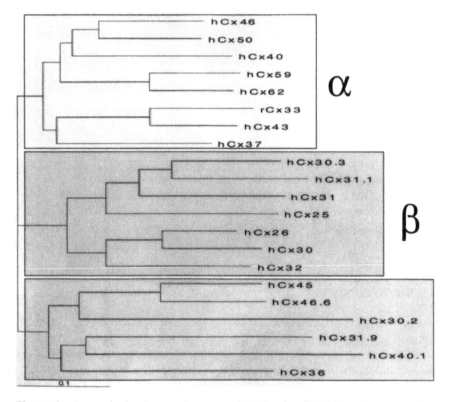

Figure 1 Connexin family tree (courtesy of D. Condorelli). Schematic representation of connexin family tree with division into alpha, beta, and non-alpha–non-beta groups.

from the endolymphatic space by tight junctions in the marginal cell layer, which is coupled to gap junctions. Immunohistochemical and ultrastructural analysis of some members of this protein family (connexin 26) in the rat cochlea showed that gap junctions in both epithelial and connective tissue cells are involved in recycling endolymphatic potassium ions (3).

The identification of mutations in several connexin genes in patients with sensorineural hearing loss definitively confirmed the involvement of gap junctions in the endocochlear potential of audition. Mutations in the gap junction genes encoding the connexins have also been shown to cause epidermal disease and peripheral neuropathy (4, 5; Connexin-Deafness Homepage at http://www.iro.es/deafness/).

II. CONNEXINS AND NONSYNDROMIC AUTOSOMAL RECESSIVE DEAFNESS (NSRD)

Approximately 80% of cases of congenital deafness are inherited in an autosomal recessive fashion or are apparently sporadic (2). Despite the fact that more than 30 loci have been described for nonsyndromic autosomal recessive deafness (DFNB) (see Hereditary Hearing Loss Homepage at http://dnalab-www.uia.ac.be/dnalab/hhh/), a single locus, DFNB1 (MIM 220290), accounts for a high proportion of the cases, with variability depending on the population. The gene involved in this type of deafness is *GJB2*, which encodes the gap junction protein connexin 26 (Cx26).

DFNB1 was mapped to 13q12 in two consanguineous Tunisian families (6) and further confirmed by linkage in large series of patients (7,8). In 1997, two independent studies demonstrated the role of the *GJB2* gene in this type of deafness. In the first study, two nonsense mutations were found in three families from Pakistan linked to DFNB1 (9). In the second study, 35 Mediterranean families with autosomal recessive NSHL were used to refine the DFNB1 interval to 5 cM between markers D13S175 and D13S232, which contains the *GJB2* gene. The following mutational search of the *GJB2* coding region in these families showed that 19 of 35 patients were homozygous for a specific deletion, named 35delG (10). Hearing-impaired individuals from another family were found to be compound heterozygotes for 35delG and another deletion named 167delT. Both sequence variants produce a frameshift in the *GJB2* mRNA, leading to a premature truncated protein and loss of function. The above-mentioned deletions show a worldwide distribution that can be dependent on the ethnic background.

The 35delG mutation appears to be more frequent in Caucasians of European origin (10–16), being particularly frequent in South European countries (12). Conversely, 35delG mutation was absent in patients and controls of Japanese origin (17–19). Since 35delG is located within a stretch of G, a mutational hot spot was hypothesized; however, the fluctuation in carrier status of 35delG in normal-hearing populations from different ethnic groups (1 in 35 in southern Europe and 1 in 79 in northern Europe) suggests a possible founder effect and positive selection for 35delG heterozygote status (20,21).

Mutation 167delT, originally reported in 2.3% of GJB2 mutant alleles of Mediterranean origin (10), was then found to be very common in Ashkenazi Jews. The presence of a conserved haplotype suggests a founder event for its origin (22–24). Several additional mutations have been identified so far in the *GJB2* gene (25). Figure 2 reports the localization of CX26 missense mutations, which are scattered along the protein apart from the

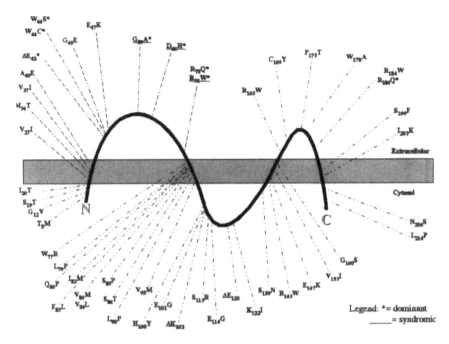

Figure 2 Distribution of missense mutations along CX26 gene and protein. Mutations detected in autosomal dominant forms as well as those identified in syndromic cases of hearing loss are clearly identified.

few dominant and syndromic mutations (see below), which are clustered in a specific domain. The density along GJB2 protein of missense mutation (a), of frameshift mutations (b), and of nonsense mutations (c) is graphically shown in Figure 3a, b, and c. While missense mutations are, more or less, distributed with an equal density along the protein, frameshift mutations are clustered in two major areas and nonsense mutations are more frequent in the first half of the gene itself.

Among *GJB2* mutations it is worthwhile to annotate mutation 235delC, which has been detected only in individuals of Japanese origin (17–19). An updated list of all mutations detected in *GJB2* is also available at the Connexin-Deafness Homepage, while a schematic representation of their localization along GJB2 protein is shown in Figure 2.

The audiological phenotype observed in individuals with *GJB2* mutations is variable, depending largely on the type of the mutation present in each affected patient. Usually, the onset is during early childhood and in most cases hearing loss is present at birth (congenital). In our experience patients homozygous for the 35delG mutation are characterized by a severe to profound bilateral sensorineural hearing loss (12). This finding has been also reported by other researchers (13,26,27), and in a few cases progression of the sensory deficit in some 35delG homozygotes has also been observed (28). Patients heterozygous compound for 35delG and missense mutation or compound for other mutations present in the mayority of cases with a progressive hearing loss of mild to severe degree. In patients homozygous for 167delT mutation, a trend in the variability of the degree of hearing loss was also evident (23). The variability of the degree of hearing loss can be explained either by a different functional role of each mutated allele and its possible residual activity or by the possible presence of environmental and genetic factors.

After *GJB3* (see below) had been found to be associated with autosomal dominant deafness, 25 Chinese families with autosomal recessive NSRD were screened for *GJB3* mutations. Two unrelated families were identified with

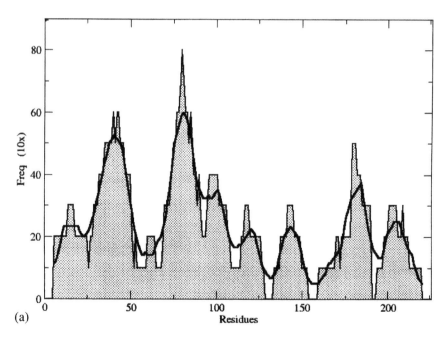

(a)

Figure 3 Graphic distribution of the density of *GJB2* missense (a), frameshift (b), and nonsense (c) mutations along the protein. The Y scale is 10×. The residue window is 12 amino acids; thus a value of 60 means the presence of six different mutations in a portion of 12 residues. (Courtesy of S. Volinia.)

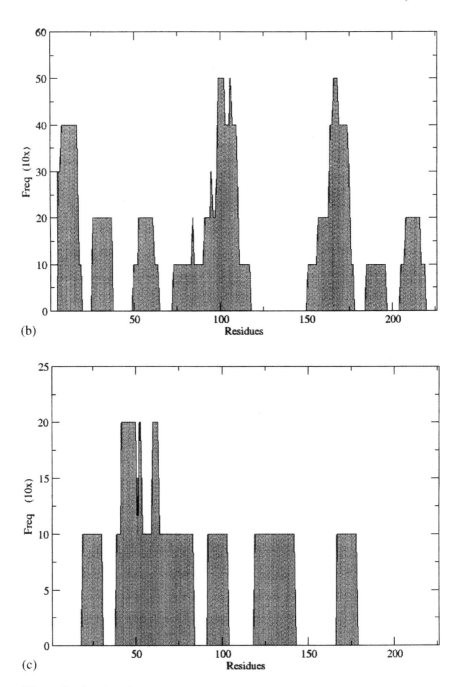

Figure 3 Continued.

compound heterozygous *GJB3* mutations, indicating that, like *GJB2,* recessive *GJB3* mutations are also associated with NSRD (29).

Finally, mutations in connexin 43 (*GJA1*), a member of the connexin family expressed in cochlear tissues, have recently been identified in African American deaf patients. Four patients of 26 were homozygous for a missense mutation, named L11F, while another one was homozygous for a V24A mutation. These data suggest a possible major role of this gene in black people (30).

The recent identification of a recessive mutation in *GJB6* and the possible presence of digenic inheritance is described in the following section.

III. CONNEXINS AND NONSYNDROMIC AUTOSOMAL DOMINANT DEAFNESS (NSAD)

About 40 loci have been described for nonsyndromic autosomal dominant deafness (DFNB) (see Hereditary Hearing Loss Homepage at http://dnalab-www.uia.ac.be/dnalab/hhh/), and 16 different genes have been identified so far. Three of them belong to the connexin family.

Few *GJB2* mutations have been described as causing dominant deafness (9,31; Connexin-Deafness Homepage). *M34T* has been found in heterozygosity in a family with a few affected subjects (9), but also in normal subjects (13,15,32) and in a recessive family (13). It is believed that *M34T* is a dominant mutation with reduced penetrance, and functional studies performed on some mutations by expression in *Xenopus laevis* oocytes showed that *M34T* had a dominant negative effect, whereas the recesive mutation W77R did not (33). W44C was identified as the cause of deafness in several families with nonsyndromic autosomic dominant deafness (31). The localization of dominant mutations within *GJB2* is shown in Figure 2. These mutations are clustered in the first extracellular domain of the protein.

Mutation analysis of the *GJB3* (*CX31*) gene, mapping at 1p33–p35, revealed that a missense mutation and a nonsense mutation were associated with high-frequency hearing loss in two families. Moreover, expression of *Gjb3* was identified in rat inner ear tissue by RT-PCR, further confirming that mutations in *GJB3* may be responsible for bilateral high-frequency hearing impairment (34).

Grifa et al. (35) cloned the human connexin 30 (*GJB6*) gene, localized it in the same YAC contig of *GJB2* on 13q11, and showed expression of *GJB6* in the mouse cochlea. Analysis of deaf patients led to the identification of a missense mutation in a family with dominant hearing impairment, although with phenotypic variation. The authors have demonstrated by studies in *Xenopus laevis* that the *GJB6* T5M mutation has a dominant negative effect

(35). Moreover, a deletion encompassing exon 1 of *GJB6* that is the cause of deafness in seven patients from four families carrying another recessive mutation in the *GJB2* gene in trans was recently identified (36). Recently a 342-kb deletion in *GJB6* was identified (37). The deletion extended distally to *GJB2*, which remained intact. Twenty-two of the 33 subjects were heterozygous for both the *GJB6* and *GJB2* mutations. Two subjects were homozygous for this new *GJB6* mutation. This deletion is the second most frequent mutation causing prelingual deafness in the Spanish population. These findings suggest that mutations in the complex locus DFNB1, which contains two genes (*GJB2* and *GJB6*), can result in a monogenic or a digenic pattern of inheritance of prelingual deafness (37).

IV. CONNEXINS AND OTHER DISEASES WITH OR WITHOUT HEARING LOSS

Connexins have been found to be mutated in several other diseases. In most of the cases mutated connexins depending on their tissue expression pattern, led to skin diseases with or without hearing loss. In particular, mutations in four connexins have been demonstrated in epidermal disorders. In three of these connexins, certain mutations may also result in syndromic or nonsyndromic sensorineural hearing loss. In addition to skin disorders, peripheral neuropathies may be the result of connexin mutations.

A. Erythrokeratodermas

Erythrokeratodermas represent a group of disorders characterized by the presence of fixed or slowly moving erythematous hyperkeratotic plaques (38). Erythrokeratoderma variabilis [EKV (MIM 133200)] is an autosomal dominant disorder presenting with diffuse palmoplantar keratoderma and transient red figurata at other epidermal sites. The erythematous patches affect the whole body but are more often found on the face, buttocks, and extensor surfaces of the limbs. With increasing age, the areas of the body affected by EKV become more restricted to the palmoplantar epidermis. In a number of families EKV is linked to the chromosomal region 1p34–p35, where a gene cluster of connexins map (39–41). Subsequently, mutations in affected members from a number of these pedigrees were identified in the gap junction -3 gene [*GJB3* (MIM 603324)] encoding connexin 31 (42). Five *GJB3* mutations causing EKV have been described throughout the Cx31 protein, occurring in the intracellular, extracellular, and transmembrane domains (43,44). Although EKV in all families described to date is linked to the chromosomal region 1p34–1p35, not all have mutations in *GJB3*.

Recently, a missense mutation in *GJB4*, encoding for the epidermally ex-pressed Cx30.3 and mapping to 1p34–35, was identified in the affected mem-bers of a family with EKV (44). The mutated residue (F137L) lies in the third transmembrane domain of the protein. The same missense mutation has also been demonstrated in *GJB3* in another individual with EKV (45). Additional families with EKV that have Cx30.3 mutations have then been identified.

B. Hidrotic Ectodermal Dysplasia

Hidrotic ectodermal dysplasia (HED), or Clouston syndrome (MIM 129500), is inherited as an autosomal dominant disorder characterized by changes in the epidermis and the appendages, including diffuse palmoplantar kerato-derma, nail dystrophy, and sparse scalp and body hair. In addition, hearing impairment of variable degree is also observed in some cases. A first locus for HED was mapped to the long arm of chromosome 13 (q11–q12) in a large kindred of French Canadian descent (46). Successively, the presence of genetic heterogeneity was demonstrated (47–49). Recently, in a study of a group of families affected by HED, the presence of mutations (G11R or A88V) in *GJB6* encoding Cx30 and mapping at HED locus has been dem-onstrated (50).

C. Vohwinkel Syndrome

Vohwinkel syndrome (MIM 124500) is an autosomal dominant condition classified as a "mutilating" diffuse keratoderma in which hyperkeratosis may develop around the circumference of the digits at points of flexion, such as the knuckle. These may form constrictions (or pseudoainhum) sometimes leading to autoamputation of the digit. Another classic epidermal feature is a honeycomb pattern of keratoderma with starfish-like keratoses on the knuckles. Mild to moderate sensorineural hearing loss is often associated with the skin disease. A specific missense mutation, named D66H, in the Cx26 gene (*GJB2*), causes Vohwinkel syndrome (51,52). In one of these families the Vohwinkel pattern of keratoderma was of a mild form and as-sociated with varying types of hearing impairment. Two D66H-heterozy-gous individuals with the keratoderma in this family were also profoundly deaf and had previously been shown to be heterozygous for another Cx26 variant, M34T (9). Mutation R75W has been described in two members of an Egyptian family affected by a skin disease similar to Vohwinkel syn-drome (53). Additional individuals carrying the R75W mutation have been identified presenting with a variable phenotype (54) including a variable degree of severity of the palmoplantar keratoderma. This finding (also noted among D66H heterozygotes) may be explained by the presence of other genetic or environmental factors that may modify the disease penetrance.

D. Autosomal Dominant Palmoplantar Keratoderma and High-Frequency Hearing Loss

Autosomal dominant palmoplantar keratoderma and high-frequency hearing loss (MIM 148350) is characterized by a diffuse palmoplantar hyperkeratosis and high-tone hearing loss. In a family affected by this disease a missense *GJB2* mutation named G59A was identified (55). A heterozygous 3-bp deletion of the residue E42 (E42) has also been associated with deafness and palmoplantar keratoderma (56). As shown in Figure 2, GJB2 mutations leading either to Vohwinkel syndrome or to autosomal dominant palmoplantar keratoderma and high-frequency hearing loss are clustered in the first extracellular domain. This location is the same as that for mutations leading to autosomal dominant deafness alone. Thus, it would be interesting to further investigate why similar mutations located in the same domain of the protein lead to different clinical phenotype with or without skin involvement.

E. Peripheral Neuropathy

The identification of a dominant *GJB3* mutation, named 66delD, in a family with peripheral neuropathy and sensorineural hearing loss (57) increases to three the number of disorders resulting from *GJB3* mutations. The amino residue at position 66 is highly conserved across species and most likely plays a functionally important role also in other connexins. As previously reported, the mutation D66H in *GJB2* causes Vohwinkel syndrome (51), whereas 66delD in the gene for another connexin, *GJB1* encoding Cx32, results in the peripheral neuropathy disorder X-linked Charcot-Marie-Tooth disease. Some additional Cx32 mutations are also associated with hearing loss in combination with peripheral neuropathy (58).

V. CONCLUSION

Most of the genes for the most common syndromic forms of hearing loss have already been identified as well as some for nonsyndromic forms, including the gene underlying the most common form of NSRD. Among them, connexins play a major role as a number of genes belonging to this family are involved in hearing loss and they have implications in terms of early molecular diagnosis, genetic counseling, and possible prevention. A simple DNA test can now be provided in NSRD cases to ascertain whether or not one is a carrier of a common mutated allele within the *GJB2* gene, making risk calculations and genetic counseling more accurate. The identification of specific mutations within connexin genes leading either to hearing impairment and/or a skin disease has further confirmed the importance of gap junction intercellular communication in both the epidermis and the inner ear. Moreover, it has revealed unexpected genotype-phenotype correlations that need further investigation. To really understand why some mutations in the same connexin protein cause skin disease whereas others cause hearing impairment, functional studies of these mutants in affected tissues and normal tissues are required. In this way, it would be possible, for example, to understand why recessive mutations in Cx26, which has a wide tissue distribution, cause only hearing loss, suggesting that, in other tissues, other connexins can compensate for loss of the Cx26 protein. Studies of the role of the different connexins in the inner ear will also be greatly facilitated by the development of animal models, which should be useful not only for studying pathophysiology but also for the development of new therapeutic strategies including gene therapy. So far, the only published connexin knockout mice are those for Cx26, which, because of placental failure, result in embryonic lethality at day 9.5 (59). This phenotype is different from that observed in humans, in which recessive protein-truncating *GJB2* mutations are associated with hearing impairment. Recently, a conditional CX26 and a CX30 knockout mouse model have been reported to the scientific community, but not yet published. The availability of these two new mouse models will give researchers new insights into the function of *GJB2* and *GJB6*, thus assisting the understanding of pathogenetic mechanisms leading to hearing loss and/ or skin involvement and of gap junction biology.

REFERENCES

1. Pitts JD. The discovery of metabolic co-operation. Bioessays 1998; 20:1047–1051.
2. Choudhry R, Pitts JD, Hodgins MB. Changing patterns of gap junctional intercellular communication and connexin distribution in mouse epidermis and hair follicles during embryonic development. Dev Dyn 1997; 210:417–430.
3. Kikuchi T, Kimura RS, Paul DL, Adams JC. Gap junctions in the rat cochlea: immunohistochemical and ultrastructural analysis. Anat Embryol 1995; 191:101–118.
4. White TW, Paul DL. Genetic diseases and gene knockouts reveal diverse connexin functions. Annu Rev Physiol 1999; 61:283–310.
5. Rabionet R, Gasparini P, Estivill X. Molecular genetics of hearing impairment due to mutations in gap junction genes encoding beta connexins. Hum Mutat 2000; 16:190–202.

6. Guilford P, Ayadi H, Blanchard S, Chaïb H, Le Paslier D, Weissenbach J, Petit C. A human gene responsible for neurosensory, non-syndromic recessive deafness is a candidate homologue of the mouse *sh-1* gene. Hum Mol Genet 1994; 3:989–993.

7. Maw MA, Allen-Powell DR, Goodey RJ, Stewart IA, Nancarrow DJ, Hayward NK, Gardner RJ. The contribution of the DFNB1 locus to neurosensory deafness in a Caucasian population. Am J Hum Genet 1995; 57:629–635.

8. Gasparini P, Estivill X, Volpini V, Totaro A, Castellvi-Bel S, Govea N, Mila M, Della Monica M, Ventruto V, De Benedetto M, Stanziale P, Zelante L, Mansfield ES, Sandkuijl L, Surrey S, Fortina P. Linkage of DFNB1 to non-syndromic neurosensory autosomal-recessive deafness in Mediterranean families. Eur J Hum Genet 1997; 5:83–88.

9. Kelsell DP, Dunlop J, Stevens HP, Lench NJ, Liang JN, Parry G, Mueller RF, Leigh IM. Connexin 26 mutations in hereditary non-syndromic sensorineural deafness. Nature 1997; 387:80–83.

10. Zelante L, Gasparini P, Estivill X, Melchionda S, D'Agruma L, Govea N, Mila M, Monica MD, Lutfi J, Shohat M, Mansfield E, Delgrosso K, Rappaport E, Surrey S, Fortina P. Connexin26 mutations associated with the most common form of non-syndromic neurosensory autosomal recessive deafness (DFNB1) in Mediterraneans. Hum Mol Genet 1997; 6:1605–1609.

11. Denoyelle F, Weil D, Maw MA, Wilcox SA, Lench NJ, Allen-Powell DR, Osborn AH, Dahl HH, Middleton A, Houseman MJ, Dode C, Marlin S, Boulila-ElGaied A, Grati M, Ayadi H, BenArab S, Bitoun P, Lina-Granade G, Godet J, Mustapha M, Loiselet J, El-Zir E, Aubois A, Joannard A, Petit C. Prelingual deafness: high prevalence of a 30delG mutation in the connexin 26 gene. Hum Mol Genet 1997; 6:2173–2177.

12. Estivill X, Fortina P, Surrey S, Rabionet R, Melchionda S, D'Agruma L, Mansfield E, Rappaport E, Govea N, Mila M, Zelante L, Gasparini P. Connexin-26 mutations in sporadic and inherited sensorineural deafness. Lancet 1998; 351:394–398.

13. Kelley PM, Harris DJ, Comer BC, Askew JW, Fowler T, Smith SD, Kimberling WJ. Novel mutations in the connexin 26 gene (*GJB2*) that cause autosomal recessive (DFNB1) hearing loss. Am J Hum Genet 1998; 62:792–799.

14. Lench N, Houseman M, Newton V, Van Camp G, Mueller R. Connexin-26 mutations in sporadic non-syndromal sensorineural deafness. Lancet 1998; 351: 415.

15. Scott DA, Kraft ML, Carmi R, Ramesh A, Elbedour K, Yairi Y, Srisailapathy CR, Rosengren SS, Markham AF, Mueller RF, Lench NJ, Van Camp G, Smith RJ, Sheffield VC. Identification of mutations in the connexin 26 gene that cause autosomal recessive nonsyndromic hearing loss. Hum Mutat 1998; 11: 387–394.

16. Lucotte G, Mercier G. Meta-analysis of GJB2 mutation 35delG frequencies in Europe. Genet Test 2001; 5:149–152.

17. Fuse Y, Doi K, Hasegawa T, Sugii A, Hibino H, Kubo T. Three novel connexin26 gene mutations in autosomal recessive non-syndromic deafness. Neuroreport 1999; 10:1853–1857.

18. Abe S, Usami S, Shinkawa H, Kelley PM, Kimberling WJ. Prevalent connexin 26 gene (*GJB2*) mutations in Japanese. J Med Genet 2000; 37:41–43.
19. Kudo T, Ikeda K, Kure S, Matsubara Y, Oshima T, Watanabe K, Kawase T, Narisawa K, Takasaka T. Novel mutations in the connexin 26 gene (*GJB2*) responsible for childhood deafness in the Japanese population. Am J Med Genet 2000; 90:141–145.
20. Gasparini P, Rabionet R, Barbujani G, Melchionda S, Petersen M, Brondum-Nielsen K, Metspalu A, Oitmaa E, Pisano M, Fortina P, Zelante L, Estivill X. High carrier frequency of the 35delG deafness mutation in European populations. Genetic Analysis Consortium of *GJB2* 35delG. Eur J Hum Genet 2000; 8:19–23.
21. Van Laer L, Coucke P, Mueller RF, Caethoven G, Flothmann K, Prasad SD, Chamberlin GP, Houseman M, Taylor GR, Van de Heyning CM, Fransen E, Rowland J, Cucci RA, Smith RJ, Van Camp G. A common founder for the 35delG *GJB2* gene mutation in connexin 26 hearing impairment. J Med Genet 2001; 38:515–518.
22. Morell RJ, Kim HJ, Hood LJ, Goforth L, Friderici K, Fisher R, Van Camp G, Berlin CI, Oddoux C, Ostrer H, Keats B, Friedman TB. Mutations in the connexin 26 gene (*GJB2*) among Ashkenazi Jews with nonsyndromic recessive deafness. N Engl J Med 1998; 339:1500–1555.
23. Lerer I, Sagi M, Malamud E, Levi H, Raas-Rothschild A, Abeliovich D. Contribution of connexin 26 mutations to nonsyndromic deafness in Ashkenazi patients and the variable phenotypic effect of the mutation 167delT. Am J Med Genet 2000; 95:53–56.
24. Sobe T, Vreugde S, Shahin H, Berlin M, Davis N, Kanaan M, Yaron Y, Orr-Urtreger A, Frydman M, Shohat M, Avraham KB. The prevalence and expression of inherited connexin 26 mutations associated with nonsyndromic hearing loss in the Israeli population. Hum Genet 2000; 106:50–57.
25. Rabionet R, Zelante L, Lopez-Bigas N, D'Agruma L, Melchionda S, Restagno G, Arbones ML, Gasparini P, Estivill X. Molecular basis of childhood deafness resulting from mutations in the *GJB2* (connexin 26) gene. Hum Genet 2000; 106:40–44.
26. Denoyelle F, Marlin S, Weil D, Moatti L, Chauvin P, Garabedian EN, Petit C. Clinical features of the prevalent form of childhood deafness, DFNB1, due to a connexin-26 gene defect: implications for genetic counselling. Lancet 1999; 353:1298–1303.
27. Murgia A, Orzan E, Polli R, Martella M, Vinanzi C, Leonardi E, Arslan E, Zacchello F. Cx26 deafness: mutation analysis and clinical variability. J Med Genet 1999; 36:829–832.
28. Cohn ES, Kelley PM, Fowler TW, Gorga MP, Lefkowitz DM, Kuehn HJ, Schaefer GB, Gobar LS, Hahn FJ, Harris DJ, Kimberling WJ. Clinical studies of families with hearing loss attributable to mutations in the connexin 26 gene. Pediatrics 1999; 103:546–550.
29. Liu XZ, Xia XJ, Xu LR, Pandya A, Liang CY, Blanton SH, Brown SD, Steel KP, Nance WE. Mutations in connexin31 underlie recessive as well as dominant non-syndromic hearing loss. Hum Mol Genet 2000; 9:63–67.

30. Liu XZ, Xia XJ, Adams J, Chen ZY, Welch KO, Tekin M, Ouyang XM, Kristiansen A, Pandya A, Balkany T, Arnos KS, Nance WE. Mutations in *GJA1* (connexin 43) are associated with non-syndromic autosomal recessive deafness. Hum Mol Genet 2001; 10:2945–2951.

31. Denoyelle F, Lina-Granade G, Plauchu H, Bruzzone R, Chaib H, Levi-Acobas F, Weil D, Petit C. Connexin 26 gene linked to a dominant deafness. Nature 1998; 393:319–320.

32. Scott DA, Kraft ML, Stone EM, Sheffield VC, Smith RJ. Connexin mutations and hearing loss. Nature 1998; 391:32.

33. Xia JH, Liu CY, Tang BS, Pan Q, Huang L, Dai HP, Zhang BR, Xie W, Hu DX, Zheng D, Shi XL, Wang DA, Xia K, Yu KP, Liao XD, Feng Y, Yang YF, Xiao JY, Xie DH, Huang JZ. Mutations in the gene encoding gap junction protein beta-3 associated with autosomal dominant hearing impairment. Nat Genet 1998; 20:370–373.

34. White TW, Deans MR, Kelsell DP, Paul DL. Connexin mutations in deafness. Nature 1998; 394:630–631.

35. Grifa A, Wagner CA, D'Ambrosio L, Melchionda S, Bernardi F, Lopez-Bigas N, Rabionet R, Arbones M, Monica MD, Estivill X, Zelante L, Lang F, Gasparini P. Mutations in *GJB6* cause nonsyndromic autosomal dominant deafness at DFNA3 locus. Nat Genet 1999; 23:16–18.

36. Lerer I, Sagi M, Ben-Neriah Z, Wang T, Levi H, Abeliovich D. A deletion mutation in *GJB6* cooperating with a *GJB2* mutation in trans in non-syndromic deafness: a novel founder mutation in Ashkenazi Jews. Hum Mutat 2001; 18:460.

37. del Castillo I, Villamar M, Moreno-Pelayo MA, del Castillo FJ, Alvarez A, Telleria D, Menendez I, Moreno F. A deletion involving the connexin 30 gene in nonsyndromic hearing impairment. N Engl J Med 2002; 346:243–249.

38. Rook A, Wilkinson D, Ebling F, Champion R, Burton J. Textbook of Dermatology. 6th ed. London: Blackwell Scientific, 1998.

39. van der Schroeff JG, Nijenhuis LE, Meera Khan P, Bernini LF, Schreuder GMT, van Loghem E, Volkers WS, Went LN. Genetic linkage between erythrokeratrodermia variabilis and Rh locus. Hum Genet 1984; 68:165–168.

40. van der Schroeff JG, van Leeuwen-Cornelisse I, van Haeringen A, Went LN. Further evidence for localisation of the gene of erythrokeratodermia variabilis. Hum Genet 1988; 80:97–98.

41. Richard G, Lin JP, Smith L, Ehyte YM, Itin P, Wollina U, Epstein EJ, Hohl D, Giroux JM, Charnas L, Bale SJ, DiGiovanna JJ. Linkage studies in erythrokeratodermias: fine mapping, genetic heterogeneity and analysis of candidate genes. J Invest Dermatol 1997; 109:666–671.

42. Richard G, Smith LE, Bailey RA, Itin P, Hohl D, Epstein EH, DiGiovanna JJ, Compton JG, Bale SJ. Mutations in the human connexin gene *GJB3* cause erythrokeratodermia variabilis. Nat Genet 1998; 20:366–369.

43. Wilgoss A, Leigh IM, Barnes MR, Dopping-Hepenstal P, Eady RA, Walter JM, Kennedy CT, Kelsell DP. Identification of a novel mutation R42P in the gap junction protein beta-3 associated with autosomal dominant erythrokeratoderma variabilis. J Invest Dermatol 1999; 113:1119–1122.

44. Richard G, Brown N, Smith LE, Terrinoni A, Melino G, Mackie RM, Bale SJ, Uitto J. The spectrum of mutations in erythrokeratodermias-novel and de novo mutations in *GJB3*. Hum Genet 2000; 106:321–329.

45. Macari F, Landau M, Cousin P, Mevorah B, Brenner S, Panizzon R, Schorderet DF, Hohl D, Huber M. Mutation in the gene for connexin 30.3 in a family with erythrokeratodermia variabilis. Am J Hum Genet 2000; 67:1296–1301.

46. Kibar Z, Der Kaloustian VM, Brais B, Hani V, Fraser FC, Rouleau GA. The gene responsible for Clouston hidrotic ectodermal dysplasia maps to the pericentromeric region of chromosome 13q. Hum Mol Genet 1996; 5:543–547.

47. Radhakrishna U, Blouin JL, Mehenni H, Mehta TY, Sheth FJ, Sheth JJ, Solanki JV, Antonarakis SE. The gene for autosomal dominant hidrotic ectodermal dysplasia (Clouston syndrome) in a large Indian family maps to the 13q11–q12.1 pericentromeric region. Am J Med Genet 1997; 71:80–86.

48. Taylor TD, Hayflick SJ, McKinnon W, Guttmacher AE, Hovnanian A, Litt M, Zonana J. Confirmation of linkage of Clouston syndrome (hidrotic ectodermal dysplasia) to 13q11–q12.1 with evidence for multiple independent mutations. J Invest Dermatol 1998; 111:83–85.

49. Stevens HP, Choon SE, Hennies HC, Kelsell DP. Evidence for a single genetic locus in Clouston's hidrotic ectodermal dysplasia. Br J Dermatol 1999; 140: 963–964.

50. Lamartine J, Munhoz Essenfelder G, Kibar Z, Lanneluc I, Callouet E, Laoudj D, Lemaitre G, Hand C, Hayflick SJ, Zonana J, Antonarakis S, Radhakrishna U, Kelsell DP, Christianson AL, Pitaval A, Der Kaloustian V, Fraser C, Blanchet-Bardon C, Rouleau GA, Waksman G. Mutations in *GJB6* cause hidrotic ectodermal dysplasia. Nat Genet 2000; 26:142–144.

51. Maestrini E, Korge BP, Ocaña-Sierra J, Calzolari E, Cambiaghi S, Scudder P, Hovnanian A, Monaco A, Munro C. A missense mutation in connexin26, D66H, causes mutilating keratoderma with sensorineural deafness (Vohwinkel's syndrome) in three unrelated families. Hum Mol Genet 1999; 8:1237–1243.

52. Kelsell DP, Wilgoss AL, Richard G, Stevens HP, Munro CS, Leigh IM. Connexin mutations associated with palmoplantar keratoderma and profound deafness in a single family. Eur J Hum Genet 2000; 8:141–144.

53. Richard G, White TW, Smith LE, Bailey RA, Compton JG, Paul DL, Bale SJ. Functional defects of Cx26 resulting from a heterozygous missense mutation in a family with dominant deaf-mutism and palmoplantar keratoderma. Hum Genet 1998; 103:393–399.

54. Loffeld A, Kelsell DP, Moss C. Palmoplantar keratoderma and sensorineural deafness in an 8-year-old boy: a case report. Br J Dermatol 2000; 143:38.

55. Heathcote K, Syrris P, Carter ND, Patton MA. A connexin 26 mutation causes a syndrome of sensorineural hearing loss and palmoplantar hyperkeratosis (MIM 148350). J Med Genet 2000; 37:50–51.

56. Bale SJ, White TW, Munro C, Taylor AEM, Richard G. Functional defects of Cx26 due to mutations in two families with dominant palmoplantar keratoderma and deafness. J Invest Dermatol 1999; 112:A550.

57. Lopez-Bigas N, Olive M, Rabionet R, Ben-David O, Martinez-Matos JA,

Bravo O, Banchs I, Volpini V, Gasparini P, Avraham KB, Ferrer I, Arbones ML, Estivill X. Connexin 31 (*GJB3*) is expressed in the peripheral and auditory nerves and causes neuropathy and hearing impairment. Hum Mol Genet 2001; 10:947–952.

58. Young P, Grote K, Kuhlenbaumer G, Debus O, Kurlemann H, Halfter H, Funke H, Ringelstein EB, Stogbauer F. Mutation analysis in Chariot-Marie-Tooth disease type 1: point mutations in the MPZ gene and the *GJB1* gene cause comparable phenotypic heterogeneity. J Neurol 2001; 248:410–415.

59. Gabriel HD, Jung D, Butzler C, Temme A, Traub O, Winterhager E, Willecke K. Transplacental uptake of glucose is decreased in embryonic lethal connexin26-deficient mice. J Cell Biol 1998; 140:1453–1461.

15
Myosin VI

Nadav Ahituv, Orit Ben-David, and Karen B. Avraham
Sackler School of Medicine, Tel Aviv University, Tel Aviv, Israel

Paolo Gasparini
Second University of Naples and Telethon Institute of Genetics and Medicine, Naples, Italy

I. INTRODUCTION

Movement of cells or their components is a fundamental activity of eukaryotic cells. The segregation of chromosomes, transport of organelles, and movement of ciliated cells are all possible owing to the large repertoire of molecular motors. Three superfamilies of motor proteins exist—myosins, kinesins, and dyneins—all of which convert chemical energy into mechanical work. Myosins are further defined by their ability to bind actin, to hydrolyze adenosine triphosphate (ATP), and to translocate along actin filaments. The function of this group of molecular motors includes many crucial cellular activities such as membrane trafficking, cell locomotion, signal transduction, and vesicle transport (reviewed in Refs. 1,2). Myosins have historically been divided into two groups: the conventional myosins (myosin II), which include the two-headed, filament-forming dimeric myosins of skeletal muscle, smooth muscle cells; and nonmuscle cells; and the unconventional myosins (myosin I, III–XVIII).

Mutations in five myosins lead to human hearing loss. These include myosin IIIA (3), myosin VI (4), myosin VIIA (5–7), MYH9 (8), and myosin XVA (9). Mouse models for three of these human deafness loci exist, and have provided much information regarding the pathophysiology of the inner ear due to mutations in these genes. The shaker 1 (*sh1*) and shaker 2 (*sh2*) mice are associated with mutations in myosin VIIa and myosin XVa, respectively

(10,11). Mutations in myosin VI are found in the deaf and circling mouse mutant, Snell's waltzer (12). Before delving into the main subject of this chapter, myosin VI in human and mouse hearing loss, we will describe myosins in general.

II. MYOSIN: A MOLECULAR MOTOR

The unconventional myosins are divided into several classes based on analysis of their motor and tail domains. To date at least 18 classes of conventional myosins have been defined and they are numbered in the order in which they were discovered (for complete list, see Myosin Homepage, http://www.mrc-lmb.cam.ac.uk/myosin/myosin.html).

The myosins are comprised of a heavy chain with a conserved ~80-kDa catalytic domain (the head or motor domain), and most are followed by an α-helical light-chain-binding region (the neck region). Most myosins contain a C-terminal tail and, in some cases, an N-terminal extension as well. The amino acid sequence of the head domain is conserved within each class-specific myosin. All myosins contain an actin-binding domain and an ATP-binding domain in their head region, allowing them to move along actin filaments. The tail domains diverge from one another between myosin classes and are believed to confer the function of each different myosin. The myosin VIIA and myosin XVA tail share MyTH4 (myosin tail homology 4) domains and FERM membrane-binding domains (13,14), whereas the myosin VI tail is unique among the myosins. Both myosin XVA and myosin IIIA contain N-terminal extensions; the latter is a kinase domain that has been shown to play an important role in phototransduction in *Drosophila* (15).

The neck domain in almost all myosins consists of a variable number (1–6) of light-chain-binding motifs, called IQ motifs. These motifs are usually formed from six tandem repeats of a basic and hydrophobic ~23 amino acid sequence (reviewed in Ref. 16). Calmodulin is used most frequently as a light chain, as well as other members of the EF hand superfamily. Many calmodulins have been shown to bind to different myosins in this region, suggesting that certain calmodulins were formed to bind different myosins throughout evolution. The actual presence of calmodulin light chains in many unconventional myosins suggests that their activity may be regulated by calcium. Finally, many myosins share a coiled-coil α-helix motif in the tail region that is predicted to form dimers.

Myosins have a class-specific tail domain, which is the main feature that distinguishes between them. It is hypothesized that this variation in structure is what dictates the varied cellular localization and function of each class of myosin (17). One myosin I, myoB, for example, is thought to control the activity of the actin-rich cortex of the cell and has a Src-homology 3 (SH3) domain at its C-terminus, suggesting that it might be regulated through tyrosine-kinase-associated receptors (18). Evidence from yeast and slime demonstrates that the SH3 domain recruits the Arp complex and may play a role in regulating actin polymerization (19). Myosin Va, associated with neurological and melanosome defects in dilute mice and Griscelli disease in humans, possesses a tail that specifies its localization to various organelles in yeast and targets it to the melanosome in vertebrate melanocytes (reviewed in Ref. 20).

III. MYOSIN VI

Myosin VI was first discovered in *Drosophila* (21) but has since been identified in pig (22), bullfrog (23), mice (12), humans (24), *C. elegans* (25), striped bass (26), sea urchin (27), and zebrafish (K.B. Avraham and T. Nicolson, unpublished observations). Myosin VI, like other unconventional myosins, has a class-conserved head, neck, and tail region (Fig. 1). Myosin VI has a number of defined features in the head region, including a ~25-amino-acid insertion at the position of a surface loop (16) and a conserved threonine residue (residue 405 in humans and 406 in mice) (24). Studies suggest that myosin VI may be activated by a heavy-chain kinase at this conserved threonine residue (28). In the neck domain, myosin VI has a 53-amino-acid segment adjacent to its single IQ motif that differs from any known N-terminal junction of the neck domain of other myosins. The tail domain has a coiled-coil domain, like a number of other myosins, followed by a globular domain that is unique and highly conserved between the different organisms' myosin VI.

The presence of a unique domain in the neck region of myosin VI led to the suspicion that myosin VI moves in the opposite direction along actin relative to other myosins, toward the "minus" end of actin filaments (29). By use of in vitro motility assays, myosin VI was shown to move toward the pointed (minus) end of actin. Cryoelectron microscopy and image analysis demonstrated that the lever arm, the putative calmodulin light-chain-binding

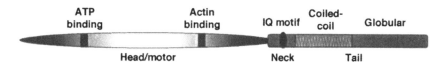

Figure 1 The myosin VI protein is composed of a head or motor domain, a neck region containing one IQ motif, and a tail composed of a coiled-coil region and a globular domain.

domain, is indeed in the opposite orientation in myosin VI relative to other myosins. The rotation of the lever arm may determine direction of movement, and thus enable this molecule to move "backward" along actin. Other reports have suggested that the motor core domain of myosin VI determines its directionality (30); this is further supported by the fact that myosin IXb was recently found to also move toward the pointed end of actin, although it does not possess an insert in its head domain (31). Regardless of what portion of the protein determines its directionality, this feature may have significance in polarized cells, where the pointed ends of actin are in the center of the cell, and in hair cells, where the pointed ends of actin face the rootlets of the stereocilia. Myosin VI is expressed in both types of cells (see Sec. VI.A).

IV. MYOSIN VI MUTATIONS IN ANIMAL MODELS

The most informative information regarding myosin VI function has been obtained from either blocking myosin VI function or studying spontaneous or induced mutations.

A. Myosin VI in *Drosophila* and *C. elegans*

The *Drosophila* myosin VI, also named 95F, was found to be required for the normal formation and organization of the syncytial blastoderm. It was shown that when 95F function was inhibited by injecting inhibitory-95F antibodies into syncytial blastoderm *Drosophila* embryos, profound defects in syncytial blastoderm organization occurred, including colliding mitotic spindles that resulted in misassortment of chromosomes and fused multipolar nuclei (32). 95F is located in cytoplasmic domains around the nuclei during interphase and is found concentrated in the region where actin-based invaginations will form during metaphase (33). It is thought that 95F myosin may be indirectly involved in furrow formation during mitosis by delivery of required furrow-forming components. Myosin VI is associated with motile particles and this movement is inhibited by the same antibodies in both *Drosophila* oocytes and embryos; this was the first discovery that led to speculation that myosin VI might play a role in vesicle trafficking.

Myosin VI also appears to have a conserved role in sperm development. *C. elegans* myosin VI deletion mutants do not properly segregate cell components, leading to aberrant spermatogenesis (34). Mitochondria, endoplasmic/ reticulum/Golgi-derived fibrous-body membranous organelle complexes, actin filaments, and microtubules are not properly sorted to developing spermatids. These data suggest that in addition to playing a role in the segregation of organelles, myosin VI may also participate in the organization of both microtubules and actin. Two *Drosophila* myosin VI mutants are known to have defects in spermatid individualization, a process where each spermatid is enclosed in its own membrane (35). Myosin VI is therefore required for transport and reorganization of membranes in the individualization complex within *Drosophila* developing spermatids.

Recent experiments in *Drosophila* demonstrate that myosin VI is required for E-cadherin-mediated border cell migration (36). Myosin VI is expressed in the outer migratory border cells of *Drosophila*, and depletion of this protein is associated with a reduction of E-cadherin, which is required for migration of these cells. This finding demonstrates yet more evidence of a function for myosin VI in cell motility.

B. Myosin VI in the Mouse

Mutations in the unconventional myosin VI gene, *Myo6*, are associated with deafness and vestibular dysfunction in the Snell's waltzer mouse (12). The Snell's waltzer mouse mutant was discovered in the late 1960s in Dr. George Snell's colony at the Jackson Laboratory in Bar Harbor, Maine. Crosses set up to identify the chromosomal location of the defective locus determined that Snell's waltzer was located on chromosome 9, within the dilute-short-ear region (37). Twenty years later, a positional cloning approach was undertaken to identify the causative gene for deafness in this mouse. Fortunately, one of the Snell's waltzer alleles, se^{sv}, had an inversion on chromosome 9 that led to access of the *sv* region (Fig. 2). Yeast artificial chromosome (YAC) clones were obtained from this region and used in an exon-trapping approach to identify an exon that shared 87% homology to the pig myosin VI (22). Myosin VI was an excellent candidate for hearing loss since mutations in the unconventional myosin VIIa had been found a short time earlier in the deaf shaker 1 mouse (10). Soon thereafter, a 130-bp deletion was found in the myosin VI coding region in the second Snell's waltzer allele, *sv* (12). This deletion leads to a frameshift in the neck portion of the protein that results in a stop codon (Fig. 1). Consequently, no myosin VI protein has been detected in any tissues examined in the *sv* allele. The inversion in the se^{sv} allele leads to a reduction in myosin VI expression. The "break" does not occur within the *sv* gene; rather, it occurs between 30 and 220 kb upstream of the first coding exon. Presumably, promoter regulatory sequences associated with controlling myosin VI expression levels are lost owing to the inversion. Despite the almost ubiquitous expression pattern of myosin VI, the only phenotypes of the Snell's waltzer mice are deafness and circling.

The major advantage of the mouse myosin VI mutant is the ability to have a mouse model for hearing loss caused by myosin VI mutations. Mice are proving to be an invaluable tool for researchers to study the morphology

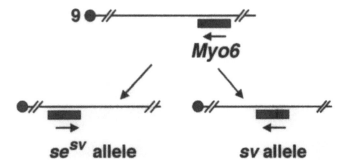

Figure 2 Myosin VI mutations lead to deafness and circling in two Snell's waltzer alleles, *sv* and *se^{sv}*. The *sv* mouse mutant arose spontaneously and contains an intragenic deletion in the *Myo6* gene. The *se^{sv}* mouse arose by radiation; the *Myo6* gene is inverted, presumably leading to the loss of regulatory sequences. The gray box depicts the myosin VI gene, the arrow under the gray boxes shows transcriptional orientation of the gene, and the black rectangle in the *sv* allele gene (*Myo6^{sv}*) demonstrates *Myo6* deletion.

and physiology of the inner ear owing to the similarity between the mouse and human genomes and the physiology and morphology of the auditory system (reviewed in Ref. 38). With use of a variety of techniques, such as the generation of transgenic mice, scanning electron microscopy (SEM), patch clamping on individual hair cells, and culturing of the organ of Corti, much can be learned about the function of a protein in the inner ear.

V. HUMAN MYOSIN VI

A. The Human Myosin VI Gene and Protein

Since myosin VIIA was involved in both mouse and human deafness, it seemed plausible that the same would be the case for myosin VI. The human myosin VI (*MYO6*) human cDNA was isolated and characterized (24). Human *MYO6* has a 3789-bp open reading frame coding for the human myosin VI protein that shares 90.2% identity with the mouse myosin VI protein. With fluorescent in situ hybridization (FISH), human myosin VI was mapped to chromosome 6q13 (24). At this time, no deafness loci had been identified in this region, suggesting that myosin VI mutations may be rare in the human deaf population or, alternatively, may be found in a population not yet examined. As this gene was still an attractive candidate for human deafness, the map position of human *MYO6* was refined by radiation hybrid mapping and its genomic structure was characterized (39).

Human myosin VI is composed of 32 coding exons, spanning a genomic region of approximately 70 kb. Exon 30, which contains a putative CKII phosphorylation site, was found to be alternatively spliced and expressed in fetal and adult human brain and testis. Another alternatively spliced exon was discovered in the tail region of myosin VI following the coiled-coil domain (40). This exon is highly conserved when compared to chicken and rat and was found to be expressed in tissues such as kidney, liver, and small intestine, all of which have a high proportion of polarized cells with microvilli at their apical surface. The myosin VI isoform containing this exon is localized to clathrin-coated vesicles, suggesting a role for myosin VI in clathrin-mediated endocytosis.

B. Human Myosin VI–Associated Hearing Loss

The successful use of a mouse model in predicting human disease was shown when a mutation in the *MYO6* gene was found to be associated with hearing loss in a large Italian family (4). Affected members of this family suffer from progressive autosomal dominant sensorineural hearing loss, with a variable age of onset mainly during childhood (8–10 years old) (Fig. 3). Audiograms showed different degrees of hearing impairment, ranging from moderate to profound sensorineural hearing loss. A genome scan revealed linkage to an 11-cM region on human chromosome 6. This locus was named DFNA22, since it was the twenty-second autosomal dominant locus to be identified (for a list of all loci, see the Hereditary Hearing Loss Homepage, http://dnalab-www.uia.ac.be/dnalab/hhh/). The human *MYO6* gene maps within this region and was an excellent candidate based on its chromosomal location,

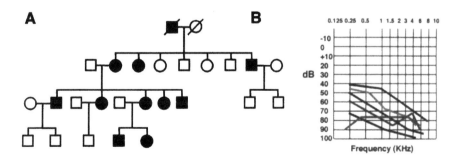

Figure 3 A myosin VI mutation leads to progressive hearing loss in an Italian family (9). (A) Pedigree of family, demonstrating dominant inheritance of hearing loss. (B) Representative pure-tone thresholds of affected members of the Italian family with a myosin VI mutation. Only the left ear is shown. (Adapted with permission from Ref. 4.)

cochlear expression, and function. The entire *MYO6* coding sequence and all exon-intron boundaries were scanned for mutations both by sequencing and by single-strand conformation polymorphism (SSCP) analysis (39). A G→A transition was detected in exon 12 at position 1325 of the cDNA sequence (relative to the ATG, designated + 1), which replaces a cysteine (TGT) with a tyrosine (TAT) at residue 442 of the protein (C442Y) (Fig. 4). All affected members of this family carried the C442Y mutation. The C442Y mutation was not identified in 200 normal chromosomes derived from Italian individuals with no family history of hearing loss.

The C442Y mutation affects a cysteine residue in the motor domain that is conserved across other myosin VI species, including human, mouse, chicken, pig, striped bass, and sea urchin. The nematode and fruitfly myosin VI each have a similar hydrophilic amino acid, serine, at this position (Fig. 4). In addition, a pairwise alignment of 143 myosins revealed no changes to tyrosine. Owing to the high homology between the motor domains of myosin VI and myosin II, for which a 3D structure was known (41), a three-dimensional model of myosin VI was made to predict what kind of damage the tyrosine could inflict (Fig. 5A). According to the model constructed, the cysteine is partly buried in the protein core, and resides at the beginning of the α-helix HO (Fig. 5B). The α-helix HG, which ends with an arginine, lies antiparallel to the cysteine. Replacing C442 with a tyrosine, which is a much bulkier amino acid, may cause a collision between this tyrosine and arginine (Fig. 5C). This collision may lead to either binding through cation-pie

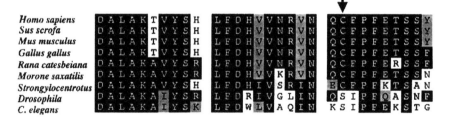

Figure 4 Alignment of a portion of human myosin VI C442 with myosin VI from various species. Note conservation of cysteine (arrow) in *Homo sapiens* (human; Accession no. U90236) through *Strongylocentrotus* (sea urchin; Accession no. AF248485) and a similar hydrophilic residue in *Drosophila* (fruitfly; Accession no. NM_079754) and *C. elegans* (worm; Accession no. NM_067528). Other accession numbers are as follows: *Sus scrofa* (pig; Accession no. Z35331), *Mus musculus* (mouse; U49739); *Gallus gallus* (chicken; Accession no. AJ278608), *Rana catesbeiana* (bullfrog, Accession no. U14370), *Morone saxatilis* (striped sea bass, Accession no. AF017304). (Adapted with permission from Ref. 4.)

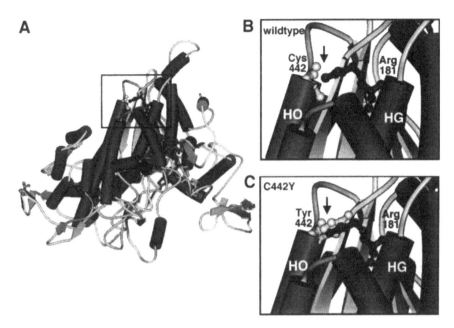

Figure 5   Three-dimensional model of human myosin VI. (A) Schematic representation of a model of the myosin VI motor domain. (B) Wild-type structure showing C442 amino acid. The α-helix HO and the α-helix HG is at approximately amino acid residue 178–184 and 412–442, respectively (see Myosin Homepage Multiple Alignment, http://www.mrc-lmb.cam.ac.uk/myosin/trees/txalign.html). Arrow depicts space between C442 and A181. (C) Mutant structure showing altered amino acid to tyrosine, with arrow depicting potential collision between T442 and A181. The model was built using the automatic homology modeling facility, Swiss Model (http://www.expasy.ch/swissmod/SWISS-MODEL.html), and the three-dimensional structures of several myosin motor domains. The mutated model was created using the "Modeler" module in Insight (Accelyrs).

interactions (42) or repulsion, both of which will disrupt the protein structure. It is important to stress that this is a model and these theories are speculative based on this model.

VI. MYOSIN VI AND THE INNER EAR

Myosin VI clearly plays a vital role in the inner ear, since mutations in both humans and mice lead to severe to profound hearing loss. Expression has been studied on both an RNA and protein level in a range of organisms.

A. Myosin VI Expression

Human *MYO6* is present in heart, brain, placenta, lung liver, skeletal muscle, kidney, pancreas, spleen, thymus, prostate, testis, ovary, small intestine, and colon, demonstrating its ubiquitous expression (24). In the striped bass, two isoforms of myosin VI (FMVIA and FMVIB) are expressed in the photo-receptors, horizontal cells, and Müller cells in fish, suggesting that myosin VI may play a role in retinal motility events (26). Fish myosin VI seems to have a more restricted expression pattern than that of mouse or rat myosin VI. Despite the fact that myosin VI is found in retina of fish and primates (rhesus monkey) (26), no retinal phenotype has been found in animal models or humans with myosin VI mutations. Several expression studies suggest that myosin VI is a general membrane transport motor and has an essential role in membrane trafficking (reviewed in Ref. 43). Myosin VI is expressed in the intermicrovillar (IMV) coated-pit region of the rat kidney brush border, suggesting a role in the function of the endocytic process of the proximal tubule (44). In fibroblasts, myosin VI is localized to the Golgi complex and the leading, ruffling edge of these cells (28).

In the inner ear, myosin VI is specifically expressed in the sensory hair cells. Using antibodies directed against a portion of the pig myosin VI tail, immunochemical studies in the mouse and guinea pig cochlea localized myosin VI to the outer and inner hair cells of the cochlea (24,45). Myosin

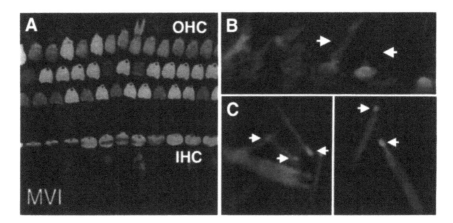

Figure 6 Localization of myosin VI in frog and guinea pig hair cells. (A) Antibodies against myosin VI label the cytoplasm of the hair cells. MVI, myosin VI labeling; OHC, outer hair cells; IHC, inner hair cells. (B) No expression of myosin VI is detected in guinea pig stereocilia (arrows). (C) Myosin VI is expressed in the tapered ends of frog stereocilia (arrows). (Adapted with permission from Ref. 45.)

VI is present in the cell body, and in particular, in the cuticular plate, the actin-rich structure underlying the stereocilia (Fig. 6A). No labelling was observed in the stereocilia (Fig. 6B). Extensive analysis has been performed on the expression of myosin VI in the adult American bullfrog (*Rana catesbeiana*) hair cells (45). Myosin VI was observed in hair cells but not in supporting cells or peripheral cells of the saccule and the cochlea (Fig. 6C). In the saccule and cochlear hair cell, myosin VI is enriched in the cuticular plate and pericuticular necklace and appears throughout the cell. In the bullfrog, myosin VI is present in the tapered ends of the stereocilia, unlike in mammals.

B.   The Consequences of Myosin VI Mutations on the Hair Cell

While we cannot determine the fate of the hair cells in humans with myosin VI–associated deafness, we can make predictions by studying the mutants with unconventional myosin mutations. Scanning and transmission electron microscopy on *sv* mice cochleas revealed severe stereocilia disorganization, with stereocilia fusing shortly after birth (46) (Fig. 7). The fusion begins at the base of the stereocilia and by 7 days after birth, only a few giant and/or fused stereocilia are found on the top of the cells. By 20 days after birth, all hair cells in the cochlear duct possess abnormal stereocilia. Fewer hair cells are seen, demonstrating degeneration of hair cells. Histological sections of the cochlear duct from *sv/sv* mice indicate a complete loss of hair cells by 6–8 weeks of age (12).

Based on the study on the *sv* mutants, it was suggested that myosin VI is involved in anchoring the apical hair cell membrane to the underlying actin-rich cuticular plate. Without myosin VI, the plasma membrane is unstable and leads to a "zipping up" of the membrane, observed as stereocilia fusion (46). How does this role coincide with the observation that myosin VI is an actin minus end-directed motor? There may be two roles for myosin VI in

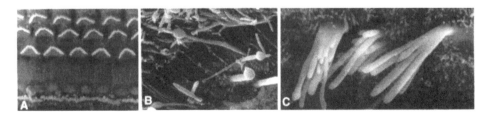

Figure 7   Morphology of stereocilia in hair cells of *sv/sv* mice. (A) In wild-type cells, there are three rows of outer hair cells and one row of inner hair cells. (B) Disorganization of stereocilia is apparent in 20-day-old mice. (C) Fusion at base of stereocilia can be seen at 7 days after birth. (Adapted with permission from Ref. 46.)

stereocilia organization (reviewed and suggested by Ref. 47). The first possible molecular function for myosin VI is as a transporter of cargo through the cell and the second function is to generate cell expansion force (Fig. 8). These molecular functions may act in several biological processes where myosin VI is required, i.e., pseudocleavage in embryo blastoderm, sperm individualization, and border cell migration in *Drosophila*, and stereocilia development in mice. In the hair cell, myosin VI may function to transport plasma membrane, thereby stabilizing the stereocilia by transporting a component that strengthens the stereocilia rootlets. This movement would occur toward actin filaments minus ends in the stereocilia rootlets. A second possible role is in generating expansion force. This is manifested as myosin VI pushing (expansion force) between adjacent stereocilia rootlets, maintaining the stereocilia in place.

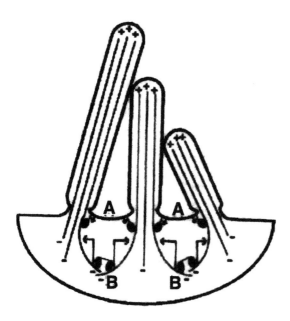

Figure 8 Two proposed functions for myosin VI, based on mutant studies in *Drosophila*, *C. elegans*, and mice. (A) Myosin VI may act as a motor to transport cargo, in this case plasma membrane, toward the minus ends of actin filaments lying near the stereocilia rootlets. (B) Myosin VI may act to generate a cell expansion force, by pushing on actin filaments and causing them to slide; this "pushing" force will allow stereocilia to remain in their proper location. (Adapted with permission from Ref. 47.)

VII. CONCLUDING REMARKS

Myosin VI clearly plays a crucial role in the auditory system, as mutations in this gene lead to both human and mouse hearing loss. A missense mutation in myosin VI leads to progressive hearing loss in humans, transmitted as a dominant trait, while in the Snell's waltzer mouse model, both a frameshift mutation in myosin VI and a chromosomal inversion (with loss of putative myosin VI regulatory sequences) lead to congenital deafness, inherited in a recessive mode. Studies of model systems are providing critical information about the function of myosin VI. A number of proteins that interact with myosin VI have been identified recently [e.g., GLUT1CBP (48); DOC-2/DAB2 (49); SAP97 (50)]. The identification of interacting molecules, coupled with phenotypic analyses and localization studies, has provided insight into myosin VI function in endocytosis and vesicle trafficking. Once more molecules are identified, we will begin to obtain a global picture of the network that myosin VI is involved in, particularly as it relates to auditory and vestibular dysfunction.

ACKNOWLEDGMENTS

The authors wish to thank the many collaborators and laboratory members who have contributed to work described in this chapter. We would like to thank Margaret Titus and Tama Sobe for reviewing the chapter. Research in the K.B.A. laboratory is supported by the European Commission (QLG2-1999-00988), the NIH/Fogarty International Center Grant 1 R03 TW01108-01, the Israel Science Foundation, the F.I.R.S.T. Foundation of the Israel Academy of Sciences and Humanities, the Israel Ministry of Health, and the Israel Ministry of Science, Culture, and Sport.

REFERENCES

1. Cheney RE, Mooseker MS. Unconventional myosins. Curr Opin Cell Biol 1992; 4:27–35.
2. Mermall V, Post PL, Mooseker MS. Unconventional myosins in cell movement, membrane traffic, and signal transduction. Science 1998; 279:527–533.
3. Walsh T, Walsh V, Vreugde S, Hertzano R, Shahin H, Haika S, Lee MK, Kanaan M, King MC, Avraham KB. From flies' eyes to our ears: mutations in a human class III myosin cause progressive nonsyndromic hearing loss DFNB30. Proc Natl Acad Sci USA 2002; 99:7518–7523.

4. Melchionda S, Ahituv N, Bisceglia L, Sobe T, Glaser F, Rabionet R, Arbones ML, Notarangelo A, Di Iorio E, Carella M, Zelante L, Estivill X, Avraham KB, Gasparini P. *MYO6*, the human homologue of the gene responsible for deafness in Snell's waltzer mice, is mutated in autosomal dominant nonsyndromic hearing loss. Am J Hum Genet 2001; 69:635–640.

5. Weil D, Blanchard S, Kaplan J, Guilford P, Gibson F, Walsh J, Mburu P, Varela A, Levilliers J, Weston MD, et al. Defective myosin VIIA gene responsible for Usher syndrome type 1B. Nature 1995; 374:60–61.

6. Liu XZ, Walsh J, Mburu P, Kendrick-Jones J, Cope MJ, Steel KP, Brown SD. Mutations in the myosin VIIA gene cause non-syndromic recessive deafness. Nat Genet 1997; 16:188–190.

7. Liu XZ, Walsh J, Tamagawa Y, Kitamura K, Nishizawa M, Steel KP, Brown SD. Autosomal dominant non-syndromic deafness caused by a mutation in the myosin VIIA gene. Nat Genet 1997; 17:268–269.

8. Lalwani AK, Goldstein JA, Kelley MJ, Luxford W, Castelein CM, Mhatre AN. Human nonsyndromic hereditary deafness DFNA17 is due to a mutation in nonmuscle myosin *MYH9*. Am J Hum Genet 2000; 67:1121–1128.

9. Wang A, Liang Y, Fridell RA, Probst FJ, Wilcox ER, Touchman JW, Morton CC, Morell RJ, Noben-Trauth K, Camper SA, Friedman TB. Association of unconventional myosin *MYO15* mutations with human nonsyndromic deafness DFNB3. Science 1998; 280:1447–1451.

10. Gibson F, Walsh J, Mburu P, Varela A, Brown KA, Antonio M, Beisel KW, Steel KP, Brown SD. A type VII myosin encoded by the mouse deafness gene shaker-1. Nature 1995; 374:62–64.

11. Probst FJ, Fridell RA, Raphael Y, Saunders TL, Wang A, Liang Y, Morell RJ, Touchman JW, Lyons RH, Noben-Trauth K, Friedman TB, Camper SA. Correction of deafness in shaker-2 mice by an unconventional myosin in a BAC transgene. Science 1998; 280:1444–1447.

12. Avraham KB, Hasson T, Steel KP, Kingsley DM, Russell LB, Mooseker MS, Copeland NG, Jenkins NA. The mouse Snell's waltzer deafness gene encodes an unconventional myosin required for structural integrity of inner ear hair cells. Nat Genet 1995; 11:369–375.

13. Weil D, Levy G, Sahly I, Levi-Acobas F, Blanchard S, El-Amraoui A, Crozet F, Philippe H, Abitbol M, Petit C. Human myosin VIIA responsible for the Usher 1B syndrome: a predicted membrane-associated motor protein expressed in developing sensory epithelia. Proc Natl Acad Sci USA 1996; 93:3232–3237.

14. Liang Y, Wang A, Belyantseva IA, Anderson DW, Probst FJ, Barber TD, Miller W, Touchman JW, Jin L, Sullivan SL, Sellers JR, Camper SA, Lloyd RV, Kachar B, Friedman TB, Fridell RA. Characterization of the human and mouse unconventional myosin XV genes responsible for hereditary deafness DFNB3 and shaker 2. Genomics 1999; 61:243–258.

15. Porter JA, Montell C. Distinct roles of the *Drosophila* ninaC kinase and myosin domains revealed by systematic mutagenesis. J Cell Biol 1993; 122:601–612.

16. Mooseker MS, Cheney RE. Unconventional myosins. Annu Rev Cell Dev Biol 1995; 11:633–675.

17. Hasson T, Mooseker MS. Molecular motors, membrane movements and physiology: emerging roles for myosins. Curr Opin Cell Biol 1995; 7:587–594.

18. Novak KD, Titus MA. The myosin I SH3 domain and TEDS rule phosphorylation site are required for in vivo function. Mol Biol Cell 1998; 9:75–88.

19. Lechler T, Shevchenko A, Li R. Direct involvement of yeast type I myosins in Cdc42-dependent actin polymerization. J Cell Biol 2000; 148:363–373.

20. Provance DW, Mercer JA. Myosin-V: head to tail. Cell Mol Life Sci 1999; 56: 233–242.

21. Kellerman KA, Miller KG. An unconventional myosin heavy chain gene from *Drosophila melanogaster*. J Cell Biol 1992; 119:823–834.

22. Hasson T, Mooseker MS. Porcine myosin-VI: characterization of a new mammalian unconventional myosin. J Cell Biol 1994; 127:425–440.

23. Solc CF, Derfler BH, Duyk GM, Corey DP. Molecular cloning of myosins from the bullfrog saccular macula: a candidate for the hair cell adaptation motor. Audit Neurosci 1994; 1:63–75.

24. Avraham KB, Hasson T, Sobe T, Balsara B, Testa JR, Skvorak AB, Morton CC, Copeland NG, Jenkins NA. Characterization of unconventional *MYO6*, the human homologue of the gene responsible for deafness in Snell's waltzer mice. Hum Mol Genet 1997; 6:1225–1231.

25. Baker JP, Titus MA. A family of unconventional myosins from the nematode *Caenorhabditis elegans*. J Mol Biol 1997; 272:523–535.

26. Breckler J, Au K, Cheng J, Hasson T, Burnside B. Novel myosin VI isoform is abundantly expressed in retina. Exp Eye Res 2000; 70:121–134.

27. Sirotkin V, Seipel S, Krendel M, Bonder EM. Characterization of sea urchin unconventional myosins and analysis of their patterns of expression during early embryogenesis. Mol Reprod Dev 2000; 57:111–126.

28. Buss F, Kendrick-Jones J, Lionne C, Knight AE, Cote GP, Paul Luzio J. The localization of myosin VI at the Golgi complex and leading edge of fibroblasts and its phosphorylation and recruitment into membrane ruffles of A431 cells after growth factor stimulation. J Cell Biol 1998; 143:1535–1545.

29. Wells AL, Lin AW, Chen LQ, Safer D, Cain SM, Hasson T, Carragher BO, Milligan RA, Sweeney HL. Myosin VI is an actin-based motor that moves backwards. Nature 1999; 401:505–508.

30. Homma K, Yoshimura M, Saito J, Ikebe R, Ikebe M. The core of the motor domain determines the direction of myosin movement. Nature 2001; 412:831–834.

31. Inoue A, Saito J, Ikebe R, Ikebe M. Myosin IXb is a single-headed minus-end-directed processive motor. Nat Cell Biol 2002; 4:302–306.

32. Mermall V, McNally JG, Miller KG. Transport of cytoplasmic particles catalysed by an unconventional myosin in living *Drosophila* embryos. Nature 1994; 369:560–562.

33. Mermall V, Miller KG. The 95F unconventional myosin is required for proper organization of the *Drosophila* syncytial blastoderm. J Cell Biol 1995; 129: 1575–1588.

34. Kelleher JF, Mandell MA, Moulder G, Hill KL, L'Hernault SW, Barstead R,

Titus MA. Myosin VI is required for asymmetric segregation of cellular components during *C. elegans* spermatogenesis. Curr Biol 2000; 10:1489–1496.

35. Hicks JL, Deng WM, Rogat AD, Miller KG, Bownes M. Class VI unconventional myosin is required for spermatogenesis in *Drosophila*. Mol Biol Cell 1999; 10:4341–4353.

36. Geisbrecht ER, Montell DJ. Myosin VI is required for E-cadherin-mediated border cell migration. Nat Cell Biol 2002; 4:616–620.

37. Deol MS, Green MC. Snell's waltzer, a new mutation affecting behaviour and the inner ear in the mouse. Genet Res 1966; 8:339–345.

38. Ahituv N, Avraham KB. Mouse models for human deafness: current tools for new fashions. Trends Mol Med 2002; 8:447–451.

39. Ahituv N, Sobe T, Robertson NG, Morton CC, Taggart RT, Avraham KB. Genomic structure of the human unconventional myosin VI gene. Gene 2000; 261:269–275.

40. Buss F, Arden SD, Lindsay M, Luzio JP, Kendrick-Jones J. Myosin VI isoform localized to clathrin-coated vesicles with a role in clathrin-mediated endocytosis. EMBO J 2001; 20:3676–3684.

41. Rayment I, Rypniewski WR, Schmidt-Base K, Smith R, Tomchick DR, Benning MM, Winkelmann DA, Wesenberg G, Holden HM. Three-dimensional structure of myosin subfragment-1: a molecular motor. Science 1993; 261:50–58.

42. Gallivan JP, Dougherty DA. Cation-pi interactions in structural biology. Proc Natl Acad Sci USA 1999; 96:9459–9464.

43. Tuxworth RI, Titus MA. Unconventional myosins: anchors in the membrane traffic relay. Traffic 2000; 1:11–18.

44. Biemesderfer D, Mentone SA, Mooseker M, Hasson T. Expression of myosin VI within the early endocytic pathway in adult and developing proximal tubules. Am J Physiol Renal Physiol 2002; 282:F785–F794.

45. Hasson T, Gillespie PG, Garcia JA, MacDonald RB, Zhao Y, Yee AG, Mooseker MS, Corey DP. Unconventional myosins in inner-ear sensory epithelia. J Cell Biol 1997; 137:1287–1307.

46. Self T, Sobe T, Copeland NG, Jenkins NA, Avraham KB, Steel KP. Role of myosin VI in the differentiation of cochlear hair cells. Dev Biol 1999; 214:331–341.

47. Cramer LP. Myosin VI: roles for a minus end-directed actin motor in cells. J Cell Biol 2000; 150:F121–126.

48. Bunn RC, Jensen MA, Reed BC. Protein interactions with the glucose transporter binding protein GLUT1CBP that provide a link between *GLUT1* and the cytoskeleton. Mol Biol Cell 1999; 10:819–832.

49. Inoue A, Sato O, Homma K, Ikebe M. DOC-2/DAB2 is the binding partner of myosin VI. Biochem Biophys Res Commun 2002; 292:300–307.

50. Wu H, Nash JE, Zamorano P, Garner CC. Interaction of SAP97 with minus-end directed actin motor myosin VI: implications for AMPA receptor trafficking. J Biol Chem 2002; 5:5.

16
K$^+$-Channel Gene *KCNQ4*

Paul Coucke
University Hospital Ghent, Ghent, Belgium

Patrick J. Willems
GENDIA, Antwerp, Belgium

I. SUMMARY

Mutations in the K$^+$-channel gene *KCNQ4* are responsible for the most frequent form of nonsyndromic autosomal dominant hearing loss, affecting at least nine families originating from the Netherlands (4 families), the United States (2 families), Belgium, France, and Japan. The *KCNQ4*-associated hearing loss is nonsyndromic, sensorineural, and progressive. It starts between the age of 5 and 15 years with high-tone loss, and deteriorates gradually over several decades affecting also the middle and lower tones. By the age of 70 most patients have severe to profound hearing loss. The hearing impairment is completely penetrant, whereas intra- and interfamilial variability is small. The *KCNQ4* gene represents the DFNA2 locus on chromosome 1p34, and encodes a K$^+$ channel that is probably involved in the K$^+$ homeostasis in the cochlea, which is essential for normal hearing.

II. THE DFNA2 LOCUS

Until 1994 only one locus (DFNA1) for nonsyndromic hearing loss (HL) had been localized on the human genome. However, in that year three more loci (DFNA2, DFNB1, and DFNB2) were mapped, marking the start of a successful hunt for genes involved in human HL (for review, see Refs. 1–4). The DFNA2 locus was originally mapped to chromosome 1p32 by a genome screen in two extended families with an autosomal dominant progressive HL originating from Indonesia and the United States (5). Afterward the original chromosomal location was corrected for 1p34 (6). Seven additional families with a similar HL were later linked to the DFNA2 locus. This includes a family from Belgium (7), a family from the Netherlands (7,8), a second Dutch family (7,9), a second U.S. family (10), a third Dutch family (11,12), a Japanese family (13), and a fourth Dutch family (14; Van Camp et al., unpublished results).

Surprisingly, the DFNA2 locus was found to represent more than one gene responsible for autosomal dominant nonsyndromic progressive HL starting in the high frequencies. The gap junction protein GJB3, which encodes connexin 31 and is located in the DFNA2 linkage region, was shown to cause HL in two small Chinese families (15). Soon thereafter, mutations in the K^+-channel gene *KCNQ4* were identified in a small French family (16), the U.S. 1, Belgian, Dutch 1 and 2 families (17), the U.S. 2 family (10), the Dutch 3 family (12), the Japanese family (13), and the Dutch 4 family (Van Camp et al., unpublished results) (Table 1). However, in the original Indonesian family (5,7) no mutation in the *KCNQ4* or *GJB3* gene has yet been found despite intensive mutation analysis. This suggests that a third and unknown gene responsible for postlingual autosomal dominant HL is located in the DFNA2 region (18). The cluster of connexin genes located in the linkage region of the Indonesian family represents good candidate genes for the HL in this family (19). Another unexplained observation is the digenic inheritance pattern of a Swedish family showing both suggestive linkage to the DFNA2 locus (lod score: 2.7) and significant linkage to the DFNA12

Table 1   *KCNQ4* Mutations in DFNA2 Hearing Loss

Family	Origin	Mutation	Type	Location	Ref.
1	French	G285S	Missense	Pore (exon 6)	16
2	Belgian	211del13	Deletion	Amino terminus (exon 1)	17
3	USA 1	G285C	Missense	Pore (exon 6)	17
4	Dutch 1	W276S	Missense	Pore (exon 5)	17
5	Dutch 2	G321S	Missense	S6 (exon 7)	17
6	USA 2	L281S	Missense	Pore (exon 6)	10
7	Dutch 3	L274H	Missense	Pore (exon 5)	12
8	Japanese	W276S	Missense	Pore (exon 5)	13
9	Dutch 4	W276S	Missense	Pore (exon 5)	Van Camp et al., unpublished results

locus (lod score: 3.9) (20). Although neither of these lod scores definitively proves linkage, the concept of digenic inheritance is supported by the observation that the HL is more severe in individuals having both disease-associated haplotypes (21). DFNA12 HL can be caused by mutations in the alpha-tectorin (22), but it is hard to imagine an interaction between alpha-tectorin, on one hand, and *KCNQ4* or connexin 31, on the other hand. Mutation analysis of these three genes in the Swedish family has not yet been reported, and is necessary to prove the digenic inheritance.

III. THE *KCNQ4* GENE

A.   Isolation and Localization

The *KCNQ4* gene was identified by Kubisch et al. (16) when screening a human retina cDNA library with a cDNA clone from another member of the *KCNQ* gene family (*KCNQ3*). The gene was mapped to chromosome 1p34 by FISH, and found to be located in the immediate vicinity of the D1S432 marker (16). As the latter marker is located in the DFNA2 linkage region (5,7), the *KCNQ4* gene was a good positional candidate gene for DFNA2.

B.   Structure

The *KCNQ4* gene is a member of a family of K⁺-channel subunits charac-terized by six transmembrane domains that anchor the protein in the cell membrane, and a single pore loop that forms the ion-specificity filter of the channel (for review, see Ref. 23). The pore loop is located between the fifth and sixth transmembrane domain, and encoded by exons 5 and 6. The fourth transmembrane domain functions as a voltage sensor. Both the short amino- and the long carboxy-terminus are located inside the cell. The *KCNQ4* gene contains 14 exons encoding for 695 amino acids with a predicted molecular weight of 77 kDa (16).

C.   Tissue Expression

KCNQ4 is expressed in the cochlea, the vestibular system, and the central auditory pathway (Fig. 1). In the mouse cochlea, *KCNQ4* expression is found in the basal membrane of the outer hair cells, but not in the inner hair cells (24). However, Beisel et al. (25) found expression in both the inner and the outer hair cells in rat cochlea. These authors also showed that the *KCNQ4* expression in inner hair cells and the spiral sensory neurons

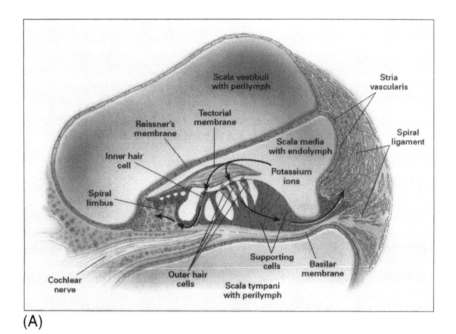

(A)

Figure 1   (A) The organ of Corti. *KCNQ4* is expressed in the hair cells of the organ of Corti, which act as mechanoelectrical transducers transforming the mechanical movements of their stereocilia into electrical signals transmitted through the cochlear nerve to the auditory cortex. The mechanical vibrations of the endolymph produced by sound lead to deflection of the stereocilia, resulting in influx of K^+ ions. These ions leave the hair cells probably through K^+ channels formed by the *KCNQ4* gene. They then recirculate to the spiral limbus and stria vascularis, where they are secreted back into the endolymph through K^+ channels formed by *KCNQ1/KCNE1*. K^+ homeostasis is essential for normal hearing. (B) Sound oscillations cause deflection of the stereocilia of the hair cells, leading to influx of K^+ ions, resulting in de-polarization of the hair cells. This leads to entry of Ca^{2+} ions, leading to neu-rotransmitter release from synaptic vesicles, which activates the acoustic nerve. Repolarization of the hair cell occurs when the K^+ ions leave the hair cell through K^+ channels at the basolateral side of the cell. The K ions than recirculate to the endolymph through connexins expressed in the membranes of the supporting cells. (From N Engl J Med 2000; 342:1101–1109.)

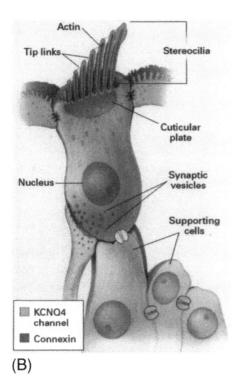

Figure 1 Continued.

decreased from the base to the apex of the cochlea, whereas the expression in outer hair cells increases from base to apex. The *KCNQ4* gene is also expressed in the vestibular organ (in type 1 vestibular hair cells and their afferent neurons), and in many nuclei of the central auditory pathway (24).

D. Function

Based on the selective expression of the *KCNQ4* channel in the outer hair cells and the type 1 vestibular hair cells, Jentsch and colleges suggested that *KCNQ4* generates the K⁺-selective "leak" current [termed I (K⁺,n) current in outer hair cells and I (K⁺,L) current in type 1 vestibular hair cells] (16,24). However, this was questioned by Trussell (26). Furthermore, the observation that *KCNQ4* is also expressed in inner hair cells, in which this leak current is not present, argues against this hypothesis. The function of the *KCNQ4* channel, therefore, is not yet completely clear. As *KCNQ4* is specifically expressed at the basolateral side of hair cells (Fig. 1), it might be involved there in the removal of the K^+ ions that accumulated in the hair cells after entering these cells at the apical side (16,24).

E. *KCNQ4* Homologs and Their Involvement in Human Disease

Five different family members *KCNQ1–5* have been identified so far, four of them being implicated in genetic disease in man (Table 2). The homology of these genes is high, certainly in the transmembrane domains and the pore region (16). The actual K^+ channels are formed by four homomers or heteromers of *KCNQ* gene products that juxtaposition their pore loops to form the actual K^+ channel. *KCNQ4* forms tetramers only with itself or with *KCNQ3*.

1. *KCNQ1*

The *KCNQ1* subunits associate with *KCNE1* subunits to form a K^+ channel expressed in the heart and the cochlea, that is the molecular correlate of the cardiac-delayed rectifier-like K^+ current. This current is involved in repolarization of action potentials in the heart, with *KCNQ1* and *KCNE1* mutations leading to a prolonged QT interval in the long-QT syndrome, also called the Romano-Ward syndrome (27). Severe functional impairment of this K^+ channel leads to Jervell and Lange-Nielsen syndrome, a combination of long-QT syndrome with congenital deafness (28). In the cochlea, K^+ homeostasis is maintained not only by the *KCNQ4* gene product and several connexins, but also by the *KCNQ1/KCNE1*-encoded K^+ channel, which allows secretion of K^+ ions from the stria vascularis back into the endolymph.

2. *KCNQ2* and *KCNQ3*

These two subunits form a heteromeric K^+ channel involved in the M-current in neurons, which is important for neuronal excitability. Mutations

Table 2 *KCNQ4* Genes Involved in Human Disease

Gene	Location	Disease	Inheritance	Ref.
KCNQ1	11p15	Romano-Ward syndrome	AD and AR	27
		Jervell and Lange-Nielsen syndrome	AR	28
KCNQ2	20q13	Epilepsy (BFNC)	AD	29
KCNQ3	8q24	Epilepsy (BFNC)	AD	30
KCNQ4	1p34	Hearing loss (DFNA2)	AD	16
				17

in either of these genes are responsible for benign familial neonatal convulsions (BFNC), a form of congenital epilepsy (29,30). HL has never been described in BFNC.

3. *KCNQ5*

This subunit is expressed in brain and muscle, and forms multimers with itself and *KCNQ3*. Mutations in this gene have not yet been identified.

F. *KCNQ4* Mutations

KCNQ4 mutations have been identified in nine unrelated families (Table 1, Fig. 2 and 3). Although the pore region of the *KCNQ4* gene only represents approximately 3% of the open reading frame, it harbors the disease-causing mutation in seven of these nine families, reflecting the importance of this domain in the function of this K^+ channel. One of the pore region mutations

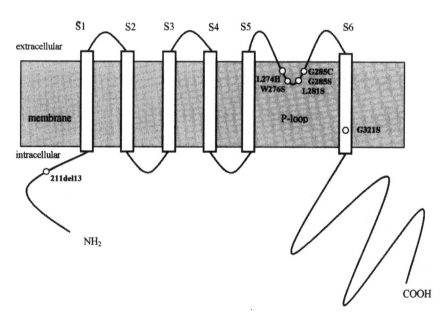

Figure 2 Schematic representation of the genomic structure of the *KCNQ4* gene with exons indicated as boxes (above), and the *KCNQ4* protein with six transmembrane domains, with a pore region between the fifth and sixth transmembrane regions, (below). The seven *KCNQ4* mutations in the nine families (the *W276S* mutation is present in three unrelated families) are indicated.

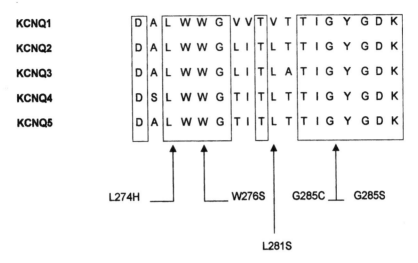

Figure 3   Alignment of the amino acid sequence of the pore region of the different members from the *KCNQ* gene family. The five missense mutations in the pore region of *KCNQ4* typically involve amino acids strongly conserved between the different members of the *KCNQ* gene family. The W276S mutation is present in three unrelated families.

(W276S) was found in three different families (the Dutch 1, Japanese, and Dutch 4 families). As these three families are not related, and the W276S mutation is present on different genetic backgrounds in these families, the W276S mutation probably represents a mutational hot spot in the *KCNQ4* gene (15). The pore region mutations are all missense mutations substituting amino acids that are strongly conserved between different members of the *KCNQ* gene family (Fig. 3). Functional studies of the K$^+$ channel with such a heterozygous mutation in the pore region (G285S) expressed in *Xenopus* oocytes showed severe reduction of K$^+$ currents to only 10% of normal, indicating a dominant-negative effect of this mutation (17). As the K$^+$ channel is formed by a tetramer of *KCNQ4* subunits, any given mutation with a dominant-negative effect can cause a severe reduction in K$^+$-channel activity, which is compatible with the autosomal dominant inheritance pattern and complete penetrance of the hearing loss. In the eighth family (Dutch 2) a missense mutation in the sixth transmembrane domain has been identified. The nineth *KCNQ4* mutation is an out-of-frame deletion of 13 bp causing a frameshift at amino acid 71, resulting in 63 novel amino acids with a premature stop codon at position 134. Most likely, the short mutant protein is degraded rapidly as it does not contain transmembrane regions.

Apart from these disease-associated mutations, 11 neutral polymorphisms and one polymorphic amino acid substitution have been identified in the *KCNQ4* gene (10).

IV. HEARING LOSS CAUSED BY *KCNQ4* MUTATIONS

Mutations in the *KCNQ4* gene have been identified in nine different families with a nonsyndromic, sensorineural, and progressive HL that is inherited in an autosomal dominant mode with complete penetrance. The clinical features of these families are summarized in Table 3, and age-related typical audiograms made by De Leenheer et al. (31) are shown in Figure 4. The clinical features of eight of the nine families have been analyzed and compared by different authors (31–33).

A. The French Family

In this small family with autosomal dominant progressive HL in three patients belonging to three consecutive generations the first *KCNQ4* mutation (G285S) was identified (16). The family is known with HL starting in the first decade progressing to severe losses between 90 and 120 dB in the 2000–4000 Hz interval. Although hearing impairment was always more

Table 3   Clinical Features of Hearing Loss Due to *KCNQ4* Mutations

Family	Origin	Threshold (dB)				Tinnitus	Ref.
		250 Hz		8000 Hz			
		20 years	60 years	20 years	60 years		
1	French	NR	NR	NR	NR	+	16
2	USA 1	30–35	45–50	70–75	100–105	+	5
3	Belgian	15–20	20–25	>120	>120	+	7
4	Dutch 1	15–20	50–55	70–75	100–105	–	8
5	Dutch 2	10–15	45–50	55–60	100–105	–	9
6	USA 2	20–25	45–50	65–70	100–105	+	10
7	Dutch 3	15–20	40–45	70–75	95–100	–	11
8	Japanese	30–35	60–65	65–70	110–115	–	13
9	Dutch 4	25–30	60–65	70–75	110–115	–	14

NR, not reported.
Source: Data derived from Ref. 31.

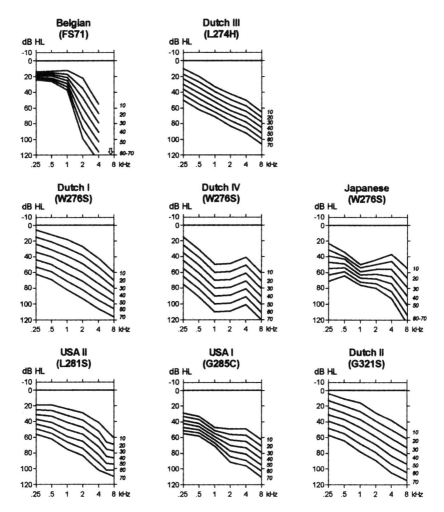

Figure 4 Typical age-related audiograms of eight of the nine families with a *KCNQ4* mutation (no data were available on the small French family). The initial high-tone loss in younger individuals, and the progressive hearing loss with age in older patients, with loss of the middle and eventually low frequencies, are evident in all families. Note that at the age of 10 years significant HL already exists, indicating that the DFNA2 HL probably is prelingual, and not postlingual. The age-related audiograms of eight of the nine families are very similar, but different from that of the Belgian family. In the latter family the HL of the high tones is more pronounced, but low tones are conserved throughout life. The data have been published before by De Leenheer et al. (31).

severe in the high frequencies, the lower tones also showed significant losses (50–90 dB at 500 Hz) (16). Detailed audiological studies of this family have not been reported.

B. The U.S. 1 Family

This five-generation family was used together with the original Indonesian family to map DFNA2 to chromosome 1p by linkage analysis (5). At that time it contained 27 patients with nonsyndromic HL, which started before the age of 10. Tinnitus was reported by a fraction of the affected family members (Table 3). Mutation analysis of the *KCNQ4* gene identified a G285C mutation in the pore region of the gene (17).

C. The Belgian Family

This four-generation pedigree contains at least 27 family members affected by a progressive hearing loss of the high frequencies (7), whereas the low tones remain relatively spared in comparison with the other families with a *KCNQ4* mutation (31–33). This family is the only one of the nine with such conservation of the low tones. Below 1000 Hz the average annual threshold increase (ATI) was only between 0.2 and 0.5 dB, whereas the ATI was very high, above 1000 Hz (2–5 dB). This family was used, together with the Dutch 1 and 2 families, to narrow down the linkage interval of the *DFNA2* gene (7). A deletion of 13 bp (FS71) was found in the *KCNQ4* gene, leading to a premature stop codon resulting in truncation of the protein (18). This is the only definite loss-of-function mutation in the *KCNQ4* gene, as all the other *KCNQ4* mutations in the other families are missense mutations, which most likely have a dominant-negative effect.

D. The Dutch Family 1

This large family contains at least 41 affected patients in six generations. The HL is similar to that of the other families, but clearly different from that of the Belgian family (8,31–33). About one-third of the patients show vestibular hyperreactivity in response to rotatory stimulation tests. A missense mutation (W276S) was identified in the pore region of *KCNQ4*. The W276S mutation is also present in the Japanese and the Dutch 4 family.

E. The Dutch Family 2

This is an extended six-generation family with at least 24 affected members. The audiological features are very similar to these of the other *KCNQ4* families, and have been described in detail (9,31–33). Coucke et al. (17) found a missense mutation (G321S) in the sixth transmembrane domain of the *KCNQ4* gene.

F. The U.S. Family 2

This large U.S. family of Austrian ancestry consists of 51 patients in five generations with a HL that is very similar to that of the other families. The majority of patients have tinnitus. The family shows linkage to the DFNA2 locus, and a L281S missense mutation was identified in the pore region of the *KCNQ4* gene (10).

G. The Dutch Family 3

In this five-generation family 20 family members are affected by a typical *KCNQ4*-associated HL (11,31–33). The family was shown to be linked to the DFNA2 locus and a missense mutation (L274H) was found in the pore region of the *KCNQ4* gene (12).

H. The Japanese Family

In this family the W276S mutation, which was also present in the Dutch 1 and Dutch 4 families, was found (13). The clinical picture is not different from that of the other families (13,31).

I. The Dutch 4 Family

This is a five-generation family with 33 affected patients. The clinical picture of this family was studied extensively by De Leenheer et al. (14). The HL is typical for *KCNQ4*-associated pathology. Although the HL starts early, possibly congenitally, speech recognition only starts to deteriorate significantly in the third decade. Although none of the patients had vertigo, two of 11 patients who underwent vestibular testing showed motion sickness. These two patients, together with a third patient, had hyperactive vestibulo-ocular reflexes. Also in this family the W276S mutation is present (Van Camp et al., unpublished results).

V. GENOTYPE-PHENOTYPE CORRELATION

Nine different families with a *KCNQ4* mutation have been described (Tables 1 and 3). In all cases the HL is autosomal dominant, nonsyndromic, and sensorineural, affecting both ears equally. Tinnitus has been reported in the Belgian, French, and both U.S. families (17,31–33). Vertigo has not been reported, but an increased vestibulo-ocular reflex activity has been found in a minority of the Dutch patients with the W276S mutation (8,31). Visualization of the middle and inner ear by CT scan or MRI has been performed in the French and Dutch 4 family, but could not reveal morphological anomalies. A detailed comparison of the audiological features of eight of the nine different DFNA2 families in which a *KCNQ4* mutation has been found (excluding the French family, for which only limited information was available) has been made by several authors (31–33). These comparative studies indicated that the hearing loss of all the families but the Belgian family is very similar in age of onset, rate of progression, and affected frequencies (Table 3, Fig. 4). Regression analysis of the HL of these families in function of time and frequency shows a linear progression of all frequencies with an average annual threshold deterioration of approximately 1 dB per year. The offset values are close to zero for the low frequencies, but increase progressively with higher frequencies. Although hardly any audiology data are available from very young affected children, it is conceivable that there is high-tone loss already at birth in these families (11,31–33). In most patients with a *KCNQ4* mutation a hearing aid becomes necessary between the age of 20 to 40 years, whereas HL is severe to profound by the age of 70. Although DFNA2 is classified with the postlingual types of HL, it is likely that prelingual HL occurs, as significant HL is already present at the age of 10 years. This probably remains undetected in most patients as only the high tones are affected at that young age.

The Belgian family shows greater loss in the high frequencies than the other families, but the low tones are relatively spared (Fig. 4). The Belgian family, therefore, represents the purest form of inherited high-tone loss. In this family a loss-of-function mutation was identified that might have a less severe impact on the residual activity of the *KCNQ4* channel activity than the missense mutations that are present in all the other families. At first sight this might explain the relative conservation of the low tones, but it is difficult to reconcile this with the more pronounced losses of the high tones in the Belgian family as compared to the other families.

VI. DISCUSSION

Progressive HL is a normal process of ageing, and hearing impairment to the level of limitation of communication is the most frequent sensory handicap present in half of the population by the age of 80. It is unclear why our auditory system does not seem to endure for a complete life span.

Other sensory systems such as the eye also show progressive malfunctioning with age, but the proportion of elderly in whom the aging process leads to real functional impairment is considerably smaller than in the case of HL. It is possible that the paucity of auditory sensory cells (a mere 30–40,000 hair cells) makes the auditory system more vulnerable than other sensory systems, such as the visual system and the olfactory system, which each contain millions of sensory cells. Therefore, it is not surprising that many of the inherited forms of progressive HL involve the cochlea, in particular the hair cells. The typical progressive HL of the elderly (presbycusis) is a gradual loss of high tones with conservation of the middle tones and the low tones. Presbycusis most likely is a multifactorial disorder caused by a complex interaction between multiple genetic factors and many environmental factors such as noise, ear infections or trauma, ototoxic medication such as aminoglycosides, etc. Many postlingual forms of monogenic HL due to mutation in a single gene offer paradigms to study presbycusis.

Among the Mendelian forms of postlingual, progressive HL of the high tones, HL due to mutations in the *KCNQ4* gene is probably the most frequent type of postlingual HL, certainly in Western Europe. Nine extended and unrelated families with a *KCNQ4* mutation have now been described, and it is remarkable that four of these families are of Dutch descent. The inheritance pattern in all families is autosomal dominant with full penetrance. The HL in these nine families is very similar, and always nonsyndromic, sensorineural, postlingual, and progressive, affecting the high tones first, the middle tones later, and the low tones in a final stage. It is likely that the HL starts in the prelingual period in most patients, and proceeds to severe HL by the age of 70. In three of the nine families tinnitus is present. Vertigo has never been reported, but vestibular studies revealed abnormalities in about a third of the patients. This is not unexpected as the *KCNQ4* gene is expressed in the type 1 hair cells of the vestibular organ. The *KCNQ4* gene is also expressed in several auditory nuclei and the outer hair cells of the organ of Corti, but controversy still exists around the presence of *KCNQ4* in the inner hair cells. Also, the function of the *KCNQ4* gene is still a matter of debate. It encodes a tetrameric K^+ channel that is involved in K^+ homeostasis in the cochlea. In view of its localization at the basolateral side of cochlear hair cells, it is possible that the K^+ channel formed by *KCNQ4* is involved in the outflux of K^+ ions that accumulate in hair cells where they lead to repolarization (16,23,24,34).

Influx of K^+ ions from the K^+-rich endolymph is triggered by mechanical stimulation when the vibrations of the basilar membrane induce shearing of the tectorial membrane (Fig. 1). This leads to bending of the stereocilia of the hair cells in the cochlea, resulting in the opening of unidentified K^+ channels involving the action of unconventional myosins such as myosin 6, 7A, and 15. The influx of potassium ions leads to depolarization of the hair cells, and subsequent Ca^{2+} influx triggering the release of the neurotransmitter glutamate, which stimulates the nerve endings of the acoustic nerve. The accumulated K^+ ions in the outer hair cells leave these cells through K^+ channels at the basolateral side, and are recirculated through the gap junctions between the supporting cells and cochlear fibrocytes to end up in the marginal cells of the stria vascularis. Here the K^+ ions reenter the endolymph through K^+ channels formed by the associated gene products of *KCNQ1* and *KCNE1*. The K^+ ions from the inner hair cells recirculate to the interdental cells of the spiral limbus, where they are taken up again by the endolymph (Fig. 1A). Mutations in many of the genes involved in cochlear K^+ homeostasis lead to hereditary HL, including the K^+ channels *KCNQ4* (DFNA2), *KCNQ1*, and *KCNE1* (Jervell and Lange-Nielsen syndrome), the gap junction proteins GJB2 (DFNA3 and DFNB1), GJB3 (DFNA2), GJB6 (DFNA3), and the tight junction protein claudin 14 (DFNB9) (for review, see Ref. 1).

Although treatment of genetic disease in general represents more "hype" than hope, it is not impossible that HL due to deficient *KCNQ4* channel activity might be prevented or even treated by drugs that activate *KCNQ4* channel activity. Components such as retigabine and BMS-204352, which are in clinical trials now to treat epilepsy and stroke, have been shown to activate *KCNQ4* channels in vivo (35).

REFERENCES

1. Willems PJ. Genetic causes of hearing loss. N Engl J Med 2000; 342:1101–1109.
2. Resendes BL, Williamson RE, Morton CC. At the speed of sound: gene discovery in the auditory system. Am J Hum Genet 2001; 69:923–935. Review.
3. Steel KP, Kros CJ. A genetic approach to understanding auditory function. Nat Genet 2001; 27:143–149. Review.
4. Tekin M, Arnos KS, Pandya A. Advances in hereditary deafness. Lancet 2001; 358:1082–1090. Review.
5. Coucke P, Van Camp G, Djoyodiharjo B, Smith SD, Frants RR, Padberg GW, Darby JK, Huizing EH, Cremers CWRJ, Kimberling WJ, Oostra BA, Van de Heyning PH, Willems PJ. Linkage of autosomal dominant hearing loss to the short arm of chromosome 1 in two families. N Engl J Med 1994; 331:425–431.
6. Van Camp G, Coucke P, Speleman F, Van Roy N, Beyer EC, Oostra BA, Willems PJ. The gene for human gap junction protein connexin37 (*GJA4*) maps to chromosome 1p35.1, in the vicinity of D1S195. Genomics 1995; 30:402–403.
7. Van Camp G, Coucke PJ, Kunst H, Schatteman I, Van Velzen D, Marres H, van Ewijk M, Declau F, Van Hauwe P, Meyers J, Kenyon J, Smith SD, Smith

RJH, Djelantik B, Cremers CWRJ, Van de Heyning PH, Willems PJ. Linkage analysis of progressive hearing loss in five extended families maps the DFNA2 gene to a 1.25-Mb region on chromosome 1p. Genomics 1997; 41:70–74.

8. Marres H, van Ewijk M, Huygen P, Kunst H, van Camp G, Coucke P, Willems P, Cremers C. Inherited nonsyndromic hearing loss: an audiovestibular study in a large family with autosomal dominant progressive hearing loss related to DFNA2. Arch Otolaryngol Head Neck Surg 1997; 123:573–577.

9. Kunst H, Marres H, Huygen P, Ensink R, Van Camp G, Van Hauwe P, Coucke P, Willems P, Cremers C. Nonsyndromic autosomal dominant progressive sensorineural hearing loss: audiologic analysis of a pedigree linked to DFNA2. Laryngoscope 1998; 108:74–80.

10. Talebizadeh Z, Kelley PM, Askew JW, Beisel KW, Smith SD. Novel mutation in the *KCNQ4* gene in a large kindred with dominant progressive hearing loss. Hum Mutat 1999; 14:493–501.

11. Ensink RJ, Huygen PL, Van Hauwe P, Coucke P, Cremers CW, Van Camp G. A Dutch family with progressive sensorineural hearing impairment linked to the DFNA2 region. Eur Arch Otorhinolaryngol 2000; 257:62–67.

12. Van Hauwe P, Coucke PJ, Ensink RJ, Huygen P, Cremers CWRJ, Van Camp G. Mutations in the *KCNQ4* K(+) channel gene, responsible for autosomal dominant hearing loss, cluster in the channel pore region. Am J Med Genet 2000; 93:184–187.

13. Akita J, Abe S, Shinkawa H, Kimberling WJ, Usami S. Clinical and genetic features of nonsyndromic autosomal dominant sensorineural hearing loss: *KCNQ4* is a gene responsible in Japanese. J Hum Genet 2001; 46:355–361.

14. De Leenheer EMR, Huygen PLM, Coucke PJ, Admiraal RJC, Van Camp G, Cremers CWRJ. Longitudinal and cross-sectional phenotype analysis in a new, large Dutch DFNA2/*KCNQ4* family. Ann Otol Rhinol Laryngol 2002; 111:267–274.

15. Xia J, Liu C, Tang B, Pan Q, Huang L, Dai H, Zhang B, Xie W, Hu D, Zheng D, Shi X, Wang D, Xia K, Yu K, Liao X, Feng Y, Yang Y, Xiao J, Xie D, Huang J. Mutations in the gene encoding gap junction protein beta-3 associated with autosomal dominant hearing impairment. Nat Genet 1998; 20:370–373.

16. Kubisch C, Schroeder BC, Friedrich T, Lutjohann B, El-Amraoui A, Marlin S, Petit C, Jentsch TJ. *KCNQ4*, a novel potassium channel expressed in sensory outer hair cells, is mutated in dominant deafness. Cell 1999; 96:437–446.

17. Coucke PJ, Van Hauwe P, Kelley PM, Kunst H, Schatteman I, Van Velzen D, Meyers J, Ensink RJ, Verstreken M, Declau F, Marres H, Kastury K, Bhasin S, McGuirt WT, Smith RJH, Cremers CWRJ, Van de Heyning P, Willems PJ, Smith SD, Van Camp G. Mutations in the *KCNQ4* gene are responsible for autosomal dominant deafness in four DFNA2 families. Hum Mol Genet 1999; 8:1321–1328.

18. Van Hauwe P, Coucke PJ, Declau F, Kunst H, Ensink RJ, Marres HA, Cremers CWRJ, Djelantik B, Smith SD, Kelley P, Van de Heyning PH, Van Camp G. Deafness linked to DFNA2: one locus but how many genes? (Letter). Nat Genet 1999; 21:263.

19. Coucke PJ, Van Laer L, Meyers J, Van Hauwe P, Ottschytsch N, Wauters JG, Kelley P, Willems PJ, Van Camp G. Identification of a new connexin gene *GJA11* (CX59) using degenerate primers. GeneScreen 2000; 1:35–40.

20. Balciuniene J, Dahl N, Borg E, Samuelsson E, Koisti MJ, Pettersson U, Jazin EE. Evidence for digenic inheritance of nonsyndromic hereditary hearing loss in a Swedish family. Am J Hum Genet 1998; 63:786–793.

21. Borg E, Samuelsson E, Dahl N. Audiometric characterization of a family with digenic autosomal, dominant, progressive sensorineural hearing loss. Acta Otolaryngol 2000; 120:51–57.

22. Verhoeven K, Van Laer L, Kirschhofer K, Legan PK, Hughes DC, Schatteman I, Verstreken M, Van Hauwe P, Coucke P, Chen A, Smith RJ, Somers T, Offeciers FE, Van de Heyning P, Richardson GP, Wachtler F, Kimberling WJ, Willems PJ, Govaerts PJ, Van Camp G. Mutations in the human alpha-tectorin gene cause autosomal dominant non-syndromic hearing impairment. Nat Genet 1998; 19:60–62.

23. Jentsch TJ. Neuronal KCNQ potassium channels: physiology and role in disease. Nat Rev Neurosci 2000; 1:21–30. Review.

24. Kharkovets T, Hardelin JP, Safieddine S, Schweizer M, El-Amraoui A, Petit C, Jentsch TJ. *KCNQ4*, a K+ channel mutated in a form of dominant deafness, is expressed in the inner ear and the central auditory pathway. Proc Natl Acad Sci USA 2000; 97:4333–4338.

25. Beisel KW, Nelson NC, Delimont DC, Fritzsch B. Longitudinal gradients of *KCNQ4* expression in spiral ganglion and cochlear hair cells correlate with progressive hearing loss in DFNA2. Brain Res Mol Brain Res 2000; 82:137–149.

26. Trussell L. Mutant ion channel in cochlear hair cells causes deafness. Proc Natl Acad Sci USA 2000; 97:3786–3788.

27. Wang Q, Curran ME, Splawski I, Burn TC, Millholland JM, VanRaay TJ, Shen J, Timothy KW, Vincent GM, de Jager T, Schwartz PJ, Toubin JA, Moss AJ, Atkinson DL, Landes GM, Connors TD, Keating MT. Positional cloning of a novel potassium channel gene: *KVLQT1* mutations cause cardiac arrhythmias. Nat Genet 1996; 12:17–23.

28. Splawski I, Tristani-Firouzi M, Lehmann MH, Sanguinetti MC, Keating MT. Mutations in the *hminK* gene cause long QT syndrome and suppress IKs function. Nat Genet 1997; 17:338–340.

29. Biervert C, Schroeder BC, Kubisch C, Berkovic SF, Propping P, Jentsch TJ, Steinlein OK. A potassium channel mutation in neonatal human epilepsy. Science 1998; 279:403–406.

30. Charlier C, Singh NA, Ryan SG, Lewis TB, Reus BE, Leach RJ, Leppert M. A pore mutation in a novel KQT-like potassium channel gene in an idiopathic epilepsy family. Nat Genet 1998; 18:53–55.

31. De Leenheer EMR, Ensink RJH, Kunst HPM, Marres HAM, Talebizadeh Z, Declau F, Smith SD, Usami SI, Van de Heyning PH, Van Camp G, Huygen PLM, Cremers CWRJ. DFNA2/*KCNQ4* and its manifestations. In: The clinical presentation of genetic hearing impairment. Adv Otol Rhinol Laryngol. In: Basel, Karger, 2002; 61:41–46.

32. Van Hauwe P, Coucke P, Van Camp G. The DFNA2 locus for hearing

impairment: two genes regulating K+ ion recycling in the inner ear. Br J Audiol 1999; 33:285–289.

33. Kunst H, Ensink R, Marres H, Declau F, Smith S, Djelantik B, Huygen P, Wuyts F, Van Camp G, Van de Heyning P, Cremers C. Genotype-phenotype correlation in progressive non-syndromic hearing impairment linked to the DFNA2 region on chromosome 1p34. Submitted.

34. Ackerman MJ, Clapham DE. Ion channels—basic science and clinical disease. N Engl J Med 1997; 336:1575–1586. Review.

35. Schroder RL, Jespersen T, Christophersen P, Strobaek D, Jensen BS, Olesen S. *KCNQ4* channel activation by BMS-204352 and retigabine. Neuropharmacology 2001; 40:888–898.

17
COL11A2

Wyman T. McGuirt and Richard J. H. Smith
University of Iowa, Iowa City, Iowa, U.S.A.

Guy Van Camp
University of Antwerp, Antwerp, Belgium

I. INTRODUCTION

The rapidly expanding field of human genetics has uncovered a number of genes that, when mutated, lead to hereditary hearing impairment. Over 60 genes have been localized and more than 20 genes identified that are implicated in hereditary hearing impairment (1). Autosomal dominant inherited deafness genes are referred to as DFNA and autosomal recessive inherited deafness genes as DFNB. In 1997, the thirteenth locus for autosomal dominant nonsyndromic hearing loss was reported (2). We review the discovery of novel mutations in a collagen gene (*COL11A2*) that cause dominantly inherited, prelingual, nonsyndromic sensorineural hearing loss (DFNA13).

Interestingly, mutations in *COL11A2* are also associated with two syndromic forms of hearing impairment, Stickler syndrome type 3 (autosomal dominant) and otospondylomegaepiphyseal dysplasia (OSMED syndrome, autosomal recessive) (3). This degree of phenotypic variability associated with allele variants of a single gene is well known in the field of deafness research. For example, mutations in *MYO7A* cause Usher syndrome type 1B, DFNB2, and DFNA11 and mutations in *SLC26A4* cause Pendred syndrome and DFNB4 (1). Variability of inheritance patterns also has been reported for several deafness-causing genes including *TECTA* (DFNA8/12, DFNB21), *GJB2* (DFNA3, DFNB1), and *GJB3* (1). The mechanisms that determine genotype/phenotype correlation are not well understood and likely are related to both intracellular and extracellular protein interactions.

In this chapter we: (1) describe the identification of a nonsyndromic form of dominantly inherited hearing loss (DFNA13); (2) detail the DFNA13 audiometric phenotype; (3) report cochlear expression patterns of *Col11a2*; (4) characterize the histological and audiometric changes in a *Col11a2* mouse mutant model: and (5) hypothesize on the role of collagen in the tectorial membrane.

II. DFNA13 GENE LOCALIZATION AND MUTATION ANALYSIS

The original family that was studied was ascertained through the Department of Otolaryngology at the University of Iowa (2). They were Caucasian, lived in the Midwestern United States, and were of European descent. Family members underwent a history and physical examination by a clinical geneticist and otolaryngologist. Individuals had no syndromic features segregating with the hearing loss. No individuals had cleft palate and cephalometric analysis revealed normal facial proportions.

Audiometry was performed in consenting individuals and blood was available for study in 48 individuals (Fig. 1A). Linkage analysis was performed across the entire genome and produced a maximum two-point lod score of 6.4 at D6S299 (2). Reconstruction of haplotypes with markers closely linked to D6S299 allowed refinement of the DFNA13 candidate gene interval to 0.5 mega-base pairs (Mb) flanked by D6S1666 and D6S1560. A Dutch family (Fig. 1B) with a similar hearing loss phenotype was concurrently localized to the same interval with a lod score > 3.

A physical map was constructed across chromosome 6p21.3 on the centromeric side of the HLA class II region using yeast artificial chromosomes (YACs) and P1-derived artificial chromosomes (PACs). The sequence data for the majority of the critical region became available during this time as a large BAC (1033B10) was sequenced through the Sanger Centre. Three genes within the candidate region were found to be cochlear expressed: *COL11A2*, retinoic acid receptor-β (*RXRB*), and *RING1*. Mutations in *COL11A2* also were known to cause of a variant form of Stickler syndrome (STLIII) (4).

Mutation screening of *COL11A2*, *RXRB*, and *RING1* was completed by single-strand conformational polymorphism (SSCP) analysis and bidirectional sequencing of all PCR products. In the American family, a heterozygous C-to-T missense mutation in *COL11A2* was discovered in exon 42 that is predicted to cause an arginine-to-cysteine substitution (Arg549Cys) in affected individuals (Fig. 2A) (5). Segregation of the disease-causing mutation within the family was confirmed by *Sfo*I digestion of the exon 42

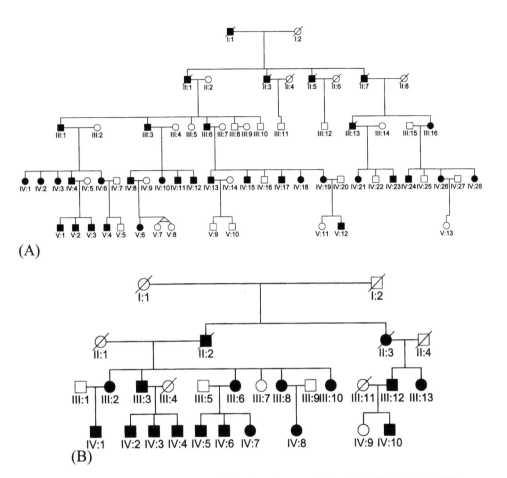

Figure 1 (A and B) Pedigree of the American and Dutch DFNA13/*COL11A2* families. Affected individuals are depicted with filled symbols. Numbers indicate individuals with available audiograms.

PCR product. All 24 affected individuals from the American DFNA13 family had hearing impairment with typical audiometric findings and were found to lack this digestion site. Analysis of the DFNA13 Dutch family revealed a heterozygous G-to-A transition in exon 31 of *COL11A2* that is predicted to cause a glycine-to-glutamate substitution (Gly323Glu) in affected individuals (Fig. 2B) (5). *BsmF1* digestion analysis of the exon 31 PCR product indicated complete cosegregation with the hearing impairment in this family. Neither *COL11A2* nucleotide change was found in an SSCP screen of 108 random individuals.

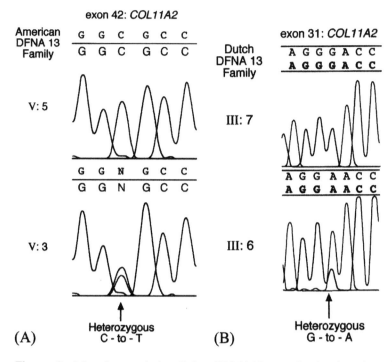

Figure 2 Mutation analysis of the *COL11A2* gene in the American (A) and Dutch (B) families revealed heterozygous missense mutations in exons 42 and 31, respectively.

III. *COL11A2* AND HEARING LOSS

Collagen is an abundant extracellular protein comprised of approximately 18 subtypes transcribed by over 32 genes. When mutated, collagens cause a wide spectrum of clinical disease (6), including a number of types of syndromic deafness such as osteogenesis imperfecta (*COL1A1, COL1A2*), Stickler syndrome type 1, 2, and 3 (*COL2A1, COL11A1,* and *COL11A2,* respectively), Alport syndrome (*COL4A3, COL4A4,* and *COL4A5*), Marshall syndrome (*COL11A1*), and OSMED syndrome (*COL11A2*) (5,6).

Type XI collagen accounts for <10% of total cartilage collagen and is believed to maintain the interfibrillar spacing and fibril diameter of type II collagen (7). It is composed of three unique gene products: α-1 (*COL11A1,* 1p21), α-2(*COL11A2,* 6p21.3), and α-3(*COL2A1,* 12q13.11-q13.2) (8). The *COL11A2* gene spans over 28 kilobases and includes 66 exons and an alternatively spliced exon in the amino terminus (8). Dominant and recessive disease-causing mutations in *COL11A2* have been described and result in a spectrum of osteochondrodysplasias (9). The phenotypes are characterized by midface hypoplasia, a short up-turned nose with a depressed nasal bridge, prominent eyes and supraorbital ridges, cleft palate, occasional micrognathia with glossoptosis, early-onset degenerative joint disease that can be severe, and often, small stature. Hearing impairment is usually present and is generally severe and sensorineural. Notably absent, however, are the ophthalmological abnormalities seen with *COL11A1* or *COL2A1* mutations, reflecting the absence of *COL11A2* expression in the ocular vitreous (4). The mutations that cause the DFNA13 phenotype are the only reported *COL11A2* mutations that are not associated with an identifiable syndrome (5).

IV. DFNA13 AUDIOMETRIC ANALYSIS

The congenital sensorineural hearing loss in the American family varied from mild to moderately severe in degree. Audiograms of affected individuals showed greater midfrequency than low- or high-frequency involvement. A detailed audiometric analysis was performed on the American DFNA13 family and revealed a mean threshold of approximately 29 dB at 0.25, 0.5, and 8 kHz (10). The mean thresholds at the frequencies between 1 and 4 kHz were higher at approximately 44 dB, producing a typical U-shaped audiogram (Fig. 3A). No significant progression of hearing impairment was noted when compared to reference levels for standardized curves. Interestingly, the rate of high-frequency hearing loss typical of presbycusis was less severe in the American DFNA13 family when compared to standardized curves. The cause of this preserved high-frequency hearing in the DFNA13 American family is unclear. The onset of hearing loss was presumed to be prelingual based on history and audiograms that revealed the typical midfrequency pattern in three children under the age of 12 years.

The hearing impairment in the Dutch family has been described as midfrequency (1–2 kHz) hearing impairment, with additional impairment at the higher frequencies (6–8 kHz) (11). There is a threshold average of approximately 25 dB at 0.25, 0.5, and 4 kHz, approximately 35–40-dB threshold at 1, 2, and 6 kHz, and approximately 50 dB at 8 kHz (Fig. 3B). Hearing impairment was documented audiometrically in one child at the age of 4 years. However, consistent with the American family, most individuals were not recognized as hearing impaired until the second or third decade of life. We believe this most likely represents a failure to diagnosis mild-to-moderate hearing impairment at a young age rather than rapid progression of hearing loss.

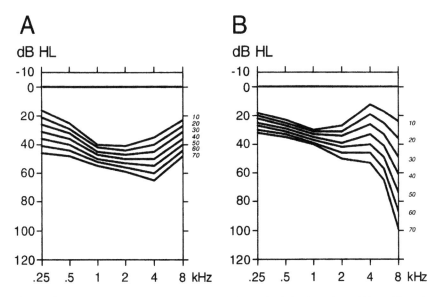

Figure 3 Age-related typical audiograms (ARTA) of the American (A) and Dutch (B) families. Left vertical axis: decibel (SPL); right vertical axis: age in years; horizontal axis: frequency (kHz).

Caloric testing of vestibular response was also performed in 17 individuals from the Dutch kindred (11). Caloric abnormalities were found in eight of 17 (47%) individuals tested. None of these individuals had substantial vestibular symptoms. Vestibular abnormalities included unilateral vestibular hyporeflexia ($n = 5$), bilateral hyporeflexia ($n = 2$), and bilateral areflexia ($n = 1$). Vestibular hyperreflexia occured in four of 17 cases tested. There was a trend for the type of vestibular dysfunction to segregate among family subgroups.

V. *COL11A2* EXPRESSION AND ANIMAL STUDIES

In situ hybridization studies of *Col11a2* in the developing murine (C57Bl/6J) cochlea were performed at E15.5, P1, and P5 (5). *Col11a2* was expressed strongly in the cartilaginous otic capsule at E15.5, with diminished hybridization at later developmental stages. Hybridization to the cochlear duct was not significantly different from that observed with the sense probe. At P5, diffuse homogeneous hybridization was observed in the spiral limbus region and lateral wall of the cochlea. *Col11a2* expression did not appear

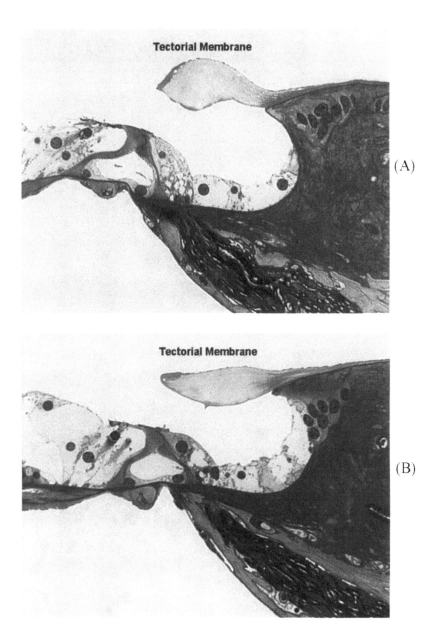

Figure 4 Light microscopy of the tectorial membrane in *Col11a2*-deficient mice (A) revealed a less compact tectorial membrane than that seen in either heterozygous or wild-type littermates (**B**).

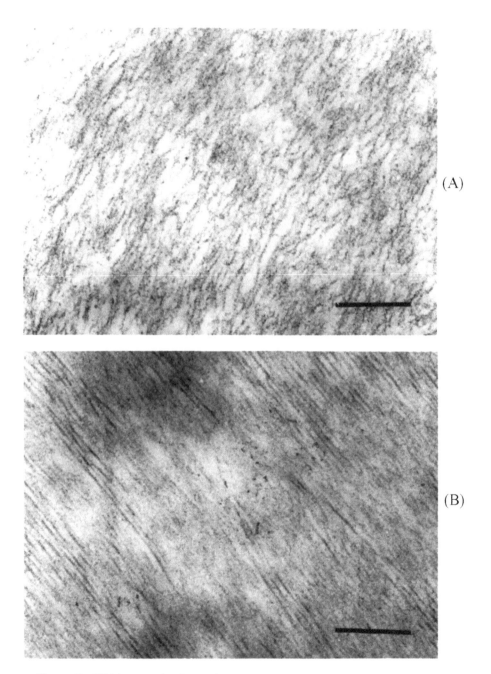

Figure 5 Widely spaced collagen fibers were evident by transmission electron microscopy level in the *Col11a2*-deficient mice (A) when compared to wild-type and heterozygous littermates (B).

to be significantly higher in the region of the inner ridge cells, the main source of type II collagen for the tectorial membrane. Hybridization was not evident in the acellular tectorial membrane. Weaker *Col11a2* RNA expression was detectable in the crista ampullaris and maculae of the saccule and utricle.

A transgenic mouse model for *Col11a2* was developed through homologous recombination in which an inverted neomycin-resistance gene was inserted between restriction sites in exons 27 and 28 (12). Transcription of shortened mRNAs was shown, but translation did not occur owing to the introduction of premature termination codons. The heterozygous mice are normal in appearance suggesting that a single copy of the *Col11a2* product is adequate to prevent detectable abnormalities. However, the homozygous *Col11a2* mice exhibit smaller snouts with a shortened midface, are smaller in size, and have abnormal hind-limb placement.

Click-evoked auditory brainstem response (ABR) testing was performed on homozygous and heterozygous *Col11a2*-deficient mice as well as their wild-type littermates (5). Animals were tested at 2 months, 6 months, and 12 months of age. Heterozygous (+ /-) and wild-type (+ / +) mice had similar hearing thresholds. The homozygous mice (-/-) were found to have an elevated hearing threshold that averaged 43 dB when compared to wild-type and heterozygous littermates. The degree of hearing impairment was not influenced by age at testing.

Histological analysis was performed on the temporal bones of 10 animals (4 homozygotes, 2 heterozygotes, and 4 wild-type mice) (5). At the light microscopic level, the tectorial membranes of the *Col11a2*-deficient mice were noted to be larger and less compact when compared to the tectorial membrane of heterozygous and wild-type mice (Fig. 4A,B). No other cochlear abnormalities were identifiable. By electron microscopy, tectorial membrane changes were more pronounced (Fig. 5A,B). Collagen fibrils in the homozygous mutants were irregular placed with widened interfibrillar distances (5), but in both the heterozygous and wild-type mice, the fibrils were in a parallel array and closely approximated.

VI. SUMMARY

To date, 16 different mutations have been described in the *COL11A2* gene and cause a diverse spectrum of phenotypic abnormalities, all with associated sensorineural hearing loss. Two mutations cause the subtlest phenotype— nonsyndromic prelingual sensorineural deafness. Three mutations have been reported to cause Stickler syndrome type 3—an exon-skipping mutation, a 27-bp in-frame deletion, and Gly955Glu. The remaining 11 mutations cause OSMED syndrome—all effectively producing a null allele (13). Consanguinity was observed in five of these cases. All parents of the OSMED patients were phenotypically normal, implying that haploinsufficiency alone does not cause a clinical effect.

The midfrequency hearing impairment associated with the DFNA13 phenotype is an unusual pattern of inherited hearing impairment. The "cookie-bite" audiometric pattern of hearing loss has classically been ascribed to genetic factors. However, of all the described nonsyndromic hearing loss loci, only the DFNA8/12, DFNB21 (*TECTA*), and DFNA21 audiometric phenotypes share the predominant midfrequency loss seen in DFNA13. The association of *TECTA* and *COL11A2* with the tectorial membrane implies that the micromechanical properties of this structure are important for effective mechanosensory transduction in the cochlea.

REFERENCES

1. Van Camp G, Smith RJH. Hereditary Hearing Loss Homepage. World Wide Web URL:http://dnalab-www.uia.ac.be/dnalab/hhh/.
2. Brown MR, et al. A novel locus for autosomal dominant nonsyndromic hearing loss, DFNA13, maps to chromosome 6p. Am J Hum Genet 1997; 6: 924–927.
3. Vikkula M, et al. Autosomal dominant and recessive osteochondrodysplasias associated with the *COL11A2* locus. Cell 1995; 80:431–437.
4. Sirko-Osadsa DA, et al. Stickler syndrome without eye involvement is caused by mutations in *COL11A2*, the gene encoding the alpha-2 (XI) chain of type XI collagen. J Pediatr 1998; 132:368–371.
5. McGuirt WT, et el. Mutations in *COL11A2* cause non-syndromic hearing loss (DFNA13). Nat Genet 1999; 23:413–419.
6. Kivirikko KI. Collagens and their abnormalities in a wide spectrum of diseases. Ann Med 1993; 25:113–126.
7. Ala-Kokko L, Prockop DJ. In: Kelly's Textbook of Rheumatology, 6th ed.
8. Vuoristo MM, et al. Complete structure of the human *COL11A2* gene: the exon sizes and other features indicate the gene has not evolved with genes for other fibriller collagens. Ann NY Acad Sci 1996; 785:343–344.
9. Spranger J. The type XI collagenopathies. Pediatr Radiol 1998; 28:745–750.
10. De Leenheer EM, Kunst HH, McGuirt WT, Prasad SD, Brown MR, Huygen PL, Smith RJ, Cremers CW. Autosomal dominant inherited hearing impairment caused by a missense mutation in *COL11A2* (DFNA13). Arch Otolaryngol Head Neck Surg 2001; 127(1):13–17.
11. Kunst H, Huybrechts C, Marres H, Huygen P, Van Camp G, Cremers C. The phenotype of DFNA13/*COL11A2*: nonsyndromic autosomal dominant midfrequency and high-frequency sensorineural hearing impairment. Am J Otol 2000; 21(2):181–187.

12. Li SW, Takanosu M, Arita M, Bao Y, Ren ZX, Maier A, Prockop DJ, Mayne R. Targeted disruption of *Col11a2* produces a mild cartilage phenotype in transgenic mice: comparison with the human disorder otospondylomegaepiphyseal dysplasia (OSMED). Dev Dyn 2001; 222(2):141–152.
13. Melkoniemi M, et al. Autosomal recessive disorder otospondylomegaepiphyseal dysplasia is associated with loss-of-function mutations in the *COL11A2* gene. Am J Hum Genet 2000; 66(2):368–377.

18
POU-Domain Transcription Factors

Ronna Hertzano and Karen B. Avraham
Sackler School of Medicine, Tel Aviv University, Tel Aviv, Israel

I. INTRODUCTION

The POU-domain genes encode for a family of transcription factors that regulate a multitude of processes and are expressed in all organ systems. This family consists of 15 known mammalian genes that are subgrouped into six families. The extensive research following their identification has created a vast body of knowledge concerning their structure, function, regulation, and interactions. A number of excellent reviews focus on different aspects of this gene family, including their role in embryonic development (1), in the neuroendocrine system (2), and in the nervous system (3).

Mutations in two different POU-domain transcription factor genes, *POU3F4* and *POU4F3*, are associated with human hereditary nonsyndromic hearing loss (NSHL). In this chapter we shall describe transcription factors in general, the POU-domain family of transcription factors, the POU genes associated with hearing loss, the proteins they encode, and their role in the pathogenesis of hearing loss.

II. TRANSCRIPTION FACTORS

Only a fraction of the 30,000 genes (4) estimated to be encoded by the mammalian genome are expressed at any given moment in any given cell type. It is the unique combination of proteins that are expressed in each cell type that gives rise to the phenotypic diversity of the tissues in our body. Transcription factors are proteins that, upon binding to a DNA segment in the nucleus, either induce or repress transcription of other genes, thus controlling the expression of other proteins.

Gene regulation in eukaryotes occurs at the level of transcriptional regulation, as well as RNA processing, mRNA stability, efficiency of translation of the mRNA into a polypeptide, and other posttranscriptional mechanisms. Transcriptional regulation involves binding of a general transcription machinery to the basal promoter that lies adjacent to the transcription start site, as well as binding of different transcription factors to specific DNA sequences that are at variable distances from the basal promoter (Fig. 1). The general transcription machinery consists of various proteins, among them transcription Factor IID, a multiprotein complex that binds to a DNA stretch containing an AT-rich region, named the TATA box. The specific transcription factors can bind to distant locations and probably draw the chromatin into a loop to establish protein-protein interactions with the basal promoter. The unique combination of transcription factors bound to the regulatory

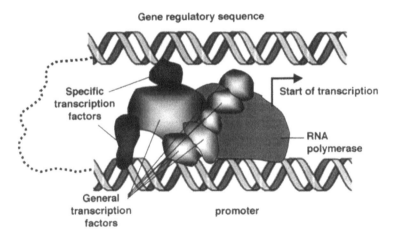

Figure 1 Eukaryotic gene expression depends on both general and specific transcription factors. The general transcription factors, which are the same for all genes, are involved in the positioning of the RNA polymerase II at the promoter; separation of the two DNA strands so that transcription can begin; and release of the RNA polymerase once transcription has begun. Specific transcription factors, such as the POU-domain transcription factors, can bind to regulatory sequences at a variable distance from the promoter, even thousands of base pairs away. Regulation of spatiotemporal gene expression is mediated by the combination of specific transcription factors bound the regulatory sequences of a gene and their interaction with the proteins at its promoter. (Adapted with permission from Ref. 67.)

regions of a gene determines whether its transcription will be turned on or off in a particular cell at any given time.

Transcription factors can be classified according to the structure of their DNA-binding domain (e.g., helix-turn-helix, helix-loop-helix, zinc fingers, and leucine zipper), their function in transcriptional regulation (e.g., activation, coactivation, repression and corepression, architectural factors, chromatin remodeling factors, and transcription elongation factors), as well as their spatiotemporal expression and involvement in specific roles in the cell cycle, cell identity and fate, developmental processes, hormone response, and more. The transcription factors themselves are regulated by modifications induced by other genes, such as kinases or phosphatases, to name a few. Most important, different transcription factors from the same family can have similar but distinct functions.

Most transcription factors regulate the expression of a myriad of genes. It is therefore not surprising that mutations in transcription factors cause a multitude of diseases. Many of these mutations affect more than one organ system, resulting in a syndrome (reviewed in Ref. 5). As key regulators of developmental processes, any of their identified targets can illuminate the pathways of cell commitment and maturation as well as represent valid candidate genes for similar or more restricted diseases (e.g., Ref. 6). A well-characterized example is that of the SOX10 pathway. Mutations in *SOX10*, a transcription modulator, underlie Shah-Waardenburg syndrome (OMIM #277580, http://www.ncbi.nlm.nih.gov/Omim), a neurocristopathy that associates intestinal aganglionosis, pigmentation defects, and sensorineural deafness (7). *GJB1* (gap junction beta 1) encodes the human connexin 32 protein and is a downstream target of *SOX10*. Both mutations in this gene, and a recently reported mutation in the promoter of this gene, underlie an autosomal dominant demyelinating disease, an X-linked form of Charcot-Marie-Tooth disease (OMIM #302800) (8). Other targets of SOX10, *PAX3* and *MITF*, cause different subtypes of Waardenburg syndrome (WS type I, OMIM #193500; WS type IIA, OMIM #193510), a disease with auditory-pigmentary abnormalities (9,10).

A selection of transcription factors play a role in pivotal steps of cell fate decision and differentiation in the mammalian inner ear, as can be learned from both mouse mutants and human disease genes (reviewed in Ref. 11). For example, the basic helix-loop-helix (bHLH) genes neurogenin-1 (*Ngn-1*) and *NeuroD* are essential for the formation of the otic ganglion (12–14), while mutations in the zinc finger protein *GATA3* cause hypomorphic development of the VIIIth cranial nerve and the whole inner ear (15). The bHLH transcription factor *Math1* is required for hair cell fate specification in mice and ectopic expression of this protein in the rat results in the development of supernumerary hair cells (16), while the sensory epithelium of a mouse knockout model of this gene never develops hair cells (17). Gene-targeted muta-genesis of another group of bHLH proteins, the hairy/enhancer of split (*Hes*) transcriptional repressors, leads to supernumerary inner and outer hair cells in *Hes1* and *Hes5* mutants, respectively (18). Last but not least, mutations in the *Pou3f4* and *Pou4f3* genes cause deafness and distinct inner ear pheno-types, as will be further discussed.

III. THE POU FAMILY OF TRANSCRIPTION FACTORS

The POU-domain family of transcription factors was identified on the basis of amino acid sequence homology in the DNA-binding domain of the tran-scription factors PIT1/GHF1, OCT1 and OCT2, and UNC86 (19). PIT1/ GHF1 is involved in controlling transcription of the growth hormone, prolactin, and other pituitary-specific genes. OCT1 activates transcription of histone H2B genes and OCT2 activates immunoglobulin genes transcrip-tion in B lymphocytes. UNC86 is a protein that determines neuroblast fate in the nematode *Caenorhabditis elegans* (20,21). Since the discovery of the first POU-domain proteins, many additional proteins have been identified in this family, sharing high sequence homology within the POU domain and differing substantially elsewhere (2). The POU domain consists of 147–156 amino acids and is comprised of two distinct DNA binding domains: a 69–78-amino-acid POU-specific domain located amino terminal to a 60-amino-acid POU homeodomain (22) (Fig. 2). The two POU domains are separated by a variable linker, a flexible stretch of amino acids that increases the repertoire of the specific sequences to which these proteins can bind to and improves the kinetics of the binding (reviewed in Ref. 23).

The three-dimensional structure of the Oct-1 POU-domain protein was the first to be resolved and shed some light on the protein-DNA interactions of this bipartite DNA-binding domain family (24,25). The POU-specific domain contains four alpha-helices surrounding a hydrophobic core, with the second and third comprising a helix-turn-helix motif. The POU-domain homeodomain motif is a homeodomain DNA-binding domain consisting of three alpha helices, creating a helix-turn-helix tertiary structure. This domain is part of the homeodomain family of transcription factors, DNA-binding motifs. Nevertheless, unlike the other transcription factors within this group (e.g., Hox and engrailed), both the POU-specific domain and POU homeo-domain are required for high-affinity sequence-specific DNA binding (26). This is done via the third helix of the POU homeodomain and the third helix of the POU-specific domain, both binding to the major groove of the DNA alpha-helix structure.

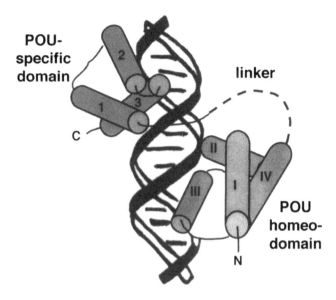

POU-specific domain

linker

POU homeo-domain

Figure 2   POU-domain transcription factors contain a bipartite DNA-binding domain, comprised of a POU-specific domain and a POU homeodomain, separated by a variable linker. A model of the position of the POU domains on DNA. The POU-specific domain contacts the DNA opposite from the POU homeodomain in the adjacent major groove. (Adapted with permission from Ref. 68.)

A.   The POU-Domain Class III Transcription Factors

The class III of POU-domain genes was identified after the initial definition of this transcription factor family. The genes of this class were identified using the polymerase chain reaction (PCR) and degenerate oligonucleotides representing codons of the nine conserved amino acids in the original POU genes. Initially, three POU-domain class III genes were isolated from cDNA derived from human brain and rat brain and testes, namely, Pou3f1 (also named Tst-1, Oct-6, SCIP, or Otf-6), Pou3f2 (also named Brn-2, N-Oct3, N-Oct5, or Otf-7), and Pou3f3 (also named Brn-1 or Otf-8) (27). The fourth member of this group, Pou3f4 (also named Brn-4, RHS2, N-Oct4, or Otf-9), was the thirteenth POU domain protein to be identified in mammals, this time via screening of a rat hypothalamic cDNA library using the Brn-2 POU domain as a probe (28). POU domain class III transcription factors have also been identified in *Drosophila melanogaster* (29), *C. elegans* (30), *Xenopus laevis* (31), *Danio rerio* (zebrafish) (32), and metazoans (33). All mammalian class III

POU-domain transcription factors are broadly expressed within the developing nervous system and assume more restricted expression patterns in the adult nervous system. Mouse knockout models for genes in this group reveal both the redundant and unique functions of these genes. For example, the functional redundancy of these genes is demonstrated by the fact that while they are broadly expressed in the neural tube, only a few neural cell types are affected in single knockout mutants. The unique functions are demonstrated by the distinct phenotypes. For example, Pou3f1 knockout mice suffer from a defect in the terminal differentiation of the Schwann cells resulting in defective peripheral myelination (34,35). Pou3f2 knockout mice do not survive beyond postnatal day 10, most probably owing to a critical loss of neurons within the hypothalamus (36). Among other abnormalities, Pou3f3 knockout mice show defects in cortical neuron migration limited in distribution to the hippocampus and extending to the entire neocortex in the Pou3f2/Pou3f3 double-knockout mice (37). Finally, Pou3f4 knockout mice suffer from an inner ear developmental defect (see Sec. III.A.2).

During development, Pou3f4 is first expressed at embryonic day (E)9.5 in the neural tube, and then in the otic capsule, the hindbrain, and the branchial arch mesenchyme (38) (Fig. 3). Pou3f4 is also expressed in the cochlea, vestibular apparatus, whisker follicles, lateral nasal recess, and cells of the pancreas (39). Although both human patients and mouse mutants suffer from defects in the formation of the bony architecture of the middle ear, the Pou3f4 protein is not expressed in the stapes. Rather, its expression in the ear is limited to the mesenchyme and the otic capsule, including the region surrounding

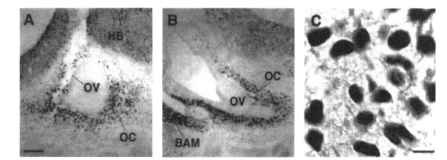

Figure 3 Immunohistochemical analyses of Pou3f4 expression during early stages of inner ear development. (A) Pou3f4 is expressed in the otic capsule (OC) and the hindbrain (HB) of a section in an E10.5 embryo. (B) Pou3f4 is expressed in the OC, HB, and in the branchial arch mesenchyme (BAM) at E11.5. (C) Pou3f4 is localized predominantly to the nucleus. OV, otic vesicle. Scale bar = 100 μm (A and B) and 5 μm (C). (Modified by permission from Ref. 38.)

the stapes, and to fibrocytes within the cochlear duct (38). Notably, the subcellular localization of the protein shifts to the cytoplasm in areas of mesenchymal remodeling that will further develop to acellular structures, demonstrating a potential mechanism for crucial silencing of the gene during normal otic development.

1. Mutations in POU3F4 Lead to DFN3 X-Linked Mixed Deafness

Identification of the POU3F4 *Mutations.* The *DFN3* locus (OMIM #304400) defines the third deafness locus to be identified on chromosome X. Although X-linked inheritance is relatively rare for nonsyndromic hearing loss (approximately 1% of inherited deafness), at least 50 DFN3 families have been identified. The DFN3 phenotype is variable, and at the very least it is characterized by profound sensorineural hearing loss. DFN3 is also often associated with conductive hearing loss and with stapes fixation. The first documented clinical description of a DFN3 family was described in 1967, and the gene for this locus was cloned almost 30 years later, in 1995 (40). This locus was initially described as a syndrome, since it is often associated with stapes fixation that may lead to a perilymphatic gusher upon surgery (gusher-deafness syndrome). Furthermore, as DFN3 maps to chromosome Xq21 in the region containing mental retardation and choroideremia as well, some patients with *POU3F4* mutations have additional symptoms due to deletions of larger portions of the chromosome. In 1988, a number of reports were published describing the mapping of the *DFN3* locus to chromosome Xq13–q21.1 (e.g., see Ref. 41). DFN3 was then localized to a 500-kb region on Xq21.1. containing the *POU3F4* gene (40). Small mutations in five unrelated individuals were identified in the coding region of this transcription factor, leading to either protein truncations or nonconservative amino acid substitutions. This established *POU3F4* as the causative gene for DFN3, and subsequently additional point mutations were identified (e.g., Ref. 42). But this left the larger deletions, duplications, and inversions of this region unexplained (43,44). These deletions account for a little over half of *DFN3* mutations and many of them do not encompass the *POU3F4* coding region (Fig. 4). A detailed molecular analysis of the region proximal to the *POU3F4* gene revealed small deletions 900 kb proximal to the gene that are associated with DFN3 deafness (44). It was suggested that the DNF3 phenotype, without coding region mutations, could be caused by the loss of the *POU3F4* enhancer, repressor, or promoter.

Clinical Phenotype of DFN3. All males with *POU3F4* deafness have profound sensorineural hearing loss, which is often accompanied by conductive hearing loss. Obligate female carriers may or may not have hearing

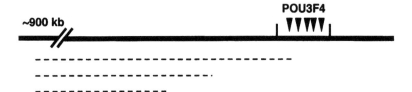

Figure 4   X-linked DFN3 is associated with mutations in the class III *POU3F4* gene. Mutations in *POU3F4* have been found both in the ~ 1 kb intronless coding region of the gene, and outside of the coding region. Deletions, inversions, and rearrangments, as far as 900 kb from the coding region, are associated with DFN3 deafness. The deletions found range in size from 8 kb to several megabases, and in some cases include the *POU3F4* coding region. Both missense and nonsense mutations have been identified in the coding region; most of the missense mutations occur in the POU homeodomain. Dashed lines indicate a few deletions; arrowheads indicate a few small substitutions and deletions in the coding region.

loss, though, when present, it is mild to moderate. Prior to the identification of the *POU3F4* mutation in DFN3, high-resolution CT scanning of individuals with X-linked deafness revealed inner ear abnormalities (45). These included a widened bulbous internal auditory meatus (IAM) and a reduced or absent bone between the lateral end of the IAM and the basal turn of the cochlea. Once *POU3F4* mutations were identified, this radiological phenotype was confirmed in DFN3 patients (Fig. 5) (42). The clinical findings included bulbous and foreshortened IAMs, widening of the labyrinth portion of the fallopian canal, and abnormal basal portion of the modiolus. It was suggested

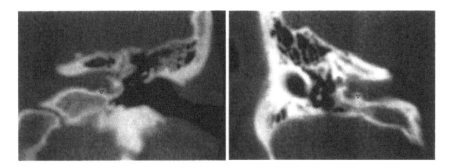

Figure 5   High-resolution computed tomography (CT) from an individual with a *POU3F4* mutation. The CT reveals abnormalities of the cochlear modiolus (arrowheads). (Reproduced with permission from Ref. 42.)

at the time that the malformations seen are consistent with there being a space between the IAM and perilymph that may lead to the perilymphatic hydrops and gusher upon stapes surgery. Since then, however, the mouse knockout has revealed another reason for the hydrops, namely that it may be due to the loss of fibrocytes in the spiral limbus, as observed in the Pou3f4 knockout (see Sec. III.A.2). The observation of this Mondini-like dysplasia of the inner ear suggests that a defect occurs between embryonic days 25 and 47 of human inner ear development (43).

2. Mouse Models for *Pou3f4* Mutations

Three mouse mutants are available for the study of the DFN3 ear phenotype. These mutants differ in both their phenotypes and the molecular mechanisms used for the silencing of the *Pou3f4* gene. The first reported targeted null allele of the *Pou3f4* gene was generated by replacing the coding sequence of the intronless *Pou3f4* gene with a *LacZ* gene and a PGK-Neo resistance cassette, through homologous recombination of embryonic stem cells (ES) (46). The expression of the LacZ protein can be visualized using a biochemical assay based on 5-bromo-4-chloro-3-indolyl-β-D-galactopyranoside (X-gal). The insertion of a *LacZ* gene under the same regulatory elements of the replaced gene creates a powerful tool for studying the expression of the replaced gene. The resulting mutant lacked *Pou3f4* gene expression in all mouse tissues in which it is known to be expressed. Shortly thereafter the same group reported the phenotype of an X-ray-induced mouse mutant, sex-linked fidget (*slf*).

Interestingly, while there is no Pou3f4 expression in the inner ear of these mice, *Pou3f4* expression in the neural tube remains normal (47). This silencing of inner ear expression is caused by a chromosomal inversion whose breakpoint lies at least a 6–10-kb stretch upstream of the *Pou3f4* coding sequence, most probably separating the *Pou3f4* gene from its inner ear–specific transcriptional regulation elements. The above two models showed indistinguishable inner ear phenotypes consisting of mild hearing loss and vertical head bobbing. The mutant mice suffered a few cochlear and temporal bone abnormalities (Fig. 6), including a constricted superior semicircular canal, widening of the internal auditory meatus, thinning of various structures in the temporal bone, a misshaped stapes footplate, and a shortening of the cochlea, demonstrated as a reduction in the number of cochlear coils in most of the mutants. In addition, the mice had a generally hypoplastic cochlea, with widening of the scala tympani, and dysplasia of fibrocytes in the spiral limbus, which may lead to the hydrops observed in these animals. Notably, no structural abnormalities were observed in the organ of Corti. Bearing in mind that the *Pou3f4* protein is expressed in mesenchymal tissue (38), the authors concluded that the widened structures result from disruption

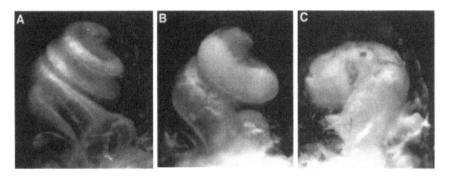

Figure 6 Cochlear hypoplasia of Pou3f4 knockout mice is demonstrated in these cleared temporal bone preparations. Cochleae from mutant mice display a reduced number of turns, which can vary from mouse to mouse and even between ears of one animal. (A) One and three-quarter turns are seen in a cochlea from a wild-type mouse. (B) The left cochlea of a mutant mouse with one and one-half turns. (C) The right cochlea of the same mutant mouse with less than one coil. (Reproduced with permission from Ref. 46.)

of mesenchymal remodeling, the shortening of the cochlea from disruption of epithelial-mesenchymal interactions, and the misshaping of the stapes from disruption of mesenchymal-mesenchymal interactions. This phenotype resembles the temporal bone phenotype of the people suffering from *POU3F4* mutations.

In contrast, the third mouse model created by a targeted deletion of the *Pou3f4* gene on a different genetic background showed no gross temporal or inner ear defect, nor in the neuroepithelium or cochlear length, while the mice displayed profound deafness and a reduced endocochlear potential (48). A transmission electron microscopy (TEM) study of these mice ears revealed ultrastructural differences in type I and type II fibrocytes that line the stria vascularis. Type I fibrocytes had fewer mitochondria and a relatively sparse surrounding mesenchyme, while type II fibrocytes suffered from a dramatically reduced number of mitochondria, a small cytoplasmic volume, and fewer cytoplasmic extensions. Both cell types are hypothesized to be involved in potassium recycling back to the endolymph (49).

B. The POU-Domain Class IV Transcription Factors

The first class IV POU-domain gene to be identified was *unc-86*, a neuronal-specific gene that is expressed in 57 of the 302 neurons in the adult nematode, *C. elegans* (50). UNC-86 protein is required for both the generation and differentiation of all six mechanosensory neurons, and loss of function mutations in *unc-86* result in a loss of the animal's ability to respond to mechanical stimulation. Since that time, class IV POU-domain proteins have been found in *Xenopus* (51), metazoans (33), and zebrafish (52). The mammalian POU-domain class IV consists of three members, namely Pou4f1 (also named Brn3a or Brn3.0), Pou4f2 (also named Brn3b or Brn3.2), and Pou4f3 (also named Brn3c or Brn3.1). This family of transcription factors was isolated using a degenerate reverse transcriptase (RT)-PCR approach (27) and then shown to be encoded by three independent genes (53,54). The class IV POU-domain proteins share high sequence similarity in their DNA-binding domains and recognition properties (53). However, in their N-terminal transactivation domains, they diverge substantially.

These three transcription factors are all expressed in cells from a neuronal origin, including the dorsal root ganglia, the retina, the inner ear, and the spinal cord. The cell type in which each gene is first expressed is associated with the most severe phenotype for that gene (54). Thus, *Pou4f1*, as the first gene within the group to be expressed in the spiral, vestibular, and geniculate ganglia, has a severe and perinatally lethal phenotype in knockout mice, including ineffective swallowing and mechanosensory defects, differential loss of neurons, defects in their migration, and reduction of neuronal soma size in these three ganglia (55–57). *Pou4f2* is first among the three to be expressed in the retinal ganglion cells and the knockout phenotype consists of a loss of approximately 60–70% of the retinal ganglion cells and defective retinal axon pathfinding (54,58,59). Mutations in the *Pou4f3* gene, which is the first reported gene among this group to be expressed in the inner ear hair cells (58), result in profound hearing loss and circling (Fig. 7).

The high similarity of these transcription factors and the critical role of their spatiotemporal control are further delineated by the fact that at least in the retina, all three class IV POU-domain proteins have a similar ability to promote retinal ganglion cell development upon misexpression (60). Nevertheless, although all three transcription factors of this group are expressed in the mammalian inner ear, to date, only mutations in the *POU4F3* gene have been associated with human hereditary hearing loss or human disease overall.

1. Mutations in *POU4F3* Lead to DFNA15 Autosomal Dominant Deafness

Identification of the POU4F3 *Mutation.* The *DFNA15* locus (OMIM #602459) defines the fifteenth dominant deafness locus to be identified, based on a large Israeli Jewish family with autosomal dominant nonsyndromic sensorineural hearing loss. A mutation in the *POU4F3* gene is associated with hearing loss in this family, named Family H (Fig. 8). Affected members of

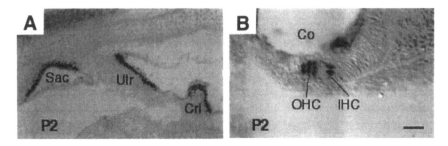

Figure 7 Immunohistochemistry with Pou4f3 antibodies reveals that Pou4f3 protein is expressed at postnatal day 2 (P2) in the sensory epithelia of the cochlea and vestibular apparatus. (A) Expression in the hair cells of the saccule (Sac), utricle (Utr), and crista (Cri). (B) Expression in the outer hair cells (OHC) and inner hair cells (IHC) of the cochlea (Co). Scale bar = 25 μm. (Reproduced with permission from Ref. 65.)

Family H suffer from progressive hearing loss that begins in the third decade of life. The genetic basis of hearing loss in this family was studied with the intention of mapping and identifying the mutated gene associated with hearing loss. This was a project that could potentially take years, but owing to advantages offered by the mouse as a research tool and technical advances in human genomics, the *DFNA15* gene was cloned in just 1 year (61). The first individual reported to lose his hearing prematurely was born in 1843 in Libya. Eventually the family migrated to Israel, settling in Tunisia and Egypt along the way. A genetic linkage study was performed on 12 affected and 11 unaffected individuals. Since only 13 dominant loci were known at the time this study was initiated, markers flanking these loci were genotyped to

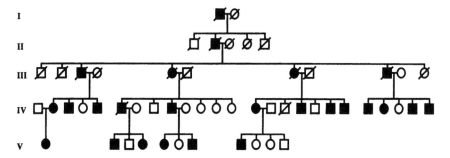

Figure 8 Pedigree of Israeli Family H showing affected (filled) and unaffected (unfilled) individuals over the age of 30. Inheritance is dominant, affecting females (circles) and males (squares) in equal proportion.

determine if deafness in Family H mapped to a chromosomal region already known to harbor a gene for hearing loss. Linkage was found to 5q31–q33, close to *DFNA1*, the first locus mapped for dominant, nonsyndromic deafness (62), but further genotyping confirmed linkage of deafness in Family H to markers distal (toward the telomere) to *DFNA1*.

Therefore, the new deafness locus was defined as *DFNA15*. Examination of this chromosomal region in humans did not reveal any interesting candidates. However, an ideal candidate was identified on mouse chromosome 18 in the region of homology to 5q31. There were two compelling reasons why the *Pou4f3* gene was a good candidate for deafness in Family H. First, targeted deletion of the entire *Pou4f3* gene leads to vestibular dysfunction and profound deafness in the knockout mice (58,63). Second, expression of murine *Pou4f3* is restricted to the cochlear and vestibular hair cells of the inner ear. Primers spanning the human gene were designed and DNA from both unaffected and affected Family H members was amplified. In hearing-impaired members of Family H, an 8-bp deletion was identified in the 3′ portion of human *POU4F3*. This deletion leads to a frameshift, causing a stop codon to be formed prematurely (Fig. 9). Presumably a truncated protein is formed, which might still have the capacity to bind to DNA, though at a lower affinity owing to the loss of the POU-specific domain and a large portion of the POU homeodomain.

Clinical Phenotype of DFNA15. A clinical study of the auditory phenotype of affected members of Family H was performed that indicated that *POU4F3* mutation-associated deafness cannot be identified through clinical evaluation, but only through molecular analysis (42,64). Hearing was measured by pure-tone audiometry (Fig. 10) on all participating relatives of Family H for whom the genome scan was performed. The thresholds were compared to the age- and gender-related median of normal-hearing standards. All individuals with a *POU4F3* mutation and who were above the age of 40 exhibited sensorineural bilateral hearing loss, ranging from mild to severe hearing loss. The shape of the audiograms ranged from flat to a sloping curve. There was no one typical audiogram for affected members of this family.

No sequential audiograms were available, although the affected individuals complained of progressive hearing loss. The rate of progression, designated as annual threshold deterioration (ATD), was calculated using cross-sectional linear regression analyses to be approximately 1.1 dB/year at 0.25–1 kHz and about 2.1 dB/year at 2–4 kHz. Correction of the hearing threshold for (median) presbyacusis was performed as well, and the results show that the hearing loss caused by the *POU4F3* mutation is progressive beyond (normal) presbyacusis. Normal ABR suggests a functional central

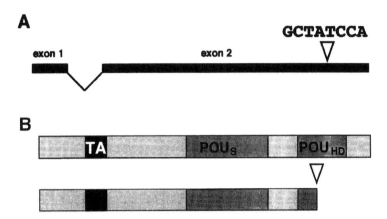

Figure 9 (A) The human *POU4F3* mutation occurs on one allele and is an 8-bp deletion in exon 2. (B) This region codes for the first alpha-helix domain of the homeodomain. The deletion forms a frameshift that produces novel amino acids and then forms a stop codon. A truncated protein is presumably translated that either prevents the wild-type form of the protein from functioning properly or causes hair cell damage on its own. TA, transactivation domain; POU$_S$, POU-specific domain; POU$_{HD}$, POU homeodomain.

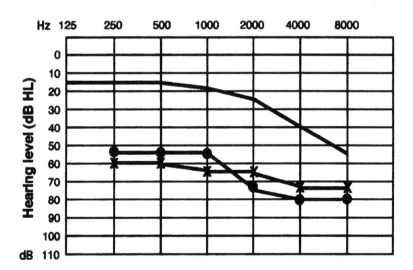

Figure 10 Hearing loss in Family H is sensorineural, affecting all frequencies by the age of 40. A representative pure-tone audiogram is shown. X, left ear; O, right ear. The unmarked line represents the age- and sex-related median of normal hearing set by the International Organization for Standardization (ISO) 7029 standard (69). (Reproduced with permission from Ref. 61.)

auditory pathway in hearing-impaired individuals with *POU4F3* mutations. Furthermore, otoacoustic emission testing (OAE) suggests that the OHCs are malfunctioning, which is consistent with *POU4F3* expression in the OHC. The clinical parameters tested demonstrate that the hearing loss due to the Family H *POU4F3* mutation is progressive, bilateral, and sensorineural. However, intrafamilial variability suggests that other genetic or environmental factors may modify the age of onset and rate of progression.

2. Mouse Models for *Pou4f3* Mutations

While very little is known to date about the bona fide targets of *Pou4f3*, the biology of the mutants of this gene can teach us a great deal about the potential cellular roles and biochemical interactions of this protein. Within the inner ear, the mammalian Pou4f3 is a hair-cell-specific protein. Pou4f3 protein expression is first noticed in scattered cells of the presumptive sensory epithelium as early as mouse E12.5 (63). By E14.5 and E15.5, when all sensory epithelia are formed (organ of Corti, saccule, utricle, and crista ampullaris), it is expressed in the hair cells of these epithelia, limited only to postmitotic hair cells. This expression pattern persists through adulthood (65).

Four mouse models are available for the study of the *Pou4f3* gene. Three groups have generated *Pou4f3* knockout mice (54,58,63), on top of an existing spontaneous mouse mutant, the dreidel (*ddl*) mouse. The *ddl* mouse mutant arose in 1995 as a phenotypic deviant at the Jackson Laboratory (Bar Harbor, Maine, USA) and was mapped to the same genetic location as the *Pou4f3* gene (http://www.informatics.jax.org/). A "TG" dinucleotide deletion was found, resulting in a premature stop codon upstream of the Pou4f3 DNA-binding domains.

The *Pou4f3* mutants suffer from congenital deafness and profound vestibular dysfunction, demonstrated by no auditory brainstem response at any level up to 114 dB SPL, hyperactivity, circling, and an inability to walk on a horizontal drum or tumbling when placed in water. The *Pou4f3* knockout phenotype is recessive, and heterozygous animals are indistinguishable from the wild types. Their viability is reported to be normal; however, most mutants are 10–20% smaller than wild type and some laboratories report that the animals suffer from low fertility (63). The most striking feature in the inner ears of the *Pou4f3* mutant mice is missing hair bundles in all of the sensory patches (Fig. 11). In the adult mice it is caused from a lack of hair cells in these patches. Instead, the sensory epithelium of the cochlea consist of a single layer of supporting cells, most probably of Hensen cells, rudimentary or variable presentation of Deiter's and Pillar cells. The vestibular system is missing the type I hair cells and both systems suffer from a secondary loss of innervation of the sensory epithelium and myelinated axons. The bony

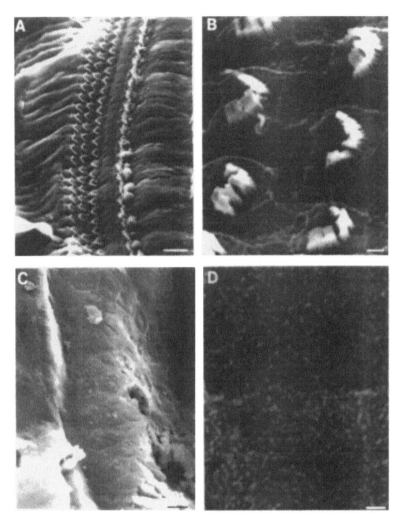

Figure 11 Scanning electron microscopy (SEM) of the organ of Corti reveals Pou4f3 knockout mouse abnormalities. (A, B) Stereocilia bundles of outer hair cells (OHC) and inner hair cells (IHC) are shown from a wild-type mouse. (C, D) There are no stereocilia bundles on the apical surface of the organ of Corti derived from Pou4f3 mutant mice. Scale bar = 10 μm (A and C) and 1 μm (B and D). (Reproduced with permission from Ref. 63.)

architecture and semicircular canal arrangement are normal (56). However, unlike the *Math1* knockout mice that never form hair cells to begin with (17), a careful look into the ears of the *Pou4f3* mutant mice at E16.5 reveals hair cell–like cells that stain positively for hair cell–specific markers such as myosin VI and myosin VIIa (65). These cells are slightly reduced in number compared with the heterozygote control, and some cells expressing hair cell markers are observed in the supporting cell layer, suggesting defective cell migration. However, all hair cells in the *Pou4f3* mutant mice are devoid of stereocilia. By E18.5, the number of hair cell–like cells reduces in the vestibular system to about 25% and by P4 even less hair cells are left. A rapid loss of the vestibular and spiral ganglia occurs as well, all dying via apoptosis (65).

IV. CONCLUDING REMARKS

The POU-domain family of transcription factors play a role in both X-linked and autosomal dominant human hereditary NSHL. While the discovery of *POU3F4* mutations in DFN3 human deafness led to the production of a mouse knockout and a study of this gene in mouse inner ear development, a detailed analysis of *Pou4f3* in the mouse preceded and actually facilitated the discovery of the human *POU4F3* human mutation. The two genes belong to the same family of transcription factors, but they are expressed in distinct cell types and time points, and their respective affected structures do not overlap.

The extensive study of the *Pou3f4* and *Pou4f3* mouse mutants sheds some light on the formation of the inner ear, as well as hair cell differentiation and survival. Compelling areas of further research include the elucidation of *POU3F4* upstream regulatory elements that are compromised in DFN3-associated deafness. There is also a need to identify the in vivo targets that take part in the mesenchymal-epithelial and mesenchymal-mesenchymal cross-talk in the formation of the otic capsule and other structures of the inner ear. The specific sequences that drive both *Pou3f4* and *Pou4f3* expression to the inner ear are yet to be found. Furthermore, the elucidation of the downstream targets for both these transcription factors, crucial for inner ear development and hair cell survival, is a key step in understanding the molecular basis of POU-domain transcription factor-associated hearing loss. With the publication of the human, mouse, and other genome sequences, as well as the development of tools for rapid characterization of global gene expression [such as microarrays (66)], these specific questions, crucial for understanding the biology and development of the inner ear, are more likely to be answered. All of these elements will aid in the development of potential remedies both for congenital deafness and for age-related hearing loss (presbycusis) affecting the majority of the elderly population.

ACKNOWLEDGMENTS

We wish to thank the many scientists who have contributed to work described in this chapter. We would like to thank E. Bryan Crenshaw III, Menging Xiang, and Nathan Fischel-Ghodsian for comments and figures. Research in our laboratory is supported by the European Commission (QLG2-1999-00988), the NIH/Fogarty International Center (Grant 1 R03 TW01108-01), the F.I.R.S.T. Foundation of the Israel Academy of Sciences and Humanities, the Israel Ministry of Science, Culture, and Sport, and the Israel Ministry of Health.

REFERENCES

1. Veenstra GJ, van der Vliet PC, Destree OH. POU domain transcription factors in embryonic development. Mol Biol Rep 1997; 24:139–155.
2. Andersen B, Rosenfeld MG. POU domain factors in the neuroendocrine system: lessons from developmental biology provide insights into human disease. Endocr Rev 2001; 22:2–35.
3. Latchman DS. POU family transcription factors in the nervous system. J Cell Physiol 1999; 179:126–133.
4. Lander ES, Linton LM, Birren B, et al. Initial sequencing and analysis of the human genome. Nature 2001; 409:860–921.
5. Semenza G.Transcription Factors and Human Disease. New York: Oxford University Press, 1998.
6. Tachibana M. A cascade of genes related to Waardenburg syndrome. J Invest Dermatol Symp Proc 1999; 4:126–129.
7. Shah KN, Dalal SJ, Desai MP, Sheth PN, Joshi NC, Ambani LM. White forelock, pigmentary disorder of irides, and long segment Hirschsprung disease: possible variant of Waardenburg syndrome. J Pediatr 1981; 99:432–435.
8. Bondurand N, Girard M, Pingault V, Lemort N, Dubourg O, Goossens M. Human connexin 32, a gap junction protein altered in the X-linked form of Charcot-Marie-Tooth disease, is directly regulated by the transcription factor SOX10. Hum Mol Genet 2001; 10:2783–2795.
9. Tassabehji M, Read AP, Newton VE, Harris R, Balling R, Gruss P, Strachan T. Waardenburg's syndrome patients have mutations in the human homologue of the *Pax-3* paired box gene. Nature 1992; 355:635–636.
10. Tassabehji M, Newton VE, Read AP. Waardenburg syndrome type 2 caused by mutations in the human microphthalmia (*MITF*) gene. Nat Genet 1994; 8:251–255.
11. Fekete DM, Wu DK. Revisiting cell fate specification in the inner ear. Curr Opin Neurobiol 2002; 12:35–42.
12. Ma Q, Anderson DJ, Fritzsch B. Neurogenin 1 null mutant ears develop fewer,

morphologically normal hair cell in smaller sensory epithelia devoid of innevation. J Assoc Res Otolaryngol 2000; 1:129–143.

13. Liu M, Pereira FA, Price SD, Chu MJ, Shope C, Himes D, Eatock RA, Brownell WE, Lysakowski A, Tsai MJ. Essential role of BETA2/NeuroD1 in development of the vestibular and auditory systems. Genes Dev 2000; 14:2839–2854.

14. Kim WY, Fritzsch B, Serls A, Bakel LA, Huang EJ, Reichardt LF, Barth DS, Lee JE. NeuroD-null mice are deaf due to a severe loss of the inner ear sensory neurons during development. Development 2001; 128:417–426.

15. Karis A, Pata I, van Doorninck JH, Grosveld F, de Zeeuw CI, de Caprona D, Fritzsch B. Transcription factor GATA-3 alters pathway selection of olivoco-chlear neurons and affects morphogenesis of the ear. J Comp Neurol 2001; 429:615–630.

16. Zheng JL, Gao WQ. Overexpression of Math1 induces robust production of extra hair cells in postnatal rat inner ears. Nat Neurosci 2000; 3:580–586.

17. Bermingham NA, Hassan BA, Price SD, Vollrath MA, Ben-Arie N, Eatock RA, Bellen HJ, Lysakowski A, Zoghbi HY. *Math1*: an essential gene for the generation of inner ear hair cells. Science 1999; 284:1837–1841.

18. Zine A, Aubert A, Qiu J, Therianos S, Guillemot F, Kageyama R, de Ribaupierre F. Hes1 and Hes5 activities are required for the normal development of the hair cells in the mammalian inner ear. J Neurosci 2001; 21:4712–4720.

19. Herr W, Sturm RA, Clerc RG, Corcoran LM, Baltimore D, Sharp PA, Ingraham HA, Rosenfeld MG, Finney M, Ruvkun G, et al. The POU domain: a large conserved region in the mammalian Pit-1, Oct-1, Oct-2, and *Caenorhabditis elegans unc-86* gene products. Genes Dev 1988; 2:1513–1516.

20. Finney M, Ruvkun G, Horvitz HR. The *C. elegans* cell lineage and differentiation gene unc-86 encodes a protein with a homeodomain and extended similarity to transcription factors. Cell 1988; 55:757–769.

21. Finney M, Ruvkun G. The *unc-86* gene product couples cell lineage and cell identity in *C. elegans*. Cell 1990; 63:895–905.

22. Rosenfeld MG. POU-domain transcription factors: pou-er-ful developmental regulators. Genes Dev 1991; 5:897–907.

23. Phillips K, Luisi B. The virtuoso of versatility: POU proteins that flex to fit. J Mol Biol 2000; 302:1023–1039.

24. Klemm JD, Rould MA, Aurora R, Herr W, Pabo CO. Crystal structure of the Oct-1 POU domain bound to an octamer site: DNA recognition with tethered DNA-binding modules. Cell 1994; 77:21–32.

25. Assa-Munt N, Mortishire-Smith RJ, Aurora R, Herr W, Wright PE. The solution structure of the Oct-1 POU-specific domain reveals a similarity to the bacteriophage lambda repressor DNA-binding domain. Cell 1993; 73:193–205.

26. Verrijzer CP, Alkema MJ, van Weperen WW, Van Leeuwen HC, Strating MJ, van der Vliet PC. The DNA binding specificity of the bipartite POU domain and its subdomains. EMBO J 1992; 11:4993–5003.

27. He X, Treacy MN, Simmons DM, Ingraham HA, Swanson LW, Rosenfeld MG. Expression of a large family of POU-domain regulatory genes in mammalian brain development. Nature 1989; 340:35–41.

28. Mathis JM, Simmons DM, He X, Swanson LW, Rosenfeld MG. Brain 4: a novel mammalian POU domain transcription factor exhibiting restricted brain-specific expression. EMBO J 1992; 11:2551–2561.

29. Johnson WA, Hirsh J. Binding of a *Drosophila* POU-domain protein to a sequence element regulating gene expression in specific dopaminergic neurons. Nature 1990; 343:467–470.

30. Burglin TR, Finney M, Coulson A, Ruvkun G. *Caenorhabditis elegans* has scores of homoeobox-containing genes. Nature 1989; 341:239–243.

31. Agarwal VR, Sato SM. *XLPOU 1* and *XLPOU 2*, two novel POU domain genes expressed in the dorsoanterior region of *Xenopus embryos*. Dev Biol 1991; 147:363–373.

32. Matsuzaki T, Amanuma H, Takeda H. A POU-domain gene of zebrafish, *ZFPOU1*, specifically expressed in the developing neural tissues. Biochem Biophys Res Commun 1992; 187:1446–1453.

33. Shah D, Aurora D, Lance R, Stuart GW. POU genes in metazoans: homologs in sea anemones, snails, and earthworms. DNA Seq 2000; 11:457–461.

34. Bermingham JR Jr, Scherer SS, O'Connell S, Arroyo E, Kalla KA, Powell FL, Rosenfeld MG. Tst-1/Oct-6/SCIP regulates a unique step in peripheral myelination and is required for normal respiration. Genes Dev 1996; 10:1751–1762.

35. Jaegle M, Mandemakers W, Broos L, Zwart R, Karis A, Visser P, Grosveld F, Meijer D. The POU factor Oct-6 and Schwann cell differentiation. Science 1996; 273:507–510.

36. Nakai S, Kawano H, Yudate T, Nishi M, Kuno J, Nagata A, Jishage K, Hamada H, Fujii H, Kawamura K, et al. The POU domain transcription factor Brn-2 is required for the determination of specific neuronal lineages in the hypothalamus of the mouse. Genes Dev 1995; 9:3109–3121.

37. McEvilly RJ, de Diaz MO, Schonemann MD, Hooshmand F, Rosenfeld MG. Transcriptional regulation of cortical neuron migration by POU domain factors. Science 2002; 295:1528–1532.

38. Phippard D, Heydemann A, Lechner M, Lu L, Lee D, Kyin T, Crenshaw EB III. Changes in the subcellular localization of the *Brn4* gene product precede mesenchymal remodeling of the otic capsule. Hear Res 1998; 120:77–85.

39. Jensen J, Heller RS, Funder-Nielsen T, Pedersen EE, Lindsell C, Weinmaster G, Madsen OD, Serup P. Independent development of pancreatic alpha- and beta-cells from neurogenin3-expressing precursors: a role for the notch pathway in repression of premature differentiation. Diabetes 2000; 49:163–176.

40. de Kok YJ, van der Maarel SM, Bitner-Glindzicz M, Huber I, Monaco AP, Malcolm S, Pembrey ME, Ropers HH, Cremers F.P.. Association between X-linked mixed deafness and mutations in the POU domain gene *POU3F4*. Science 1995; 267:685–688.

41. Brunner HG, van Bennekom A, Lambermon EM, Oei TL, Cremers WR, Wieringa B, Ropers HH. The gene for X-linked progressive mixed deafness with perilymphatic gusher during stapes surgery (DFN3) is linked to PGK. Hum Genet 1988; 80:337–340.

42. Friedman RA, Bykhovskaya Y, Tu G, Talbot JM, Wilson DF, Parnes LS, Fis-

chel-Ghodsian N. Molecular analysis of the *POU3F4* gene in patients with clinical and radiographic evidence of X-linked mixed deafness with perilymphatic gusher. Ann Otol Rhinol Laryngol 1997; 106:320–325.

43. Piussan C, Hanauer A, Dahl N, Mathieu M, Kolski C, Biancalana V, Heyberger S, Strunski V. X-linked progressive mixed deafness: a new microdeletion that involves a more proximal region in Xq21. Am J Hum Genet 1995; 56:224–230.

44. de Kok YJ, Vossenaar ER, Cremers CW, et al. Identification of a hot spot for microdeletions in patients with X-linked deafness type 3 (DFN3) 900 kb proximal to the DFN3 gene *POU3F4*. Hum Mol Genet 1996; 5:1229–1235.

45. Phelps PD, Reardon W, Pembrey M, Bellman S, Luxom L. X-linked deafness, stapes gushers and a distinctive defect of the inner ear. Neuroradiology 1991; 33:326–330.

46. Phippard D, Lu L, Lee D, Saunders JC, Crenshaw EB III. Targeted mutagenesis of the POU-domain gene Brn4/Pou3f4 causes developmental defects in the inner ear. J Neurosci 1999; 19:5980–5989.

47. Phippard D, Boyd Y, Reed V, Fisher G, Masson WK, Evans EP, Saunders JC, Crenshaw EB III. The sex-linked fidget mutation abolishes Brn4/*Pou3f4* gene expression in the embryonic inner ear. Hum Mol Genet 2000; 9:79–85.

48. Minowa O, Ikeda K, Sugitani Y, Oshima T, Nakai S, Katori Y, Suzuki M, Furukawa M, Kawase T, Zheng Y, Ogura M, Asada Y, Watanabe K, Yamanaka H, Gotoh S, Nishi-Takeshima M, Sugimoto T, Kikuchi T, Takasaka T, Noda T. Altered cochlear fibrocytes in a mouse model of DFN3 nonsyndromic deafness. Science 1999; 285:1408–1411.

49. Spicer SS, Schulte BA. The fine structure of spiral ligament cells relates to ion return to the stria and varies with place-frequency. Hearing Res 1996; 100:80–100.

50. Finney M, Ruvkun G. The *unc-86* gene product couples cell lineage and cell identity in *C. elegans*. Cell 1990; 63:895–905.

51. Hutcheson DA, Vetter ML. The bHLH factors Xath5 and XNeuroD can upregulate the expression of XBrn3d, a POU-homeodomain transcription factor. Dev Biol 2001; 232:327–338.

52. Sampath K, Stuart GW. Developmental expression of class III and IV POU domain genes in the zebrafish. Biochem Biophys Res Commun 1996; 219:565–571.

53. Gruber CA, Rhee JM, Gleiberman A, Turner EE. POU domain factors of the Brn-3 class recognize functional DNA elements which are distinctive, symmetrical, and highly conserved in evolution. Mol Cell Biol 1997; 17:2391–2400.

54. Wang SW, Mu X, Bowers WJ, Kim DS, Plas DJ, Crair MC, Federoff HJ, Gan L, Klein WH. Brn3b/Brn3c double knockout mice reveal an unsuspected role for Brn3c in retinal ganglion cell axon outgrowth. Development 2002; 129:467–477.

55. McEvilly RJ, Erkman L, Luo L, Sawchenko PE, Ryan AF, Rosenfeld MG. Requirement for Brn-3.0 in differentiation and survival of sensory and motor neurons. Nature 1996; 384:574–577.

56. Xiang M, Gan L, Zhou L, Klein WH, Nathans J. Targeted deletion of the mouse

POU domain gene *Brn-3a* causes selective loss of neurons in the brainstem and trigeminal ganglion, uncoordinated limb movement, and impaired suckling. Proc Natl Acad Sci USA 1996; 93:11950–11955.

57. Huang EJ, Liu W, Fritzsch B, Bianchi LM, Reichardt LF, Xiang M. *Brn3a* is a transcriptional regulator of soma size, target field innervation and axon pathfinding of inner ear sensory neurons. Development 2001; 128:2421–2432.

58. Erkman L, McEvilly RJ, Luo L, Ryan AK, Hooshmand F, O'Connell SM, Keithley EM, Rapaport DH, Ryan AF, Rosenfeld MG. Role of transcription factors *Brn-3.1* and *Brn-3.2* in auditory and visual system development. Nature 1996; 381:603–606.

59. Gan L, Xiang M, Zhou L, Wagner DS, Klein WH, Nathans J. POU domain factor *Brn-3b* is required for the development of a large set of retinal ganglion cells. Proc Natl Acad Sci USA 1996; 93:3920–3925.

60. Liu W, Khare SL, Liang X, Peters MA, Liu X, Cepko CL, Xiang M. All *Brn3* genes can promote retinal ganglion cell differentiation in the chick. Development 2000; 127:3237–3247.

61. Vahava O, Morell R, Lynch ED, Weiss S, Kagan ME, Ahituv N, Morrow JE, Lee MK, Skvorak AB, Morton CC, Blumenfeld A, Frydman M, Friedman TB, King M-C, Avraham KB. Mutation in transcription factor *POU4F3* associated with inherited progressive hearing loss in humans. Science 1998; 279:1950–1954.

62. Lynch E, Lee MK, Morrow JE, Welcsh PL, Leon PE, MC K. Nonsyndromic deafness DFNA1 associated with mutation of a human homolog of the *Drosophila* gene diaphanous. Science 1997; 278:1315–1318.

63. Xiang M, Gan L, Li D, Chen ZY, Zhou L, O'Malley BW Jr, Klein W, Nathans J. J. Essential role of POU-domain factor *Brn-3c* in auditory and vestibular hair cell development. Proc Natl Acad Sci USA 1997; 94:9445–9450.

64. Gottfried I, Huygen PLM, Avraham KB. The clinical presentation of DFNA15/ *POU4F3*. In: Smith RJH, Cremers CWRJ, eds. Advances in ORL. Basel: Karger AG, 2002, pp. 92–97.

65. Xiang M, Gao WQ, Hasson T, Shin JJ. Requirement for *Brn-3c* in maturation and survival, but not in fate determination of inner ear hair cells. Development 1998; 125:3935–3946.

66. Schulze A, Downward J. Navigating gene expression using microarrays—a technology review. Nat Cell Biol 2001; 3:E190–E195.

67. Purves WK, Sadava D, Orians GH, Heller HC. Life: The Science of Biology. 6th ed. Massachusets: Sinauer Associates, Inc., 2001.

68. Verrijzer CP, Van der Vliet PC. POU domain transcription factors. Biochim Biophys Acta 1993; 1173:1–21.

69. International Organization for Standardization International Standard ISO 7029, 1984.

19
α-Tectorin

P. Kevin Legan, Richard J. Goodyear, and Guy P. Richardson
University of Sussex, Brighton, England

Guy Van Camp
University of Antwerp, Antwerp, Belgium

I. INTRODUCTION

The tectorial membrane, the otoconial membranes, and the cupulae are specialized extracellular matrices of the inner ear that are associated with the apical surfaces of the sensory epithelia. The tectorial membrane lies over the organ of Corti in the cochlea, and the otoconial membranes cover the maculae of the vestibule. These membranes provide a structure against which the stereocilia bundles of the hair cells can react when the epithelia are displaced in response to sound waves, as in the cochlea, or head motion, as in the vestibule. A cupula sits on top of the crista in each of the ampullary organs of the semicircular canals and acts like a sail, transmitting the fluid motion caused by head movements to the sensory hair bundles. These three types of extracellular membrane differ considerably in their structure and molecular composition (1). The mammalian tectorial membrane contains collagenase sensitive polypeptides that react with antibodies to type II, type V, and type IX collagen (2,3), and three noncollagenous glycoproteins, α-tectorin, β-tectorin, and otogelin (4,5). The otoconial membrane contains α-tectorin, β-tectorin and otogelin (1,4). The cupula contains otogelin (1,4). Other, as yet unidentified components, either collagens or noncollagenous glycoproteins/proteoglycans, may also be present in these structures.

In this chapter we will briefly describe the structure of the mammalian tectorial membrane and provide evidence that the tectorins are major components of the noncollagenous matrix of the tectorial membrane. We will discuss the predicted molecular structures of the tectorins and how they may interact to form the observed matrix structure. The expression patterns of the tectorin genes in the inner ear will be described, and we will review the genetic evidence showing that mutations in the gene encoding human α-tectorin, *TECTA*, cause nonsyndromic hearing loss. Finally, we will describe how mice with a targeted deletion in Tecta can be used to reveal how the tectorial membrane is required for the amplification of basilar membrane motion.

II. STRUCTURE OF THE TECTORIAL MEMBRANE

The mammalian tectorial membrane is a ribbon-like sheet of extracellular matrix that spirals along the length of the cochlea. It is attached along one edge to the spiral limbus, stretches over the internal sulcus, and lies over the surface of the organ of Corti where it connects to the tips of the stereocilia bundles of the outer hair cells. Ultrastructural studies (5) reveal it contains radial bundles of 20-nm-diameter collagen fibrils that are embedded in a laminated, striated-sheet matrix formed from light- and dark-staining fila-

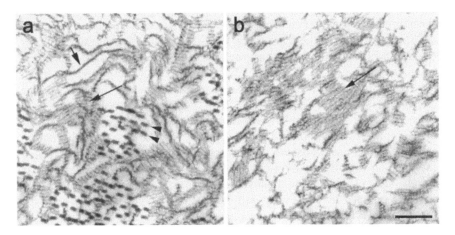

Figure 1 Transmission electron micrographs revealing the ultrastructural appearance of normal (a) and collagenase digested (b) mouse tectorial membranes. In (a), obliquely sectioned, 20-nm-diameter collagen fibrils (arrowheads) form bundles that are embedded in striated sheet matrix (large arrow). On-edge profiles of the striated sheet matrix have the appearance of wavy, irregular diameter fibrils (short arrow). In the collagenase-digested samples shown in (b), only striated-sheet matrix (large arrow) can be observed. Bar = 200 nm.

ment types (Fig. 1a). These filaments have a diameter that ranges from 7 to 9 nm, are aligned parallel to one another, and are linked together by staggered cross-bridges. The alternating arrangement of the light- and dark-staining filaments gives a striated appearance to the sheets that they form. The available evidence indicates that the striated-sheet matrix is predominantly a tectorin-based structure. It is not degraded by bacterial collagenase (Fig. 1b), it is trypsin sensitive, and its structure is unaffected in otogelin null mutant mice (5,6).

III. TECTORINS AS MAJOR NONCOLLAGENOUS COMPONENTS OF THE TECTORIAL MEMBRANE

The tectorins are pepsin-sensitive glycoproteins of the mammalian and avian tectorial membranes that are resistant to digestion with bacterial collagenase (7–9). Mouse α-tectorin is a large disulfide cross-linked complex that barely enters a 8.2% acrylamide resolving gel under nonreducing conditions (Fig. 2a). Following reduction, mouse α-tectorin generates three broad, polydisperse bands with peak apparent molecular masses (Mr) of 173,000, 60,000, and 45,000 (Fig. 2b). These have been referred to as the high-, medium-, and low-molecular-mass mouse tectorins (HMM, MMM, and LMM tectorins) (9). Chick α-tectorin resolves as a discrete band with an Mr of 196,000 under nonreducing conditions (Fig. 2c). On reduction, chick β-tectorin generates six polypeptides (α1–α6) with Mr ranging from 146,000 to 33,000. Beta-tectorin is not covalently associated with α-tectorin and has an Mr of approximately 43,000 under nonreducing conditions in both mouse and chick (Fig. 2a,c). On reduction, β-tectorin shows a small decrease in electrophoretic mobility characteristic of the presence of intra-chain disulfide bonds.

Under reducing conditions, mouse β-tectorin comigrates with the LMM tectorin derived from mouse α-tectorin, and chick β-tectorin comigrates with the chick α4-tectorin subunit (Fig. 2b,d). The tectorins react with the lectins from *Concanavalia ensiformis* and *Triticum vulgaris*, indicating the presence of mannose and *N*-acetylglucosamine (7). HMM mouse tectorin also reacts with lectin from *Glycine max*, indicating the presence of N-acetyl-galactosamine (7), can be metabolically labeled with radioactive sulfate (9), and undergoes a significant shift in electrophoretic mobility following treatment with endo-β-galactosidase (7,9), indicating it may be a sulfated glycoprotein or a keratan sulfate proteoglycan. HMM mouse tectorin has a buoyant density on cesium chloride gradients that is typical of glycoproteins (9), and if it were a proteoglycan it would be classified as a "light" proteoglycan (i.e., has relatively few or only short keratan sulfate GAG associated with it).

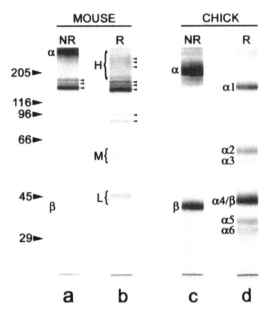

Figure 2 Coomassie-stained gels of mouse (a,b) and chick (c,d) tectorial membrane proteins separated by SDS-PAGE on 8.25% gels under nonreducing (NR) and reducing (R) conditions. The collagenase-sensitive components of the mouse tectorial membrane are indicated by small arrowheads. Collagens are not present in the chick tectorial membrane. Mouse α-tectorin (α, lane a) generates three bands on reduction, the high-, medium-, and low-molecular-mass mouse tectorins (H, M, and L, lane b). Chick α-tectorin (α, lane c) generates six bands on reduction (α1–α6, lane d). The difference in mobility of nonreduced mouse and chick α-tectorin (lanes a and c) is most likely due to a difference in glycosylation. Mouse and chick β-tectorin have a similar apparent molecular mass under nonreducing conditions (β, lanes a and c), and comigrate with α-tectorin subunits on reduction (L and β, lanes b and d).

Antibodies raised to both the chick and the mouse tectorin "subunits" prepared by gel electrophoresis (1,8,9) all react intensely with the tectorial and otolithic membranes, but most show little, if any, cross-reactivity outside the inner ear. An antiserum directed against HMM mouse α-tectorin and an antibody raised to the chick α1-tectorin subunit stain the mucus layer in the olfactory epithelium of the nose (9). An antiserum directed against the combined α5 and α6 chick tectorin subunits stains the epithelial glands supplying the respiratory epithelia of the avian nose (8). These studies suggest that the tectorins have a very restricted tissue distribution, and that α-tectorin may have properties in common with the mucins.

IV. CLONING AND MOLECULAR STRUCTURE OF THE TECTORINS

Chick and mouse tectorin cDNAs were obtained by screening cochlear cDNA libraries with antibodies and DNA probes (3,10,11). Southern blot analysis indicates the chick and mouse tectorins are the products of single-copy genes. The deduced amino acid sequences for the tectorins from these two species have ~74% similarity (73% for chick and mouse α-tectorin, 75% for chick and mouse β-tectorin) and predict virtually identical proteins in which all the major features are conserved. A composite DNA sequence for human α-tectorin derived from genomic DNA predicts a protein with 95% identity to mouse α-tectorin (12), also with all features conserved.

The cDNA for mouse α-tectorin predicts a large, modular protein of 239 kDa with an N-terminal domain that has similarity to the G1 domain of entactin (nidogen), a large central region composed of three full (D1–D3) and two partial (D0 and D4) von Willebrand factor (vWF) type D repeats, and a C-terminal region forming a zona pellucida (ZP) domain (Fig. 3a). The cDNA for mouse β-tectorin encodes a small, 36-kDa protein that is predicted to form a single zona pellucida domain (Fig. 3b). The predicted protein sequences for the chick, mouse, and human tectorins all encode proteins with hydrophobic N-terminal signal sequences characteristic of secreted proteins, and hydrophobic C-termini characteristic of proteins that are linked to the lipid bilayer via a glycosyl-phosphatidylinositol (GPI) anchor (13). The predicted sites for the addition of the C-terminal GPI anchor are preceded by extended or tetra-basic consensus sites for cleavage by furin-like endoproteinases (14,15). GPI anchors act as signals for targeting proteins to the apical membranes of polarized epithelial cells (16), so these sequence data indicate that the tectorins are most likely to be synthesized as GPI-linked, membrane-bound precursors, targeted to the apical surface of the sensory epithelia in the ear by the lipid tail, and released from the membrane either while on route to or when at the apical membrane.

The N-terminal amino acid sequence data obtained from gel-purified tectorin bands from mouse and chick (3) allow one to determine where the α-tectorin sequence from these species is cleaved to produce the various α-tectorin subunits that are observed on SDS gels under reducing conditions (Fig. 3a). This analysis indicates mouse α-tectorin is cleaved at two sites to produce the HMM, MMM, and LMM mouse α-tectorin subunits that correspond approximately to the central region containing the vWF type D repeats, the C-terminal ZP domain, and the N-terminal entactin G1-like domain, respectively. In chick, the same sites are used but the central vWF repeat region appears to be cleaved at two other points to produce the additional subunits, chick α5- and chick α6-tectorin. The sites at which the α-

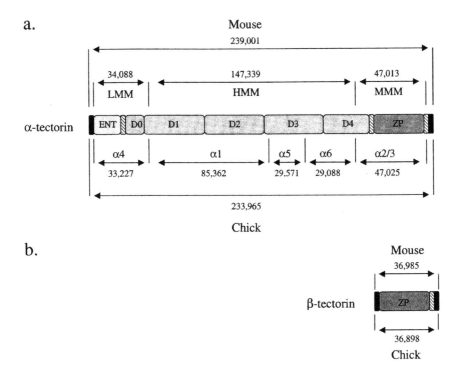

Figure 3 Diagram illustrating the predicted domain structures for (a) α- and (b) β-tectorin, and how α-tectorin (a) is cleaved to produce the LMM, HMM, and MMM fragments in the.mouse, and the α1–α6 fragments in the chick. Predicted molecular masses (in Da) are indicated for each fragment. ENT = entactin G1-like domain; D = vWF type D repeats; ZP = zona pellucida domain; black boxes = hydrophobic N- and C-termini; hatched boxes indicate regions with no similarity to other proteins.

tectorin sequence in mouse and chick is cleaved to produce these subunits are not specific for any known endoproteinases, and the extent to which the fragments observed on reduction are bona fide subunits and a consequence of active posttranslational processing or a consequence of proteolytic damage at susceptible sites remains to be determined.

The N-terminal region of α-tectorin shares sequence similarity with a part of the G1 domain of entactin (nidogen), a component of the basal lamina that is known to interact with laminin, type IV collagen, perlecan, and fibulin (17). These interactions mostly involve the G2 and G3 domains of entactin, although there is some evidence from surface plasmon resonance assays that the G1 domain of nidogen-1 interacts with fibulin-2 (17). It is hard to ascribe a function to the N-terminal entactin G1-like domain of α-tectorin, although a large deletion in this region (18) has a profound influence on the stability of the molecule or its ability to be incorporated into the matrix (see Sec. VII).

The vWF type D repeats of α-tectorin are cysteine-rich domains characteristic of a number of molecules including the mucins (19). vWF is produced by endothelial cells and megakaryocytes and is involved in hemostasis, acting as a carrier for procoagulant factor VIII and mediating platelet adhesion (20). It forms disulfide-linked dimers that can then assemble into large disulfide-linked multimers, and this multimerization process is thought to be dependent on the protein disulfide isomerase activity of vicinal cysteines present in the D1 and D2 domains of pre-pro vWF (21). Vicinal cysteines are present in the D1 and the D4 domains of α-tectorin and, although there is no evidence that α-tectorin forms disulfide cross-linked multimers, these vicinal cysteines may be involved in the assembly of the tectorin subunits.

The ZP domains of α- and β-tectorin are common to a number of other proteins, including ZP1, ZP2, and ZP3, the three major proteins of the zona pellucida, the extracellular matrix that surrounds the unfertilized egg. ZP domains are approximately 260 amino acids long, with a conserved pattern of hydrophobic, polar, and turn-forming residues and have eight highly conserved cysteine residues (22). The ZP domain is a module found in many proteins that either can or do form filamentous-based extracellular structures and is usually located at or toward the C-termini of these proteins (23). In addition to ZP1, ZP2, and ZP3, these proteins include GP2, a protein that forms a mesh-like matrix in the pancreatic acinar ducts (24), uromodulin, a major component of urine (25) that can form urinary casts under pathological conditions (26), and nompA, a protein that forms part of the dendritic cap of the insect mechanoreceptor (27). The ZP domains of α- and β-tectorin may enable these proteins to form the filamentous-based matrix of the tectorial membrane.

The vWF type D-repeats of α-tectorin show highest similarity with the vWF type D repeats of a pig sperm membrane protein known as zonadhesin that has been shown to bind to the zona pellucida in vitro (28), and may be involved in sperm-egg interactions in vivo. Zonadhesin is processed during sperm capacitation to leave a membrane-bound extracellular domain that is composed exclusively of vWF repeats with an arrangement that is identical to that found in the central core of α-tectorin.

These sequence similarities have led to the suggestion (3) that α- and β-tectorin may each form homomeric filaments via their ZP domains. These two different filament types could then interact with one another via the zonadhesin-like region of α-tectorin, possibly in conjunction with the entactin G1-like domain. Alternatively, α- and β-tectorin could form heteromeric (α/β) filaments via their ZP domains. These filaments could also self-assemble into larger structures via interactions between the ZP domains and the zonadhesin-like domain of α-tectorin.

V.   EXPRESSION OF TECTORIN mRNAs IN THE INNER EAR

Northern blot analysis of poly(A) + mRNA from eight different tissues of the 2-3 day postnatal mouse indicates that the tectorins are expressed at high levels only in the cochlea, with probes for α- and β-tectorin hybridising to single major bands of 7.5 and 2.7 kb, respectively (3). Tectorin splicing has not been systematically investigated. However, there is evidence for the use of an alternative 3' splice site in Tecta (3,12). Also in the rat cochlea, a mouse β-tectorin cDNA probe hybridizes to two bands of 2.9 and 2.6 kb (29), indicating β-tectorin splice variants may exist in this species.

In situ hybridization has been used to study the spatial and temporal aspects of tectorin mRNA expression during the development of the mouse inner ear (30). Expression of both tectorins can be detected in the basal end of the cochlear duct as early as embryonic day (E) 12.5. By E14.5 expression is detected throughout the length of the cochlea. By birth two distinct but partially overlapping expression patterns are observed for the two tectorin mRNAs (Fig. 4). α-Tectorin mRNA is expressed throughout the greater epithelial ridge and in the immature Hensen's cells that lie immediately lateral to the developing organ of Corti (Fig. 4a–c). β-Tectorin is expressed within a narrow region of the greater epithelial ridge that lies close to the inner hair cells, by the pillar cells that separate the rows of inner and outer hair cells, and by Deiter's cells surrounding the outer hair cells, with expression levels being greatest in the third, outermost row of Deiter's cells (Fig. 4d–f). Expression of α-tectorin mRNA in the cochlea as revealed by in situ hybridization decreases rapidly during the first week after birth, and can no longer be detected by P15. β-Tectorin mRNA expression can be detected by in situ hybridization in the cochlea at P15, but not at P21. A similar postnatal decrease in tectorin mRNA expression has been shown using both in situ hybridization and Northern blot analysis in the cochlea of the rat (29), where expression is no longer detectable for either tectorin by P15. A quantitative RT-PCR study confirms there is a dramatic developmental decrease in α-tectorin mRNA levels in the mouse cochlea between P3 and P15, but suggests low-level expression may persist until P67 (31). These data indicate that the tectorin mRNAs are only expressed at high levels transiently during the development of the cochlea, and imply that the tectorins may be stable proteins with very long half-lives.

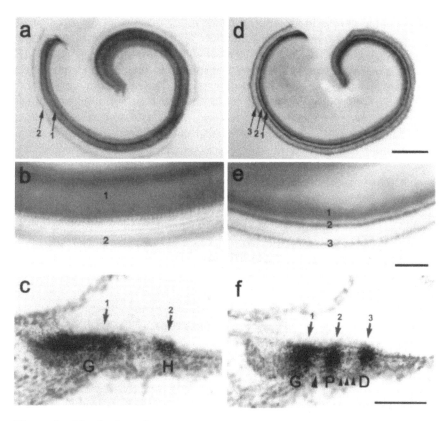

Figure 4   Distribution of mRNA for α- (a–c) and β- (d–f) tectorin mRNA in the early postnatal mouse cochlea revealed by in situ hybridization of apical-coil cochlear cultures with DIG-labeled probes (a,b,d,e), and cochlear sections with ^{35}S-labeled probes (c,f). For α-tectorin (a–c), two bands of expression are observed, one encompassing the entire greater epithelial ridge (1), and the other in the immature Hensen's cells that flank the lateral edge of the organ of Corti (2). For β-tectorin (d–f), three bands are seen, one in the region of the greater epithelial ridge (1) adjacent to the inner hair cells, one in the pillar cells (2), and one in the third row of Deiter's cells (3). In parts c and f, G = greater epithelial ridge; H = Hensen's cells; P = pillar cells; D = 3rd-row Deiters' cell; large arrowhead indicates the position of the inner hair cell, and small arrowheads indicate the positions of the three rows of outer hair cells. Bars = 200 μm (a,d), 50 μm (b,c,e,f). (Adapted from Ref. 30 with permission from the publisher.)

α- and β-tectorin are also expressed in the maculae of the saccule and utricle (30). Expression of α-tectorin mRNA is detected in the maculae of the mouse inner ear by E12.5, and expression of β-tectorin mRNA by E14.5. β-Tectorin mRNA expression is always restricted to the maculae, and within the maculae it is restricted to the striolar regions. The expression of β-tectorin mRNA persists within the striolar region until at least 5 months after birth (the latest stage examined thus far). α-Tectorin mRNA is also expressed in the epithelia that surround the sensory maculae and continues to be expressed in these flanking regions for the first 2 weeks after birth, after expression has decreased within the maculae. As in the cochlea, α-tectorin mRNA expression can no longer be detected in the vestibular organs by 3 weeks after birth. Tectorin expression has not been detected in any of the ampullary organs of the semicircular canals.

VI. MUTATIONS IN *TECTA* CAUSING HUMAN HEREDITARY DEAFNESS

The mouse gene for α-tectorin, *Tecta*, maps to mouse chromosome 9, and the human *TECTA* gene maps to a syntenic region of human chromosome 11 (32), within the interval for autosomal dominant nonsyndromic hearing loss DFNA8/12 (33–35). *Tectb* maps to mouse chromosome 19, and *TECTB* maps to a region of synteny on human 10q15 (36). *TECTB* is not a candidate for any of the deafness loci that have been reported thus far, but mutations in *TECTA* have been shown to cause autosomal, nonsyndromic deafness in a number of familes. To date six families have been identified with mutations in *TECTA* (12,37–41); the data from these studies are summarized in Table 1. Mutations in *TECTA* cause both dominant (DFNA) and recessive (DFNB) forms of deafness. The dominant mutations are at conserved residues in both the ZP (12,41) and zonadhesin-like domains (38,39) of α-tectorin. In the Belgian family there are two closely spaced missense mutations, both of which are at residues conserved within the most closely related members of the ZP domain family. It is not yet known whether one of these is a rare polymorphism or whether the two mutations interact synergistically to produce the phenotype. In the Swedish family, there is considerable phenotypic variation that may possibly be caused by modifying genes.

The various dominant mutations lead to a spectrum of phenotypes. It was originally suggested (38) that mutations in the zonadhesin-like domain of α-tectorin lead to pre- or postlingual, progressive, high-frequency hearing loss, and mutations in the ZP domain cause prelingual, stable, midfrequency hearing impairments. However, the discovery of a family with a dominant mutation in a conserved cysteine residue in the ZP domain of α-tectorin that

Table 1 Mutations in *TECTA* Leading to Nonsyndromic Hearing Loss

Family origin	Mutation	Exon	Protein mutation	Domain	Onset	Progression	Severity	Affected frequencies	Ref.
Dominant									
Swedish	3170T>A	10	C1057S	vWFD2	Postlingual	Progressive	Mild-severe	High	38
French	4857G>C	14	C1619S	vWFD4	Pre- or postlingual	Progressive	Mild-moderately severe 20–80-dB hearing loss	High	39
Belgian	5725C>T 5738G>A	17	L1820F G1824D	ZP	Prelingual	Stable	Mild-moderately severe 20–80-dB hearing loss	Mid	12
Spanish	5509T>G	17	C1837G	ZP	Postlingual	Progressive	Mild-moderately severe	Mid	41
Austrian	5876A>G	18	Y1870C	ZP	Prelingual	Stable	Moderate-moderately severe 60–80 dB hearing loss	Mid	12
Recessive									
Lebanese	G>A intron 9 donor splice site		Premature stop codon	vWFD2	Prelingual	Stable	Severe-profound 70–110-dB hearing loss	All	40

is associated with a progressive midfrequency hearing loss (41) suggests the situation may be more complex. Currently it appears that mutations at cysteine residues may underlie the progressive forms of hearing loss. Inter and intrachain disulfide bonds may be essential for the long-term stability of α-tectorin, and it is interesting that the mutation in the French family involves one of the two vicinal cysteines in the vWF D4 repeat that is thought to have protein disulfide isomerase activity.

The recessive mutation (DFNB21) is a G-to-A transition at the intron 9 donor splice site that is predicted to cause skipping of the preceding exon and introduce a premature stop codon in the vWF D2 repeat (40). The mutation causes severe to profound deafness across all frequencies, is prelingual in onset, and may essentially be a null mutation. Heterozygous carriers in the DFNB21 family have apparently normal hearing, indicating that a reduction in the α-tectorin content of the tectorial membrane as a consequence of reduced gene dosage may have little effect on hearing, and lending support to the suggestion (40) that the DFNA mutations have a dominant negative effect. However, it is not yet known at what level the tectorin content of the tectorial membrane is regulated. Halving the gene dose may not necessarily lead to a reduction in the amount of protein incorporated.

VII. HEARING IN A *Tecta* MUTANT MOUSE

Transgenic mice homozygous for a targeted deletion in the entactin (nidogen)-like G 1 domain of α-tectorin ($Tecta^{\Delta ENT/\Delta ENT}$ mice) have tectorial membranes that lack all known noncollagenous components—α-tectorin, β-tectorin, and otogelin, are composed solely of randomly organized collagen fibrils, and are completely detached from the surface of the organ of Corti and the spiral limbus (18). The tectorial membranes of mice heterozygous for this deletion are apparently normal, indicating the deletion does not act as a dominant negative. These observations indicate that α-tectorin is probably a major component and organizer of the noncollagenous striated sheet matrix of the tectorial membrane. The organ of Corti in the $Tecta^{\Delta ENT/\Delta ENT}$ mice is normal, apart from the loss of a tectorial membrane (Fig. 5), and the structure and orientation of the hair bundles are unaffected.

The basilar membrane in the high-frequency basal coil of the cochlea in these *Tecta* mutant mice with detached tectorial membranes is still tuned, but 35 dB less sensitive than the basilar membrane of a wild-type mouse. Cochlear microphonics and compound action potentials can still be recorded at high sound levels, indicating the hair bundles can be driven by fluid coupling in the absence of a tectorial membrane. However, the cochlear microphonic potentials differ in phase and symmetry relative to those recorded from wild-type mice, so the mechanical feedback from the

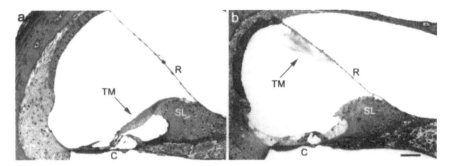

Figure 5 Cochlear sections from wild-type (a) and $Tecta^{\Delta ENT/\Delta ENT}$ (b) mice illustrating how the deletion in $Tecta$ causes detachment of the tectorial membrane (TM) from the organ of Corti (C) and the spiral limbus (SL). In the $Tecta^{\Delta ENT/\Delta ENT}$ mice the tectorial membrane is associated with Reissner's membrane (R). Bar = 100 μm.

electromotile hair cells to the basilar membrane will be largely ineffective, as it will be delivered with reduced gain and at an inappropriate time. At low frequencies, the CAP threshold in these $Tecta^{\Delta ENT/\Delta ENT}$ mice is reduced by as much as 80 dB. As $Tecta^{\Delta ENT/\Delta ENT}$ mice are effectively functional α-tectorin null mutant mice, they may provide a model for DFNB21. A recent in vitro study has shown that mutations in ZP2 equivalent to the Y1870C and C1837G mutations in α-tectorin prevent or severely reduce incorporation of the mutant proteins into the zona pellucida of mouse eggs (42). However, a real understanding of the effect the various TECTA mutations have on the structure and function of the tectorial membrane will have to await the production of knock-in mice bearing the same mutations in Tecta.

ACKNOWLEDGMENTS

Work in the authors' laboratories is supported by the Wellcome Trust (Grant ref: 057410/Z/99/Z), Defeating Deafness, The Flemish Fonds voor Wetenschappelijk onderzoek (FWO), and the University of Antwerp.

REFERENCES

1. Goodyear RJ, Richardson GP. Extracellular matrices associated with the apical surfaces of sensory epithelia in the inner ear: molecular and structural diversity. J Neurobiol 2002; 53:212–227.
2. Thalmann I, Thallinger G, Crouch EC, Comegys TH, Barret N, Thalmann R.

Composition and supramolecular organisation of the tectorial membrane. Laryngoscope 1997; 97:357–367.

3. Legan PK, Rau A, Keen JN, Richardson GP. The mouse tectorins: modular matrix proteins of the inner ear homologous to components of the sperm-egg adhesion system. J Biol Chem 1997; 272:8791–8801.

4. Cohen-Salmon M, El-Amraoui A, Leibovici M, Petit C. Otogelin: a glycoprotein specific to the acellular membranes of the inner ear. Proc Natl Acad Sci USA 1997; 94:14450–14455.

5. Hasko JA, Richardson GP. The ultrastructural organization and properties of the mouse tectorial membrane matrix. Hearing Res 1998; 35:21–38.

6. Simmler M-C, Cohen-Salmon M, El-Amraoui A, Guillard L, Benichou J-C, Petit C, Panthier J-J. Targeted disruption of *Otog* results in deafness and severe imbalance. Nat Genet 2000; 24:139–143.

7. Richardson GP, Russell IJ, Duance VC, Bailey AJ. Polypeptide composition of the mammalian tectorial membrane. Hearing Res 1987; 25:45–60.

8. Killick R, Malenczak C, Richardson GP. The protein composition of the avian tectorial membrane. Hearing Res 1992; 64:21–38.

9. Killick R, Richardson GP. Antibodies to the sulphated, high molecular mass mouse tectorin stain hair bundles and the olfactory mucus layer. Hearing Res 1997; 103:131–141.

10. Killick R, Legan PK, Malenczak, Richardson GP. Molecular cloning of chick β-tectorin, an extracellular matrix molecule of the inner ear. J Cell Biol 1995; 129:535–547.

11. Countinho P, Goodyear R, Legan PK, Richardson GP. Chick α-tectorin: molecular cloning and expression during embryogenesis. Hearing Res 1999; 130:62–74.

12. Verhoeven K, Van Laer L, Kirschhofer K, Legan PK, Hughes DC, Schatteman I, Verstreken M, van Hauwe P, Coucke P, Chen A, Smith RJH, Somers T, Offeciers FE, van de Heyning P, Richardson GP, Wachtler F, Kimberling WJ, Willems PJ, Govaerts PJ, van Camp G. Mutations in the human α-tectorin gene cause autosomal dominant non-syndromic hearing impairment. Nat Genet 1998; 19:60–62.

13. Cross GAM. Glycolipid anchoring of plasma membrane proteins. Annu Rev Cell Biol 1990; 6:1–39.

14. Molloy SS, Bresnahan PA, Leppla SH, Klimpel KR, Thomas G. Human furin is a calcium-dependent serine endoproteinase that recognizes the sequence Arg-X-X-Arg and efficiently cleaves anthrax toxin protective antigen. J Biol Chem 1992; 267:16396–16402.

15. Seidah HG, Chrétien M. Proprotein and prohormone convertases: a family of subtilases generating diverse polypeptides. Brain Res 1999; 848:45–62.

16. Lisanti MP, Sargiacomo M, Graeve L, Saltiel AR, Rodriguez-Boulan E. Polarized apical distribution of glycosyl-phosphatidylinositol-anchored proteins in a renal epithelial cell line. Proc Natl Acad Sci USA 1998; 85:9557–9561.

17. Ries A, Gohring W, Fox JW, Timpl R, Sasaki T. Recombinant domains of mouse nidogen-1 and their binding to basement membrane proteins and monoclonal antibodies. Eur J Biochem 2001; 268:5119–5128.

18. Legan PK, Lukashkina VA, Goodyear RJ, Kössl M, Russell IJ, Richardson GP. A targeted deletion in α-tectorin reveals that the tectorial membrane is required for the gain and timing of cochlear feedback. Neuron 2000; 28:273–285.

19. Gum JR, Hicks JW, Toribara NW, Siddiki B, Kim YS. Molecular cloning of human intestinal mucin (MUC2) cDNA: identification of the amino terminus and overall sequence similarity to prepro-von Willebrand factor. J Biol Chem 1994; 269:2440–2446.

20. Ruggeri ZM, Ware J. von Willebrand Factor. In: Kreis T, Vale R, eds. Guidebook to the Extracellular Matrix and Adhesion Proteins. Oxford: Oxford University Press, 1995:105–108.

21. Mayadas TN, Wagner DD. Vicinal cysteines in the prosequence play a role in von Willebrand-factor multimer assembly. Proc Natl Acad Sci USA 1992; 89: 3531–3535.

22. Bork P, Sander C. A large domain common to sperm receptor (Zp2 and Zp3) and TGF-B type III receptor. FEBS Lett 1992; 300:237–240.

23. Waserman PM, Jovine L, Litscher ES. A profile of fertilization in mammals. Nat Cell Biol 2001; 3:E59–E64.

24. Grondin G, St.-Jean P, Beaudoin AR. Cytochemical and immunocytochemical characterization of a fibrillar network (GP2) in pancreatic juice: possible role as a sieve in the pancreatic ductal system. Eur J Cell Biol 1992; 57:155–164.

25. Pennica D, Kohr WJ, Kuang WJ, Glaister D, Aggarwal BB, Chen EY, Goeddel DV. Identification of human uromodulin as the Tamm-Horsfall urinary glycoprotein. Science 1987; 236:83–88.

26. McQueen EG. Composition of urinary casts. Lancet 1966; 1:397–398.

27. Chung YD, Zhu J, Han Y-G, Kernan MJ. *NompA* encodes a PNS-specific, ZP domain protein required to connect mechanosensory dendrites to sensory structures. Neuron 2001; 29:415–428.

28. Hardy Z, Garbers DL. A sperm membrane protein that binds in a species-specific manner to the egg extracellular matrix is homologous to von Willebrand factor. J Biol Chem 1995; 270:26025–26028.

29. Knipper M, Richardson G, Mack A, Müller M, Goodyear R, Limberger A, Rohbock K, Köpschall I, Zenner H-P, Zimmermann U. Thyroid hormone deficient period prior to the onset of hearing is associated with reduced levels of β-tectorin protein in the tectorial membrane. J Biol Chem 2001; 276:39046–39052.

30. Rau A, Legan PK, Richardson GP. Tectorin mRNA is spatially and temporally restricted during mouse inner ear development. J Comp Neurol 1999; 405:271–280.

31. Maeda Y, Fukushima K, Kasai N, Maeta M, Nishizaki K. Quantification of *TECTA* and DFNA5 expression in the developing mouse cochlea. Neuroreport 2001; 12:3223–3226.

32. Hughes DC, Legan PK, Steel KP, Richardson GP. Mapping of the α-tectorin gene (*TECTA*) to mouse chromosome 9 and human chromosome 11: a candidate for human autosomal dominant nonsyndromic deafness. Genomics 1998; 48:46–51.

33. Verhoeven K, Van Camp G, Govaerts PJ, Baelemans W, Schatteman I, Verstreken M, Van Laer L, Smith RJH, Brown MR, van de Heyning P, Somer T, Offeciers FE, Willems PJ. A gene for autosomal dominant nonsyndromic hearing loss (DFNA12) maps to chromosome 11q22–24. Am J Hum Genet 1997; 60:1168–1173.

34. Govaerts PJ, De Ceular G, Daemers K, Verhoeven K, van Camp G, Schatteman I, Verstreken M, Willems PJ, Somers T, Offeciers FE. A new autosomal-dominant locus (DFNA12) is responsible for a nonsyndromic, midfrequency, prelingual and nonprogressive sensorineural hearing loss. Am J Otol 1998; 19: 718–723.

35. Kirschhofer K, Kenyon JB, Hoover DM, Franz P, Weipoltshammer K, Wachtler F, Kimberling WJ. Autosomal-dominant, prelingual, nonprogressive sensorineural hearing loss: localization of the gene (DFNA8) to chromosome 11q by linkage in an Austrian family. Cytogenet Cell Genet 1998; 82:126–130.

36. Kim HJ, Noben-Trauth K, Morell RJ. Tectorin-β (*Tectb*) maps to mouse chromosome 19. Genomics 1998; 53:419–420.

37. Balciuniene J, Dahl N, Jalonen P, Borg E, Samuelsson E, Koisti MJ, Petterson U, Jazin EE. Evidence for digenic inheritance of nonsyndromic hereditary hearing loss in a Swedish family. Am J Hum Genet 1998; 63:786–793.

38. Balciuniene J, Dahl N, Jalonen P, Verhoeven K, van Camp G, Borg E, Petterson U, Jazin EE. Alpha-tectorin involvement in hearing disabilities: one gene—two phenotypes. Hum Genet 1999; 105:211–216.

39. Alloisio N, Morle L, Bozon M, Goder J, Verhoeven K, van Camp G, Plauchu H, Muller P, Collet L, Lina-Granade G. Mutation in the zonadhesin-like domain of α-tectorin associated with autosomal dominant non-syndromic hearing loss. Eur J Hum Genet 1999; 7:255–258.

40. Mustapha M, Weil D, Chardenoux S, Elias S, El-Zir E, Beckmann JS, Loiselet J, Petit C. An α-tectorin gene defect causes a newly identified autosomal recessive form of sensorineural pre-lingual non-syndromic deafness, DFNB21. Hum Mol Genet 1999; 8:409–412.

41. Moreno-Pelayo MA, del Castillo I, Villamar M, Romero L, Hernández-Calvin FJ, Herraiz C, Barberá R, Navas C, Moreno F. A cysteine substitution in the zona pellucida domain of α-tectorin results in autosomal dominant, postlingual, progressive, mid frequency hearing loss in a Spanish family. J Med Genet 2001; 38:e13.

42. Jovine L, Qi H, Williams Z, Litscher E, Wassarman PM. The ZP domain is a conserved module for polymerisation of extracellular proteins. Nat Cell Biol 2002; 4:457–461.

20
EYA4

Sigrid Wayne and Richard J. H. Smith
University of Iowa, Iowa City, Iowa, U.S.A.

Els de Leenheer and Cor W. R. Cremers
University Hospital Nijmegen, Nijmegen, The Netherlands

I. INTRODUCTION

A. Background

Hereditary hearing loss may be classified by phenotype as syndromic, in which the hearing loss is associated with other phenotypic anomalies, or non-syndromic, in which the hearing loss is the sole manifestation of the disorder. Nonsyndromic hereditary hearing loss can be further characterized by mode of inheritance as autosomal dominant, autosomal recessive, or X-linked—denoted, respectively, by the abbreviation DFNA, DFNB, and DFN, followed by a number indicating the order of locus identification. In addition, hearing loss may adhere to a mitochondrial mode of inheritance. DFNA10 is the tenth of 39 loci identified to date for autosomal dominant nonsyndromic hearing loss (1). DFNA10 has been localized to the long arm of chromosome 6 (2); the causative gene was recently identified as *EYES ABSENT 4 (EYA4)* (3), a transcriptional activator with a role in regulating early development events.

B. Families

To date, two families, A and B, have been identified that segregate hearing loss linked to the DFNA10 locus (4) (Fig. 1). Family A is comprised of the descendants of an individual from the Alsace-Lorraine region of France who immigrated to America in 1850. Family B is Belgian in origin. Affected

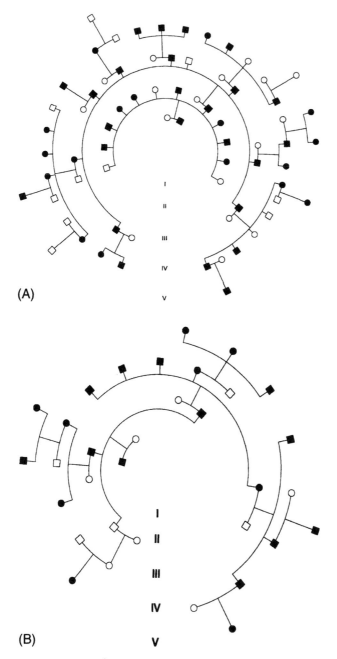

Figure 1 Pedigrees of DFNA10 affected families. (A) Simplified pedigree of American Family A. Only one branch is shown in full. (B) Belgian Family B. ■, affected male; □, unaffected male; ●, affected female; ○, unaffected female. (From Ref. 5.)

members of both families share a similar phenotype of postlingual, progressive, sensorineural hearing loss. All affected individuals have normal speech and language development.

II. AUDIOMETRIC ANALYSIS OF DFNA10 PHENOTYPE

A. Evolution of DFNA10 Phenotype with Age

1. Methods

Pure tone and speech audiograms were obtained on 27 affected individuals in Family A, age range 15–87 years. Air conduction thresholds (decibels hearing level) were used for cross-sectional linear regression analysis, to analyze progression at each frequency. Bone conduction levels were obtained to confirm sensorineural hearing loss. To explore the effects of presbyacusis on the DFNA10 phenotype, analyses were repeated with thresholds corrected for age and sex according to ISO 7029 norms.

2. Results

All affected individuals dated the onset of hearing loss within the first three decades of life (5). During the second and third decades of life, fairly rapid progression of hearing loss is seen (Fig. 2). The derived mean threshold deterioration is approximately 2–3 decibels (dB) per year over all frequencies. After age 30 years, the rate of progression of hearing loss slows to approximately 0.6 dB/year, which, when corrected for the effects of presbyacusis, is not significant. Thus, DFNA10 hearing loss is postlingual in onset, progressive over the first three decades of life, and followed by further gradual progression that can be attributed to normal presbyacusis.

B. Phenotype Comparison of Families A and B

Linear regression analysis was performed using pure tone thresholds obtained from 25 affected persons from Family A and 17 affected persons from Family B. Age-related audiograms were constructed (Fig. 3). Both families demonstrate flat-to-gently sloping audiograms, which evolve with advancing age to a steeply sloping configuration. The hearing loss in Family A appears to be slightly more severe than in Family B.

III. CLONING OF *EYA4*, THE CAUSATIVE GENE OF DFNA10

A. Linkage Mapping

The DFNA10 locus was originally mapped by linkage analysis on the American Family A in 1996 to a 15-cM interval on chromosome 6q22–23

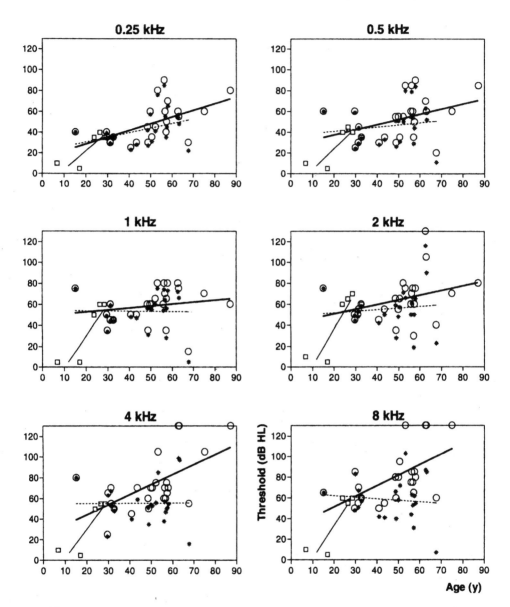

Figure 2 Cross-sectional threshold-on-age data (air conduction threshold in right ear). Circles and bold solid lines relate to the linear regression analysis in all cases (age over 15 years). Asterisks and dotted lines relate to age-corrected thresholds. Audiograms from a single individual from Family A are shown separately with squares and thin solid lines. (From Ref. 5.)

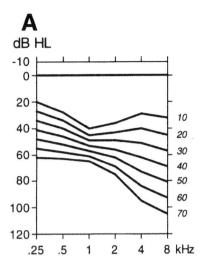

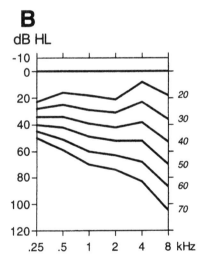

Figure 3 Age-related typical audiograms of (A) Family A and (B) Family B. Italics indicate age in years. (From Ref. 5.)

delimited by the markers D6S474 and D6S270 (2). By expanding the pedigree
to include distant branches of the family, the DFNA10 interval was refined
to 2.8 cM flanked by D6S472 and D6S975, although haplotype inconsis-
tencies in two persons prompted reanalysis of the data. These individuals
were subsequently omitted from the pedigree, thereby increasing the size of
the DFNA10 interval to a 6-cM region flanked by D6S413 and D6S292 (3).

B.   Identification of Candidate Gene

The newly refined DFNA10 interval was found to contain several known
genes, including an excellent candidate, *EYA4*, the most recently identified
member of the vertebrate *EYA* gene family (6). The *EYA* gene family encodes
a family of transcriptional activators that interact with other proteins in a
conserved regulatory hierarchy to ensure normal embryological development. Mutations in another member of this family, *EYA1*, are associated
with syndromic hearing loss in branchio-oto-renal (BOR) syndrome (7,8).

C.   Mutation Screening of DFNA10 Families (3)

1.   Mutation Screening of Family A

Family A was screened for mutations in the coding region of *EYA4* by single-
strand conformation polymorphism (SSCP) analysis of its 21 exons, revealing a striking band shift in exon 12 that segregated with the hearing loss

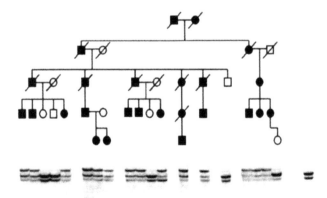

Figure 4   SSCP result of *EYA4* exon 12 for Family A. Each lane on the gel is the
SSCP result of the individual in the pedigree directly above. A dramatic shift segregates with the hearing loss. Individual on the far right is a normal-hearing, unrelated
control. ■, affected male; □, unaffected male; ●, affected female; ○, unaffected
female; /, deceased. (From Ref. 3.)

A.

B.

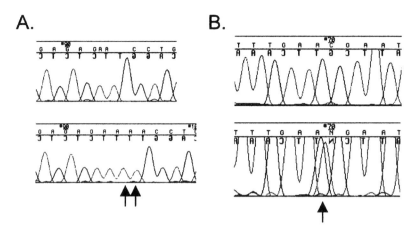

Figure 5 Sequencing results for *EYA4*. (A) In Family A, a portion of the electropherogram for *EYA4* exon 12 sequenced from subcloned PCR products demonstrates the insertion of 2 adenine residues (arrows) in one allele of the affected individual; wild-type sequence is seen in the other allele (compare to unaffected alleles). (B) In Family B, a portion of the electropherogram for *EYA4* exon 20 shows a cytosine-to-thymine transition (arrow), resulting in a premature stop codon (TGA). (From Ref. 3.)

(Fig. 4). Direct sequencing of exon 12 produced an electropherogram featuring the superimposition of two sequences, suggesting a frameshift mutation. By sequencing of subclones of exon 12 PCR products from affected and unaffected family members, the mutation was characterized as the insertion of two adenine residues at position 1468 (1468insAA) (Fig. 5A). This mutation is predicted to generate a frameshift and premature stop codon in exon 14.

2. Mutation Screening of Family B

SSCP analysis of *EYA4* in Family B revealed no band shifts segregating with the hearing loss; however, direct sequencing of all exons identified a cytosine-to-thymine transition in exon 20 at position 2200 (2200C→T) that segregated with the hearing loss. This base change converts an arginine codon (CGA) to a stop codon (TGA) (Fig. 5B).

IV. EYA PROTEIN STRUCTURE AND FUNCTION

A. General Structure of EYA Proteins

The *EYA* gene family encodes a family of transcriptional activators that interact with other proteins in a conserved regulatory hierarchy to ensure normal embryological development. The prototypical *EYA* protein structure includes a highly conserved carboxy terminus called the eya-homologous region (eyaHR; alternatively referred to as the eya domain or eya homology domain 1) and a more divergent proline-serine-threonine (PST)-rich (34–41% of amino acids) transactivation domain at the amino terminus (6,9) (Fig. 6A).

B. EYA Protein Function

Studies of *Drosophila* eya indicate that the eya-homologous region mediates interaction with the gene products of *so* (sine oculis) and *dac* (dachshund),

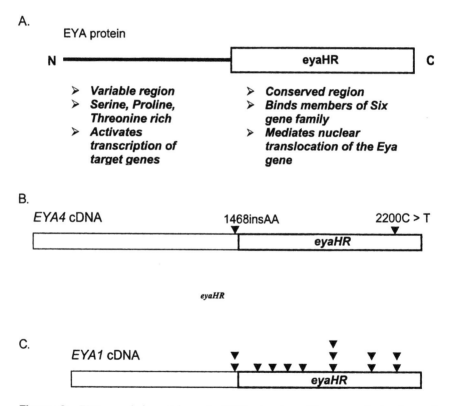

Figure 6 *EYA*-encoded protein and cDNA structure. The general structure of EYA proteins (A), a diagram of *EYA4* cDNA showing the positions (triangles) of the two mutations identified in DFNA10 families (B); and a diagram of *EYA1* cDNA showing the positions of mutations associated with BOR syndrome (C). N, amino terminus; C, carboxy terminus; eyaHR, eya-homologous region. *EYA1* and *EYA4* share 31.8% amino acid identity. (From Ref. 3.)

and that expression of both *eya* and *so* is initiated by *ey* (eyeless) (10,11). In vertebrates, members of the *Six* gene family (the orthologs of *so*) bind to Eya proteins to induce nuclear translocation of the resultant protein complex (12). Amino-terminal transcriptional activation activity has been demonstrated for the *Drosophila eya* and murine *Eya1-3* gene products, suggesting that EYA interactions and pathways are conserved across species (9–17).

C. *EYA4* Structure and Predicted Effects of DFNA10 Causing Mutations

The structure of EYA4, as deduced from its cDNA sequence, conforms to the basic pattern established by EYA1-3. The *EYA4* coding sequence is comprised of 20 exons. The mutations we identified in *EYA4* are predicted to affect the eyaHR. The 1468insAA mutation in the American family causes a frameshift and subsequent novel stop codon in exon 14. Since the eyaHR of *EYA4* is encoded by the 3′-most 6 bp of exon 12 through the 5′-most 78 bp of exon 21, this mutation effectively eliminates the entire eyaHR (Fig. 6B). The 2200C→T mutation in the Belgian family creates a premature stop codon, eliminating 52 amino acids from the C-terminal end of the eyaHR (Fig. 6B). Given the importance of the eyaHR to EYA protein function, it is not surprising that these mutations have a phenotypic correlate.

D. *EYA4* Alternative Splicing

Alternative splicing of *EYA4* mRNA has been reported for exons 5, 16, and 20 and results in several isoforms (6) (Fig. 7). Exon 5 may be spliced in or out; the first 68 bp of exon 16 may be spliced out by use of a cryptic splice acceptor site within the exon that results in a predicted truncated protein of 452 amino acids; and exon 20 may be substituted for exon 19, equal in length and with 69.3% nucleic acid identity and 66.7% amino acid identity.

1. *EYA4* Splice Variants in the Cochlea and Brain (3)

To determine which splice variants are expressed in the cochlea, RT-PCR and sequencing was performed on human fetal cochlear RNA, using primers flanking exons 5, 16, and 19/20. Human fetal and adult brain cDNA libraries were screened as well. Neither the exon 5–containing isoform of *EYA4* nor the shorter form of exon 16 was detected in the cochlea, but both exon 19– and exon 20–containing splice variants could be amplified in human fetal cochlear cDNA. Both of the latter two isoforms also were present in

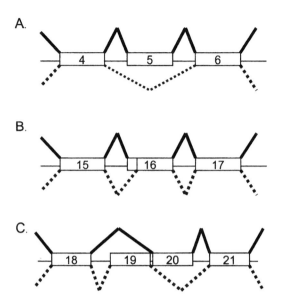

Figure 7 Alternative splicing of *EYA4* mRNA involving (A) exon 5, (B) exon 16, and (C) exon 19/20. Numbered boxes correspond to exons, thin solid lines to introns, and alternative splicing patterns are represented by heavy solid and dotted lines. (Adapted from Ref. 6.)

human brain cDNA libraries, although only the exon 19–containing variant was found in fetal brain. Adult brain had minimally detectable exon 19–containing *EYA4* transcripts and abundant expression of the exon 20–containing variant. Adult rat cochlea had only the exon 20–containing variant.

V. *Eya* GENE EXPRESSION

Eya genes are expressed in a wide range of tissues early in embryogenesis, and although each *Eya* gene has a unique expression pattern, there is extensive overlap. For example, murine studies have shown that *Eya1, Eya2,* and *Eya4* are all expressed in the presomitic mesoderm and head mesenchyme, but only *Eya1* and *Eya4* are expressed in the otic vesicle (12). *Eya3* expression is restricted to craniofacial and branchial arch mesenchyme, in regions underlying or surrounding the *Eya1-2-or-4* expressing cranial placodes (12,15).

A. *Eya4* Inner Ear Expression

In situ hybridization, performed on embryonic and postnatal rat cochleae with a probe derived from mouse *Eya4* cDNA, revealed strong *Eya4* mRNA expression in the neuroepithelium of the developing rat inner ear (Fig. 8). On embryonic day 14 (e14.5) and e16.5, moderate expression was present primarily in the upper epithelium of the cochlear duct, a region that gives rise to Reissner's membrane and the stria vascularis. Low-level expression was observed in the mesenchyme surrounding the duct. The highest levels of expression were seen on e18.5 and were found in areas of the cochlear duct destined to become the spiral limbus, organ of Corti, and spiral prominence,

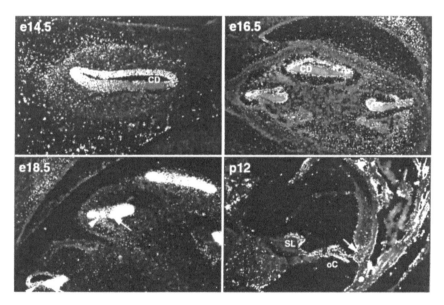

Figure 8   In situ hybridization for *Eya4* mRNA in the developing rat cochlea. Expression is greatest in the epithelium of the cochlear duct (CD). At e14.5 and e16.5, this expression is greatest in the upper half of the duct, cells destined to form the stria vascularis and Reissner's membrane. Concurrently, weak expression is observed in the mesenchyme adjacent to the cochlear duct. Cochlear expression of *Eya4* mRNA peaks at e18.5 and is found preferentially in the lower half of the duct epithelium, in the greater (arrows) and lesser (arrowheads) epithelial ridges, especially in the basal turn. At older ages, expression becomes restricted to cells derived from the spiral limbus, organ of Corti, and spiral prominence. For the first 2 weeks after birth, strong expression is also observed in cells of the developing bony cochlear capsule, as illustrated at p12. (From Ref. 3.)

especially its more rapidly maturing basal turn. These areas continued to express *Eya4* as total expression decreased. Strong expression was also observed in the developing cochlear capsule during the period of ossification, from shortly after birth until p14. In the developing vestibular system, expression was observed primarily in the developing sensory epithelia.

In situ hybridization studies in developing rodent inner ears thus reveal a spatial variability in *Eya4* expression not seen with *Eya1* expression. Both *Eya1* and *Eya4* are expressed early in the otic vesicle (6,18). However, after differentiation of the otic vesicle into auditory and vestibular components, *Eya4* is concentrated in the upper cochlear duct within cells that develop into the stria vascularis and Reissner's membrane, while *Eya1* is expressed in the floor of the cochlear duct, an area that gives rise to the organ of Corti. Throughout development of the inner ear, *Eya1* expression is maintained in derivatives of the neuropithelium of the cochlear duct floor; *Eya4* expression shifts from the upper cochlear duct to the neuroepithelim of the cochlear duct floor only at stage e18.5.

VI.   WHY IS DFNA10 HEARING LOSS POSTLINGUAL?

These data suggest an apparent disjunction between the early expression of *Eya4* and the late-onset hearing loss characteristic of DFNA10; however, it is not unusual for genes to play different roles at different times in development. *Eya4* is present in the adult rodent inner ear, where expression of the exon 20–containing splice variant has been documented. Based on the in situ data and the DFNA10 phenotype, it is tempting to speculate that *Eya4* plays a developmental role in embryogenesis and a survival role in the mature system. Although the neuroepithelial cell types that express *Eya4* have not been characterized, the apparent overlap in expression of *Eya1* and *Eya4* in embryogenesis suggests that some functions of *Eya4* may be redundant to *Eya1* during development. Creating and studying a mouse with a targeted mutation of *Eya4* would resolve many of these issues.

VII.   WHY IS DFNA10 HEARING LOSS NONSYNDROMIC?

The association of late-onset hearing loss with developmentally important transcriptional activators is not unprecedented, as mutations in *POU4F3* are known to cause postlingual hearing loss at the DFNA15 locus (14). What is surprising, however, is the limited DFNA10 phenotype, especially when one considers the clinical impact of *EYA1* mutations. Like the DFNA10-causing *EYA4* mutations, the BOR syndrome-causing mutations in *EYA1* nearly all cluster in the eyaHR (Fig. 6C), but the BOR syndrome phenotype is characterized by widespread disruption of normal embryogenesis. BOR patients have numerous congenital anomalies, including branchial fistulae or cysts, preauricular pits or tags, malformed or small auricles, external auditory canal atresia or stenosis, ossicular hypoplasia, malformed middle ear spaces, underdeveloped or absent cochleae, abnormal semicircular canals, and renal hypoplasia, dysplasia, or aplasia. In contrast, no congenital anomalies, not even hearing loss, are part of the DFNA10 phenotype, despite the wide range of tissues in which *Eya4* is expressed during embryogenesis. Possible explanations include the effect of dosage, whereby haploinsufficiency for wild-type EYA4 does not impair development or survival in extracochlear tissues, but is not tolerated in the inner ear. Another possibility is that there may be redundancy of function in tissues where *EYA* gene expression overlaps. Deficient EYA4 in extracochlear tissues may be compensated for by other EYA proteins, but cannot be compensated for in the cochlea.

REFERENCES

1. Hereditary Hearing Loss Homepage. http://hgins.uia.ac.be/dnalab/hhh/.
2. O'Neill ME, Marietta J, Nishimura D, Wayne S, Van Camp G, Van Laer L, Negrini C, Wilcox ER, Chen A, Fukushima K, Ni L, Sheffield VC, Smith RJH. A gene for autosomal dominant late-onset progressive non-syndromic hearing loss, DFNA10, maps to chromosome 6. Hum Mol Genet 1996; 5:853–856.
3. Wayne S, Robertson NG, DeClau F, Chen N, Verhoeven K, Prasad S, Tranebjarg L, Morton CC, Ryan AF, Van Camp G, Smith RJH. Mutations in the transcriptional activator EYA4 cause late-onset deafness at the DFNA10 locus. Hum Mol Genet 2001; 10(3):195–200.
4. Verhoeven K, Fagerheim T, Prasad S, Wayne S, De Clau F, Balemans W, Verstreken M, Schatteman I, Solem B, Van de Heyning P, Tranebjarg L, Smith RJH, Van Camp G. Refined localization and two additional linked families for the DFNA10 locus for nonsyndromic hearing impairment. Hum Genet 2000; 107:7–11.
5. E De Leenheer, Autosomal dominant non-syndromic hearing impairment. Thesis, 2001.
6. Borsani G, DeGrandi A, Ballabio A, Bulfone A, Bernard L, Banf S, Gattuso C, Mariani M, Dixon M, Donnai D, Metcalfe K, Winter R, Robertson M, Axton R, Brown A, van Heyningen V, Hanson I. *Eya4*, a novel vertebrate gene related to *Drosophila eyes absent*. Hum Mol Genet 1999; 8:11–23.
7. Abdelhak S, Kalatzis V, Heilig R, Compain S, Samson D, Vincent C, Weil D, Cruaud C, Sahly I, Leibovici M, Bitner-Glindzicz M, Francis M, Lacombe D, Vigneron J, Charachon R, Boven K, Bedbeder P, Van Regemorter N, Weissenbach J, Petit C. A human homologue of the *Drosophila eyes absent gene*

underlies branchio-oto-renal (BOR) syndrome and identifies a novel gene family. Nat Genet 1997; 15:157–164.

8. Abdelhak S, Kalatzis V, Heilig R, Compain S, Samson D, Vincent C, Levi-
    Acobas F, Cruaud C, Le Merrer M, Mathieu M, Konig R, Vigneron J, Weis-
    senbach J, Petit C, Weil D. Clustering of mutations responsible for branchio-
    oto-renal (BOR) syndrome in the *eyes absent* homologous region (eyaHR) of
    EYA1. Hum Mol Genet 1997; 6:2247–2255.

9. Xu PX, Cheng J, Epstein JA, Maas RL. Mouse *Eya* genes are expressed during
    limb tendon development and encode a transcriptional activation function. Proc
    Natl Acad Sci USA 1997; 94:11974–11979.

10. Bonini NM, Bui QT, Gray-Board GL, Warrick JM. The *Drosophila eyes absent*
    gene directs ectopic eye formation in a pathway conserved between flies and
    vertebrates. Development 1997; 124:4819–4826.

11. Bonini NM, Fortini ME. Surviving *Drosophila* eye development: integrating
    cell death with differentiation during formation of a neural structure. BioEssays
    1999; 21:991–1003.

12. Ohto H, Kamada S, Tago K, Tominaga SI, Ozaki H, Sato S, Kawakami K.
    Cooperation of *Six* and *Eya* in activation of their target genes through nuclear
    translocation of *Eya*. Mol Cell Biol 1999; 19:6815–6824.

13. Xu PX, Woo I, Her H, Beier DR, Maas RL. Mouse *Eya* homologues of the
    Drosophila eyes absent gene require *Pax6* for expression in lens and nasal plac-
    ode. Development 1997; 124:219–231.

14. Vahava O, Morell R, Lynch ED, Weiss S, Kagan ME, Ahituv N, Morrow JE,
    Lee MK, Skvorak AB, Morton CC, Blumenfeld A, Frydman M, Friedman TB,
    King MC, Avraham KB. Mutation in transcription factor associated with in-
    herited progressive hearing loss in humans. Science 1998; 279:1950–1954.

15. Heanue TA, Reshef R, Davis RJ, Mardon G, Oliver G, Tomarev S, Lassar AB,
    Tabin CJ. Synergistic regulation of vertebrate muscle development by *Dach2*,
    Eya2, and *Six1*, homologs of genes required for *Drosophila* eye formation. Genes
    Dev 1999; 13(24):3231–3243.

16. Zimmerman JE, Bui QT, Steingrimsson E, Nagle DL, Fu W, Genin A, Spinner
    NB, Copeland NG, Jenkins NA, Bucan M, Bonini NM. Cloning and char-
    acterization of two vertebrate homologs of the *Drosophila eyes absent gene*.
    Genome Res 1997; 7:128–141.

17. Xu PX, Adams J, Brown Peters.MC, Heaney S, Maas R. *Eya1*-deficient mice
    lack ears and kidneys and show abnormal apoptosis of organ primordia. Nat
    Genet 1999; 23:113–117.

18. Kalatzis V, Sahly I, El-Amraoui A, Petit C. *Eya1* expression in the develop-
    ing ear and kidney: towards the understanding of the pathogenesis of branchio-
    oto-renal (BOR) syndrome. Dev Dynam 1998; 213:486–499.

21
DFNA5

Lut Van Laer and Guy Van Camp
University of Antwerp, Antwerp, Belgium

Egbert H. Huizing
University Hospital of Utrecht, Utrecht, The Netherlands

I. CLINICAL FEATURES

An extended Dutch family with hereditary hearing impairment was first described in 1966 (1,2) and ever since followed up clinically (3–6). The hearing loss follows an autosomal dominant inheritance pattern with complete penetrance in more than 100 affected individuals (Fig. 1). No additional symptoms are present, indicating that the hearing loss is nonsyndromic. The hearing loss is bilateral, affecting both ears equally. None of the patients ever reported tinnitus or vertigo (1,2). The hearing impairment is sensorineural, and starts between 5 and 15 years of age in the high frequencies, with a progressive loss following a characteristic pattern. First the high-tone losses increase to approximately 80 dB, but low-frequency thresholds remain normal (Fig. 2A). Only when the high-tone thresholds further deteriorate beyond 80 dB do the lower frequencies become affected as well (Fig. 2B). A mean high-frequency loss of approximately 7 dB/year was calculated, but the progression rate significantly differs between individual patients. Fast-progressing patients exhibit their first symptoms at age 5, the lower frequencies become affected by age 15, and the endstage is reached by age 20–25. On the other hand, slowly progressing patients have their first complaints before age 15, low frequencies become affected before age 40 and the endstage is reached in the sixth decade (5,6). When the endstage is established, audiograms show profound hearing impairment at the higher frequencies and severe hearing impairment at the lower frequencies (Fig.

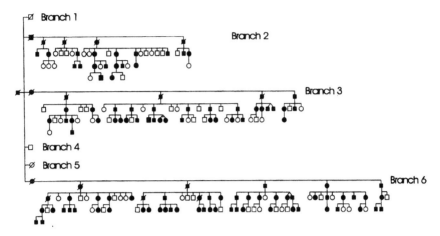

Figure 1   The extended Dutch family with hearing impairment linked to the *DFNA5* locus. The pedigree represents only those family members from whom DNA was obtained during our molecular studies in the period 1995–1998. DFNA5 genotyping defines the affection status of each family member. Affected individuals are represented by solid symbols. Spouses are omitted. Branches 1, 4, and 5 are excluded, as these contain no additional patients.

2C). Generally, most individuals use hearing aids as soon as their losses exceed 40 dB in the speech frequency range. Occasionally, CT scans have been made; however, no abnormalities have been detected. Recently, speech recognition scores were analyzed in 34 affected individuals. Surprisingly, in spite of the severity of the hearing impairment, speech recognition scores were relatively good. At age 70, the extrapolated maximum score was still more than 50%. In comparison with two other well-characterized types of progressive hearing impairment, the maximum phoneme scores for DFNA5 were between those for DFNA2 and DFNA9, DFNA9 showing the worst scores, while typical DFNA5 threshold levels were fairly similar to DFNA2 and DFNA9 threshold levels (7). Although none of the affected family members had vestibular problems, four of them were subjected to extensive vestibular testing, but the response parameter values were normal with few exceptions (8).

Figure 2   The progression of the hearing impairment in the DFNA5 family. Air conduction is represented by open circles. (A) Initially, high-tone losses increase, but low-frequency thresholds remain normal. (B) When the high-tone thresholds further deteriorate beyond 80 dB, the lower frequencies become affected as well. (C) Finally, the endstage is reached.

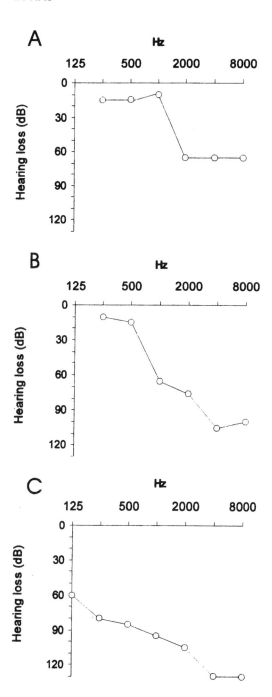

II. LOCALIZATION AND IDENTIFICATION

To localize the gene responsible for the hearing loss in this family, DNA was collected from 68 members of one familial branch. Initially, linkage to DFNA1 and 2 was ruled out (9). After exclusion of other loci known at that time (DFNA3 and 4; DFNB1–3), a genome search was performed. Fifty-one percent of the genome was excluded before linkage was detected in band 7p15 on the short arm of chromosome 7. With genetic marker D7S673 a maximum lod score of 13.53 at 0% recombination was obtained. Haplotypes were constructed and key recombinational events delineated a candidate interval of 15 cM between the flanking markers D7S493 (telomeric side) and D7S632 (centromeric side). The locus was designated DFNA5, as it was the fifth locus for autosomal dominant hearing impairment (10).

Up to now, the Dutch family remains the only one linked to the DFNA5 locus. Therefore, a refinement of the candidate region could be accomplished only by performing linkage analysis on samples from additional familial branches, and by the analysis of additional polymorphic markers. This resulted in a reduction of the candidate region to less then 2 cM between the flanking markers D7S682 (telomeric side) and D7S1791 (centromeric side) (11). Additionally, a YAC-contig covering the complete candidate region was constructed (11,12). One expressed sequence tag (EST) that was derived from a cochlear cDNA library was positioned in the candidate region using the YAC-contig. The complete cDNA sequence of the corresponding gene was determined and it was designated candidate gene 1 (CG1). Extensive mutation analysis, however, could not reveal any disease-causing mutation (11).

A further reduction of the DFNA5 critical region to 600–850 kb between the flanking markers D7S3076 (telomeric side) and D7S1821 (centromeric side) was accomplished by the analysis of additional family members and by the development of new polymorphic markers from the candidate region (13) (Fig. 3). ESTs previously mapped in the vicinity of the DFNA5 candidate region were fine-mapped using the previously established YAC-contig. Only four ESTs mapped in the candidate region, two of them belonging to one gene. Seventy to ninety percent of the candidate region was covered by BACs and PACs, which were completely sequenced as part of the Human Genome Project. By use of a combination of electronic exon trapping (Grail, Mzef, and Genscan), nucleic acid sequence database homology searches (Blast), and 5'-RACE, the full-length cDNA sequences of the genes corresponding to the ESTs were generated. Subsequently, mutation analysis was performed. In one of the genes present in the *DFNA5* candidate region, a complex deletion/insertion mutation was identified in all affected family members: a 1191-bp fragment of intron 7 was deleted and substituted with

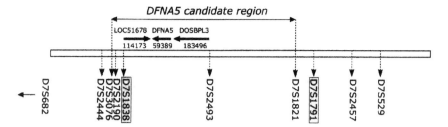

Figure 3 The 600–850-kb *DFNA5* candidate region and adjacent genetic markers. The genes identified in the candidate region are represented with bold arrows (LOC51678: MAGUK protein p55T—protein associated with Lins 2; DFNA5: autosomal dominant deafness type 5; OSBPL3: oxysterol binding protein—like 3). The genomic length of the genes is indicated underneath the arrows. The positions of the genetic markers are indicated with dashed arrows. D7S1838 and D7S1791, the two polymorphic markers preferred for linkage analysis, are indicated.

a 127-bp fragment derived from intron 8, which was inserted in the opposite direction and followed by a GCCCA stretch of unknown origin (Fig. 4). On the mRNA level, the mutation causes skipping of exon 8 (193 bp), resulting in a frameshift starting at amino acid 330, introducing an aberrant stretch of 41 amino acids followed by a stop codon. This intronic mutation does not affect intron-exon boundaries or the branchpoint, but deletes five G-triplets at the 3' end of the intron. Evidence is growing that, in addition to the intron-exon and the branchpoint consensus sequences, other sequences, in particular G-triplets, are involved in splice site selection. For this reason we assume that the deletion of five G-triplets at the 3' side of intron 7 causes skipping of exon 8. The mutation was never found in any of the 250 controls. The gene was designated *DFNA5*, as no physiological function could be deduced from extensive computational analysis. At the genomic level *DFNA5* measures approximately 60 kb and contains 10 exons. *DFNA5* encodes a protein of 496 amino acids with a molecular weight of 54,454 D. *DFNA5* expression was demonstrated by RT-PCR both in the cochlear greater epithelial ridges and in the stria vascularis, as well as in every other tissue investigated so far (13).

III. FUNCTIONAL CONSIDERATIONS

DFNA5 most probably is identical to *ICERE1* (inversely correlated with estrogen receptor expression gene 1), a gene identified during a differential display study comparing gene expression in estrogen-receptor-positive and

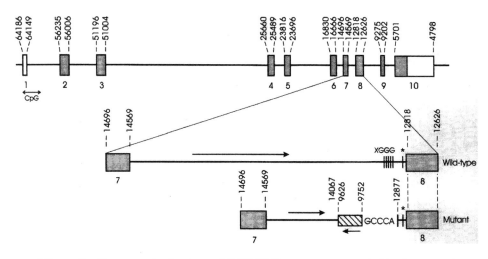

Figure 4 The genomic structure of *DFNA5*. Exons are represented by boxes, and introns by lines. The open reading frame is gray. The position of the exon borders, as derived from the genomic sequence of BAC RG385F02 (GenBank accession number: AC003093), is given above each exon. Exons and introns are drawn at different scales. The position of the CpG island is indicated. A detailed representation of the wild-type and the mutant sequence of exon 7, intron 7, and exon 8 is shown below the genomic structure of *DFNA5*. The putative branchpoint of intron 7 is indicated with an asterisk. In the wild-type chromosome the 5 XGGG-repeats at the 3'-side of intron 7 are represented by vertical lines. The direction of the gene is indicated with arrows. The inserted piece of intron 8 in the mutant chromosome is indicated with a hatched box. It is inserted in the opposite direction and followed by a GCCCA stretch of unknown origin. The borders of the deleted regions are also indicated with their respective nucleotide number. (From Ref. 13. Reproduced with permission.)

estrogen-receptor-negative breast carcinomas (14). This study showed that high expression of estrogen receptors is always accompanied by low levels of *ICERE1/DFNA5*. However, low expression levels of estrogen receptor are not sufficient to obtain high expression of *ICERE1/DFNA5*. Furthermore, transfection of an estrogen-receptor-negative breast cancer cell line with estrogen receptor does not change the *ICERE1/DFNA5* expression level, and transfection of *ICERE1/DFNA5* in an estrogen-receptor-positive breast cancer cell line does not alter the estrogen receptor expression level (14). The interactions between *ICERE1/DFNA5* and the estrogen receptor are therefore not straightforward. This could suggest the involvement of an intermediate factor (e.g., a transcription factor) that would induce one gene and repress the other. In conclusion, definite proof of the involvement of the *ICERE1/DFNA5* gene in breast cancer pathogenesis is lacking and it might be that the upregulation of *ICERE1/DFNA5* in estrogen-receptor-negative breast carcinomas is a side effect rather than a causative factor of tumor formation.

Another differential display set up aimed at studying the mechanisms of acquired drug resistance in malignant melanoma by comparing melanoma cell lines that were either resistant or sensitive to different types of antineoplastic drugs (etoposide, vindesine, fotemustine, and cisplatin). Interestingly, *DFNA5* expression levels are clearly decreased in melanoma cell lines that are highly resistant to etoposide. It was hypothesized that this decrease in *DFNA5* expression level contributes to the etoposide resistance phenotype (15). To prove this hypothesis, the etoposide-resistant melanoma cell line was stably tranfected with *DFNA5*, and it was demonstrated that the transfected cell line was more susceptible to etoposide treatment than the untransfected melanoma cell line. Furthermore, etoposide exposure of *DFNA5*-transfected cells resulted in an increase of caspase-3-mediated programmed cell death, which might indicate that the resistant melanoma phenotype may be due to a decreased cellular susceptibility to trigger apoptotic events as a result of a decreased level of *DFNA5* (16). It is unlikely that similar events take place in cochlear cells from *DFNA5*-mutated subjects, because apoptosis in terminally differentiated cells differs from apoptosis in dividing cells in many aspects. However, the data from this study (16) might indicate that *DFNA5* is involved in the receptor/transporter function that is responsible for cellular drug uptake. Association to or regulation of a cellular receptor/transporter might also be a plausible role for *DFNA5* in cochlear cells.

REFERENCES

1. Huizing EH, van Bolhuis AH, Odenthal DW. Studies on progressive hereditary perceptive deafness in a family of 335 members. I. Genetical and general audiological results. Acta Otolaryngol (Stockh) 1966; 61:35–41.
2. Huizing EH, van Bolhuis AH, Odenthal DW. Studies on progressive hereditary perceptive deafness in a family of 335 members. II. Characteristic pattern of hearing deterioration. Acta Otolaryngol (Stockh) 1996; 61:161–167.
3. Huizing EH, Odenthal DW, van Bolhuis AH. Results of further studies on progressive hereditary sensorineural hearing loss. Audiology 1972; 12:261–263.
4. Huizing EH, van den Wijngaart WSIM, Verschuure J. A follow-up study in a family with dominant progressive inner ear deafness. Acta Otolaryngol (Stockh) 1983; 95:620–626.
5. van den Wijngaart WSIM, Verschuure J, Brocaar MP, Huizing EH. Follow-up study in a family with dominant progressive hereditary sensorineural hearing impairment. I. Analysis of hearing deterioration. Audiology 1985; 24:233–240.

6. van den Wijngaart WSIM, Huizing EH, Niermeijer MF, Verschuure J, Brocaar MP, Blom W. Follow-up study in a family with dominant progressive hereditary sensorineural hearing impairment. II. Clinical aspects. Audiology 1985; 24:336–342.

7. De Leenheer EMR, van Zuijlen DA, Van Laer L, Van Camp G, Huygen PLM, Huizing EH, Cremers CWRJ. Further delineation of the DFNA5 phenotype. Results of speech recognition tests. Ann Otol Rhinol Laryngol 2002; 111:639–641.

8. De Leenheer EMR, van Zuijlen DA, Van Laer L, Van Camp G, Huygen PLM, Huizing EH, Cremers CWRJ. Clinical features of DFNA5. Adv Oto-Rhino-Laryngol 2002; 61:53–59.

9. Coucke P, Van Camp G, Djoyodiharjo B, Smith SD, Frants RR, Padberg GW, Darby JK, Huizing EH, Cremers CWRJ, Kimberling WJ, Oostra BA, Van de Heyning P, Willems PJ. Linkage of autosomal dominant hearing loss to the short arm of chromosome 1 in two families. N Engl J Med 1994; 331:425–431.

10. Van Camp G, Coucke P, Balemans W, van Velzen D, van de Bilt C, Van Laer L, Smith RJH, Fukushima K, Padberg GW, Frants RR, Van de Heyning P, Smith SD, Huizing EH, Willems PJ. Localization of a gene for non-syndromic hearing loss (*DFNA5*) to chromosome 7p15. Hum Mol Genet 1995; 4:2159–2163.

11. Van Laer L, Van Camp G, van Zuijlen D, Green ED, Verstreken M, Schatteman I, Van de Heyning P, Balemans W, Coucke P, Greinwald JH, Smith RJH, Huizing EH, Willems PJ. Refined mapping of a gene for autosomal dominant progressive sensorineural hearing loss (*DFNA5*) to a 2-cM region, and exclusion of a candidate gene that is expressed in the cochlea. Eur J Hum Genet 1997; 5:397–405.

12. Van Laer L, Van Camp G, Green ED, Huizing EH, Willems PJ. Physical mapping of the HOXA1 gene and the *hnRPA2B1* gene in a YAC contig from human chromosome 7p14–p15. Hum Genet 1997; 99:831–833.

13. Van Laer L, Huizing EH, Verstreken M, van Zuijlen D, Wauters JG, Bossuyt PJ, Van de Heyning P, McGuirt WT, Smith RJH, Willems PJ, Legan PK, Richardson GP, Van Camp G. Nonsyndromic hearing impairment is associated with a mutation in *DFNA5*. Nat Genet 1998; 20:194–197.

14. Thompson DA, Weigel RJ. Characterization of a gene that is inversely correlated with estrogen receptor expression (ICERE-1) in breast carcinomas. Eur J Biochem 1998; 252:169–177.

15. Grottke C, Mantwill K, Dietel M, Schadendorf D, Lage H. Identification of differentially expressed genes in human melanoma cells with acquired resistance to various antineoplastic drugs. Int J Cancer 2000; 88:535–546.

16. Lage H, Helmbach H, Grottke C, Dietel M, Schadendorf D. *DFNA5 (ICERE-1)* contributes to acquired etoposide resistance in melanoma cells. FEBS Lett 2001; 494:54–59.

22
COCH

Nahid G. Robertson and Cynthia C. Morton
*Brigham and Women's Hospital and Harvard Medical School,
Boston, Massachusetts, U.S.A.*

I. IDENTIFICATION OF *COCH*: ORGAN-SPECIFIC APPROACH

COCH (*c*oagulation *f*actor *C h*omology) was identified as a novel sequence isolated initially as a partial transcript from a second-trimester human fetal cochlear (membranous labyrinth) cDNA library (developmental ages 17–19 weeks) (1). Its identification was through an organ-specific approach to gene discovery in the auditory system. Subsequent chromosomal mapping of expressed sequences in the inner ear from this method provides candidate genes for deafness disorders localized in coincidental regions.

To isolate genes expressed preferentially or specifically in the inner ear, the cochlear cDNA library was first subtracted against transcripts of the brain (cortex), which is a highly complex tissue in both number and diversity of mRNAs. Subtractive hybridization reduces the number of housekeeping or other common transcripts and enriches for cochlear-specific messages. For further enrichment, subtraction of the cochlear clones was followed by differential screening, whereby a number of both known and novel cochlear transcripts were identified (1). One novel cDNA isolated was originally designated as Coch-5B2 (1) and later renamed *COCH* (GenBank accession number AF006740), based on sequence similarity of the domain of *COCH* that harbors all of its known disease-causing mutations to a region of *Limulus* (horseshoe crab) coagulation factor C (2). Subtractive hybridization techniques using a chicken inner ear cDNA library also yielded *Coch* as one of the differentially expressed transcripts in the auditory system (3).

II. EXPRESSION OF *COCH* MRNA AND PROTEIN

Northern blot analysis (Fig. 1) of human *COCH* on different organs (1,4), including fetal cochlea, vestibule (not shown), brain (cerebral cortex), eye, kidney, liver, spleen, skeletal muscle, lung, skin, thymus, adrenal, small intestine, and cartilage, revealed the presence of very high levels of *COCH* transcripts (~2.0, 2.3, and 2.9 kb) only in the cochlea and vestibule, confirming its differential expression in the inner ear. Very faint *COCH* expression is detected in fetal eye and brain, and adult skeletal muscle, with no detectable hybridization in any other organs tested. Northern blots of adult mouse tissues show messages of approximately 2.0 and 2.5 kb, consistent in size with two mouse cDNAs isolated with two polyadenylation sites, and of similar size to two of the three human messages. In the mouse, a somewhat wider range of expression is seen, including the spleen, brain (cerebrum), thymus, cerebellum, and medulla, and very faint levels in eye and lung (4). The significance of these differences in expression between the two species is not known, but may represent alternative functions of the spleen in hematopoiesis in mice as compared to humans.

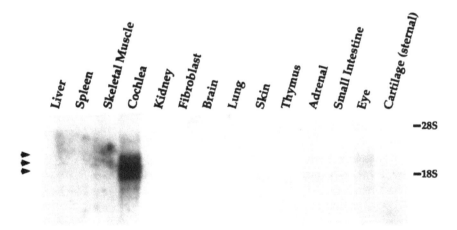

Figure 1   Autoradiograph of Northern blot of 10 µg of total RNAs extracted from human fetal cochlea, brain (cortex), liver, spleen, skeletal muscle, kidney, lung, skin, thymus, adrenal, small intestine, eye, sternal cartilage, and cultured fibroblasts hybridized with *COCH*. Differential expression of *COCH* in the cochlea as compared to other tissues tested is seen, represented by high levels of three transcripts (~2.0, 2.3, and 2.9 kb in size) in the cochlea; very faint hybridization is detected in brain and eye. Transcripts are indicated by arrowheads; the positions of 28S and 18S rRNAs are marked by lines. (From Ref. 1.)

Furthermore, diverse expression patterns of *COCH* in humans and mice may indicate some difference in the function of this gene in the two species during the developmental stages examined. Mapping in the mouse (4) shows localization of *Coch* to mouse chromosome 12 within a region of homologous synteny with the human map assignment on chromosome 14 (see Sec. IV A).

The expression profile of *COCH* throughout different organs of the body indicates that although *COCH* mRNA is not found exclusively in the inner ear, it is present at much higher levels in the cochlea and vestibule than all other organs examined. A recent proteomic analysis of bovine inner ear (5) revealed that the *COCH* protein, cochlin, constitues approximately 70% of proteins isolated from the inner ear and represents the most abundantly detected protein by this analysis. The finding of large amounts of cochlin is in agreement with the high levels of *COCH* mRNA expression, and may also be a reflection of the relative stability of the protein. This study (5) further revealed the presence of three differently sized isoforms (~40, 44, and 63 kD) of cochlin, as well as differently charged isoforms, represented by 16 unique spots on 2D gel electrophoresis. The differently sized isoforms of cochlin may arise from mRNA splice variants, or could result from posttranslational proteolytic processing. These data also suggest that cochlin may undergo other posttranslational modifications, such as glycosylation, phosphorylation, and/or deamination.

III. SEQUENCE ANALYSIS AND STRUCTURE OF *COCH*

A. cDNA and Deduced Amino Acid Sequences

Full-length protein-coding cDNAs for *COCH* (2,4) have been isolated in three species: human, mouse, and chicken (GenBank accession numbers AF006740, AF006741, and AF012252). Sequence comparison (Fig. 2) reveals a high degree of cross-species conservation of *COCH* in the coding region, showing 94% and 79% amino acid identity in the open reading frame (ORF) of the human to the mouse and chicken sequences, respectively. This homology drops abruptly after the translation stop codon, indicating lack of conservation in the 3′ untranslated region of the gene. In all three species, the predicted encoded proteins are almost the same size. The deduced amino acid sequence of human *COCH* shows an ORF of 550 amino acid residues; the mouse and chicken sequences show an ORF of 552 and 547 amino acids, respectively. The minor variation in size and the lowest degree of amino acid conservation in the three species is in the short N-terminal signal peptide, which would be cleaved off and absent in the mature protein.

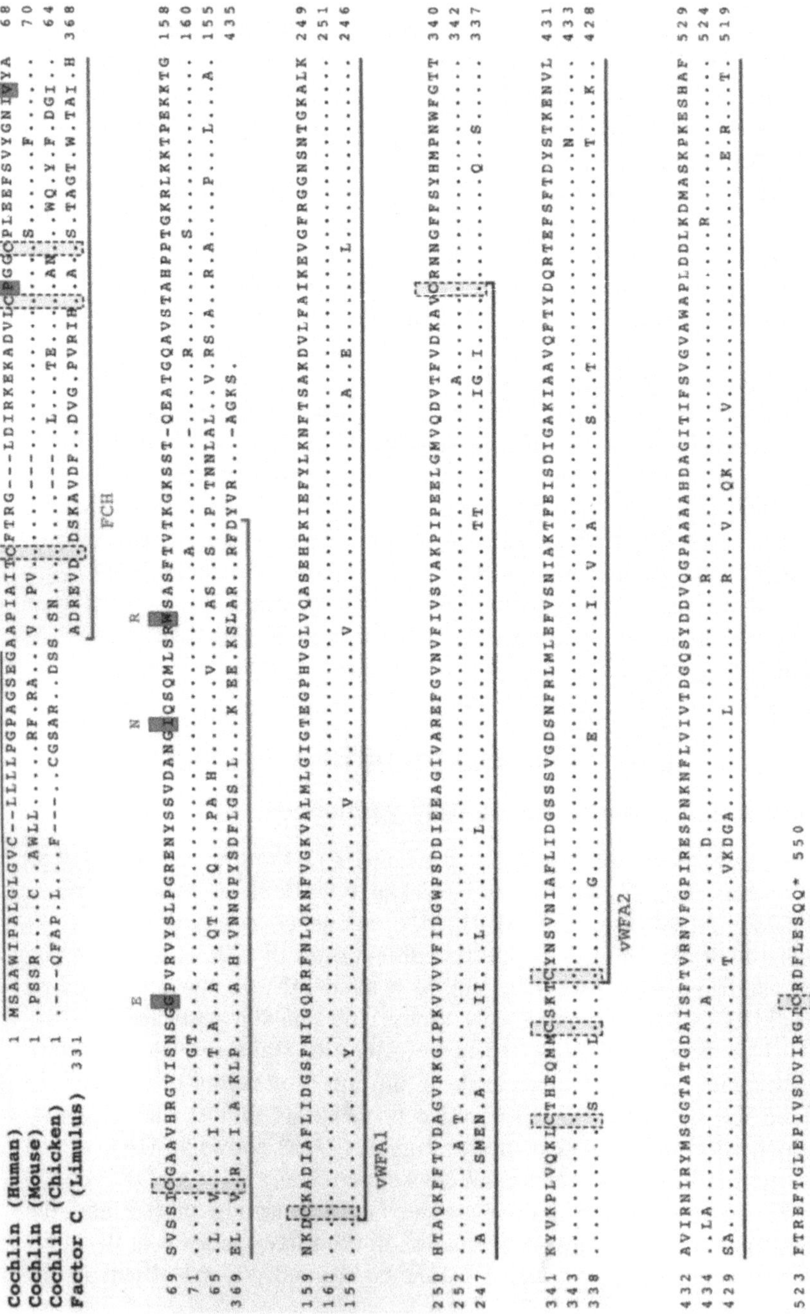

Figure 2

B. Domain Structure

The deduced amino acid sequence of *COCH* (Fig. 2 and 3) shows a mosaic molecule consisting of a secretion signal peptide followed by two different types of domains that are also found in combination with other modules in proteins with diverse functions (2,4). Such protein modules may serve similar functions in different contexts, but have been shuffled and rearranged in the course of evolution. In juxtaposition with a unique set of domains, such modules may create novel associations. *COCH*, encoding the protein cochlin, shows a predicted signal peptide (SP), characteristic of secreted proteins, followed by a region homologous to a domain in factor C of *Limulus* (factor C–homologous domain, FCH), an intervening domain (ivd1), and two von Willebrand factor A–like domains (vWFA1 and vWFA2) separated by an intervening domain (ivd2) (6).

vWFA-like domains are regions approximately 200 amino acid residues in length, often present in multiple copies (and sometimes in tandem) within a single protein. A superfamily of genes with type A domains or "modules" includes proteins, all with ligand-binding properties, involved in various functions such as hemostasis (vWF), the complement (C2, Factor B) and immune systems (integrins such as LFA-1, Mac-1, VLA-1, VLA-2, p150, 95), and the extracellular matrix (cartilage matrix protein, collagens types VI, VII, XII, and XIV) (reviewed in Refs. 7–9). With the exception of integrins, which are transmembrane proteins, the only molecules currently identified to contain type A domains are secreted proteins. The largest number of type A domains known to date are found in the extracellular matrix (ECM), in proteins such as ColVIα3, which has 11 type A–like modules, making up almost all of the protein (10).

Figure 2 Alignment of the complete deduced amino acid sequence of *COCH* in human, mouse, and chicken, and one domain of factor C in *Limulus* (horseshoe crab). A high degree of cross-species homology, including conservation of all cysteine residues (dashed boxes), is seen. Dots indicate amino acid residues that are identical to those in human *COCH*, and dashes indicate gaps introduced to align the sequences. A predicted signal peptide in the beginning of the sequence is indicated by a line above the sequence. Five missense mutations, P51S, V66G, G88E, I109N, and W117R, found in the different DFNA9 families, are indicated. Amino acid residues mutated in DFNA9 show cross-species conservation and all reside in the FCH domain, homologous to a domain in *Limulus* factor C, containing four conserved cysteines. The different domains of cochlin are underlined and labeled as FCH (factor C homologous) and vWFA1 and vWFA2 (von Willebrand factor A–like domains 1 and 2). (From Ref. 2.)

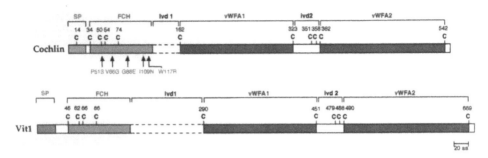

Figure 3 Schematic representation of the deduced amino acid sequence of human *COCH*, encoding the protein cochlin, shows a predicted signal peptide (SP), followed by a region homologous to a domain in factor C of *Limulus* (FCH, factor C–homologous domain), an intervening domain (ivd1), and two von Willebrand factor A–like domains (vWFA1 and vWFA2) separated by an intervening domain (ivd2). Five missense mutations in the FCH domain, causing the DFNA9 deafness and vestibular disorder, are indicated by arrows. The positions of all cysteine residues are shown. Schematic representation of the protein structure of Vit1 is shown below. Vit1 is an extracellular protein in the vitreous gel of the eye. Comparison of cochlin and Vit1 shows very similar structures of the two proteins, with utilization of the same domains in the same order (with a longer ivd1 domain in Vit1). All cysteine residues are conserved between the two proteins except for one cysteine in the signal peptide of cochlin, which would be cleaved out in the mature protein. (From Ref. 6.)

Factor A–like domains of various proteins are thought to mediate a variety of interactions between components of the ECM, cell-ECM interactions, cell-cell adhesion, and cell membrane receptor and soluble factor interactions via binding of the type A domain to proteins such as fibrillar collagens, hyaluronic acid, glycoprotein GpIb, heparin, and complement fragment iC3B (reviewed in Ref. 8). The type A domains in von Willebrand factor have been shown to bind to fibrillar collagens types I and III (11–13). Other collagens, types VI, XII, and XIV, and CMP are also thought to bind fibrillar collagens as a bridging role in ECM assembly and stabilization (8). A conserved motif within vWFA domains for protein binding has been identified and designated as a metal-ion-dependent adhesion site (MIDAS motif) (14). It is likely that cochlin may interact via its two vWFA domains with the abundant fibrillar collagens and other connective tissue elements for ECM assembly in the cochlea and vestibule where function is so tightly dependent on the highly structured architecture of these sensory organs.

All mutations so far detected in cochlin (Fig. 2 and 3), responsible for the pathology manifested in DFNA9 (see Sec. V), occur in the N-terminal region, homologous to the domain in factor C of *Limulus* (horseshoe crab). The FCH region of cochlin is distinct from the adjacent vWFA domain, suggesting it is an independent functional module. This domain is also physically well delineated in *Limulus* factor C and does not overlap with the well-characterized adjacent upstream "sushi" protein-binding domain, also present in many mammalian complement system proteins, or with the adjacent downstream lectin-like domain, also present in mammalian proteins (15,16). Factor C is a serine protease, which, in response to binding lipopolysaccharide endotoxin on a gram-negative bacterial cell surface, initiates a coagulation cascade for host defense (15,16). Although to date no function has been elucidated for this specific domain, it is located within the H chain of *Limulus* factor C, which has been shown to bind lipopolysaccharides (17). Alterations in this cysteine-containing region of cochlin may alter its overall structure and solubility or disrupt the function of this or the downstream vWFA domains.

The FCH motif appears to be quite rare among known proteins. Database homology searches (18,19) have revealed the presence of this domain in few other mammalian proteins: *Lgl1* (late gestation lung protein) (20), a partial cDNA related to a CUB domain (an extracellular module in functionally diverse proteins) (21), a predicted protein from a BAC on human chromosome 2 (GenBank accession number AC007363), and a recently identified member of the cysteine-rich secreted proteins (crisp), CocoaCrisp, described in GenBank (accession number NM031461) as a novel protein associated with the process of septation in the developing chicken midbrain. The FCH domain was referred to as the LCCL module (18,19) for its presence in *Limulus* factor C, *COCH*, and *Lgl1*. *Lgl1*, which contains two tandem FCH/LCCL motifs, is a developmentally regulated gene expressed in lung mesenchyme and involved in lung maturation, possibly through regulation of extracellular matrix degradation (20). The specific function of the FCH/LCCL motif in these newly identified proteins is not known.

Multiple alignment comparisons in various proteins and three-dimensional structure analysis by nuclear magnetic resonance (NMR) spectroscopy of the FCH/LCCL domain identified it as an autonomous folding domain (18,19). The fold is thought to be novel, consisting of a central α-helix wrapped by two β-sheets composed of a total of eight β-strands, some of which are very short (19). Most of the cochlin residues mutated in DFNA9 are located on the protein surface in the FCH/LCCL domain, but introduction of the mutations in vitro has been shown to interfere with proper folding of this domain (19).

C. New Family of "Cochlin-Related" Proteins

The predicted peptide from the human chromosome 2 BAC containing an FCH domain (18) appears to be the human homolog of a recently isolated protein, designated Vit1, from the vitreous of the bovine eye (22). Human and mouse *VIT1* cDNAs were cloned using degenerate primers to the bovine peptide sequence (22). The protein sequence of Vit1 (Fig. 3) reveals a modular structure very similar to that of cochlin: a secretion signal peptide followed by an FCH domain, an intervening domain (ivd1), and two tandem vWFA-like modules, also separated by a short intervening domain (ivd2).

The only apparent structural difference between the two proteins is the length of the ivd1 (~125 aa in Vit1, ~35 aa in cochlin). The longer ivd1 in Vit1 may represent an additional domain, but it does not contain any cysteine residues. All cysteines, including the ones in ivd2, are conserved between Vit1 and cochlin. Furthermore, *COCH* and *VIT1* possess the same exon/intron boundaries of their vWFA domains, which differ from some boundaries of other vWFA-containing genes (22). *COCH* and *VIT1* are the only genes presently reported with evolutionary utilization of the same combination of modules in the same order, indicating that they may be closely related members of the same family of proteins with similar functions.

The vitreous gel of the eye is a network of connective tissue elements, including thin collagen fibrils (predominantly type II, some types IX, V/XI), hyaluronan, and Vit1, speculated to have a bridging role between these components for stabilization of the vitreous gel (22). Cochlin and Vit1 are similar in their colocalization with collagen fibrils, suggesting possible inter-

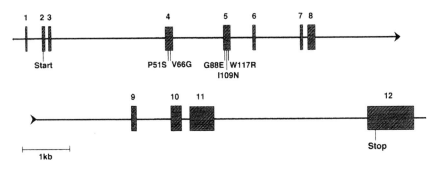

Figure 4 Schematic drawing of human *COCH* genomic structure showing intron-exon organization of the gene. The two separate lines represent continous genomic sequence. Exons are indicated by shaded boxes, separated by introns shown as lines. Positions of missense mutations P51S, V66G, G88E, I109N, and W117R, found in the different DFNA9 families, are indicated. The region of *Limulus* factor C homology (FCH) spans exons 4–5. The von Willebrand factor type A–like domain, vWFA1, is contained within exons 8–10; vWFA2 is in exons 11 and 12. Position of start and stop codons for translation are indicated. All known DFNA9 mutations are contained in exons 4 and 5 corresponding to the FCH domain of *COCH*. (From Ref. 2.)

actions with these proteins. Occurrence of these two closely related proteins in the inner ear and the eye may be a reflection of their common role in the matrices of these two sensory organs, and parallel studies of these proteins may provide valuable insight into their roles in the respective organs.

D. Genomic Structure

The human *COCH* gene consists of 12 exons (Fig. 4) with the methionine for start of translation in exon 2. The region with homology to *Limulus* factor C (FCH region) spans exons 4–5. This region contains all missense mutations known to cause DFNA9: P51S and V66G mutations are in exon 4 and G88E, I109N, and W117R mutations are in exon 5. The first vWFA-like domain, vWFA1, is contained within exons 8–10; vWFA2 is in exons 11 and 12. The stop codon for translation is present in exon 12.

IV. *COCH* MUTATIONS AND DFNA9

A. U.S. Families

The human *COCH* gene was mapped to 14q11.2–q13 (4) wholly within the interval for the DFNA9 locus, assigned by linkage analysis in one large U.S. family (23). DFNA9 (OMIM #601369) was initially described in this and another unrelated U.S. kindred as an autosomal dominant, fully penetrant sensorineural hearing loss with a postlingual age of onset (between 16 and 28 years of age), initially more profound at high frequencies, with progression to anacusis (40–50 years of age) (24–26). Some DFNA9 individuals have received cochlear implants and others use hearing aids. An accompanying feature of this type of deafness is a variable spectrum of vestibular involvement including unsteadiness, difficulty walking in the dark, vertigo, and vestibular dysfunction as assessed by electronystagmography (ENG) and other clinical tests. DFNA9 also has a strikingly characteristic histopathology as seen in temporal bone sections of affected individuals, where there is a marked loss of cellularity in the fibrocytes of the cochlea and vestibular labyrinths, accumulation of a homogeneous, eosinophilic material, and neuronal and organ of Corti degeneration (discussed further in Sect. V) (24,25,27).

Mutation analysis of three unrelated DFNA9 U.S. families (designated 1W, 1Su, and 1St) was performed by PCR amplification and direct sequencing of genomic DNAs in all coding exons and intron-exon boundaries of *COCH* (2); three different nucleotide changes were revealed in the same domain of *COCH*: T $\mapsto$ G substitution at nucleotide position 253 in exon 4 in kindred 1W, G $\mapsto$ A substitution at position 319 in exon 5 in kindred 1Su, and T ↦ C substitution at position 405 in exon 5 in kindred 1St. The three nucleotide changes cause missense mutations in *COCH* resulting in amino acid substitutions of Val ↦ Gly at codon 66 (GTA↦GGA), designated V66G; Gly ↦ Glu at codon 88 (GGA↦GAA), designated G88E; and Trp ↦ Arg at codon 117 (TGG↦CGG), designated W117R. All affected individuals were heterozygous for the mutation, as expected for an autosomal dominant mode of inheritance. The nucleotide change segregated completely with the disease phenotype and was never observed in unaffected family members (past the expected age of onset) and in a large number of unaffected individuals in the general population, supporting the conclusion that the changes are true mutations and not polymorphisms.

B. Belgian and Dutch Families

Other families with DFNA9 cochleovestibular disorder were also shown to have different point mutations in the same domain of *COCH*. Two groups (28,29) reported the finding of a C ↦T nucleotide change at position 207 in exon 4 of *COCH* resulting in a Pro ↦Ser substitution at codon 51 (CCA↦TCA), designated P51S, in a total of seven families from Belgium and the Netherlands.

In one series of reports (28,30,31), a large Dutch family (designated W98-011) and three small Dutch kindreds (designated W98-065, W98-066, and W98-094) are described with DFNA9 and found to have the P51S mutation in *COCH* (28). Members of the large family have a somewhat later age of onset (ranging from 36 to 62 years), suggesting *COCH* mutations and DFNA9 as a possible monogenic etiology or risk factor for the multifactorial age-related hearing loss presbyacusis. There is rapid progression to profound hearing loss, as well as more consistent and well-established vestibular impairment, including instability especially in the dark, head-movement-dependent oscillopsia, and vestibular areflexia or hyporeflexia. Of note, there is also a high incidence of cardiovascular disease among affected members (28,30,31).

In another series of reports (29,32–34), the disease phenotype and the finding of the P51S mutation are described in one large Belgian and two Dutch families. One of the members of the large Belgian family, who was homozygous for the P51S mutation, had an earlier age of onset of DFNA9 symptoms in comparison to most affected family members (~25 years vs. median of 42 years), and was more severely affected at age 34 than several older heterozygotes (29). In addition to progressive late-onset sensorineural hearing loss and balance problems, a significant number of affected individuals had additional vestibular symptoms, including episodes of vertigo, tinnitus, and aural fullness. Clinically, these symptoms are consistent with

the criteria for Meniere disease (OMIM #156000), which includes disturbances in inner ear fluid homeotasis. Because some DFNA9 patients
received a diagnosis of Meniere disease, and because Meniere disease is
most likely a disorder with heterogeneous and multifactorial etiologies, it
may be warranted to consider the possibility of *COCH* mutations in
individuals with symptoms of Meniere disease (29), in particular those in
which a family history of hearing loss is present.

Subsequently, a combined study of these seven families with the P51S
COCH mutation, as well as an additional 29 families or simplex cases from
Belgium and the southern region of the Netherlands, was performed to
assess whether there is an ancestral haplotype (35). Of the 29 new families or
individuals, eight were shown to have the P51S mutation, bringing the
number of DFNA9 families examined with this mutation to a total of 15.
The rest of the *COCH* gene was not screened in these patients for the
presence of other mutations. Haplotype analysis with markers flanking the
COCH gene strongly suggested a single common founder for the P51S
mutation in the DFNA9 families in this geographic region (35).

C. Australian Family

A different missense mutation was found in an Australian family (36) in the
same domain of *COCH* that contains the previously reported mutations. A
T↦A substitution at nucleotide 382 in exon 5 of *COCH* results in an Ile ↦
Asn change at codon 109, (ATC ↦ AAC), designated I109N. The clinical
features in the affected members of this family are consistent with the
DFNA9 phenotype of progressive sensorineural hearing loss starting in the
high frequencies with presence of vestibular symptoms. The age of onset is
variable but fairly early, in the second and third decades, progressing to
severe to profound loss across all frequences by the sixth to seventh decades.
Remarkably, progressive vestibular dysfunction seemed to be fully penetrant in the affected individuals in this family, seen mostly as unsteadiness,
especially in the dark, but infrequent vertigo (36).

D. Comparison of DFNA9 Families and the Different *COCH* Mutations

Although there is variability in the age of onset of hearing loss within a family
as well as between families with different *COCH* mutations, the hearing loss
in DFNA9 is fully penetrant, dominantly inherited, sensorineural with
postlingual age of onset, and progressive. Also, despite variability in the
age of onset, nature, and severity of vestibular dysfunction, it is a prominent
and defining characteristic of DFNA9 and *COCH* mutations, as also

supported by the finding of histological abnormalities in the vestibular labyrinth (see Sec. V). Even though there is a very common association of hearing and balance problems in mice, to date DFNA9 is the only autosomal dominant nonsyndromic deafness in humans that is associated with vestibular problems. Of note, several of the individuals and families with DFNA9 were identified initially on the basis of their characteristic hearing loss and vestibular abnormalities, without genetic linkage analysis, and were subsequently determined to have *COCH* mutations.

Differences in reports of balance dysfunction may be due to several factors. Vestibular problems may be underestimated or may go unnoticed because of other compensatory mechanisms provided by the visual and proprioceptive systems that may attenuate the symptoms of balance dysfunction. More careful examination, systematic and thorough testing, as is being done more frequently in DFNA9 families, will provide more accurate documentation of the extent and severity of vestibular dysfunction. It is possible that the nature and position of the different mutations in *COCH* account for phenotypic variation among different families. Also, other genetic or environmental factors may be responsible for differences in symptomatology within members of the same family.

The underlying cause of DFNA9, presence of missense mutations in *COCH*, all within its FCH domain, point toward a common mechanism of pathogenesis. A summary of the *COCH* mutations identified to date in the DFNA9 families is presented in Table 1. The five mutated cochlin amino acid residues (Fig. 2) are evolutionarily conserved among human, mouse, and chicken: all residues are identical in the deduced amino acid sequence of *COCH* in the three species except for a conservative change of valine at codon 66 to isoleucine in the chicken (2). Furthermore, of the five *COCH* residues mutated in DFNA9, Pro51, Gly88, and Ile109 are identical to the FCH domain in *Limulus*; Val66 is conserved as isoleucine, and Trp117 corresponds in *Limulus* factor C to a leucine, also an uncharged hydrophobic residue (2).

All known mutations in *COCH* result in nonconservative amino acid changes, supporting the possibility of disruption of the normal structure and function of cochlin. The FCH domain, containing all known *COCH* mutations, has four cysteine residues, which are all conserved in the human, mouse, and chicken cochlin and in *Limulus* factor C (Fig. 2 and 3). Amino acid changes in this cysteine-containing region may interfere with formation of disulfide bonds, disrupting proper folding, overall structure, and possibly secretion and solubility of the protein. Altered tertiary structure may perturb function of this and the downstream vWFA domains, which are expected to bind other molecules, including those with sugar moieties. The link to the abnormal acidophilic ground substance deposits seen in DFNA9

Table 1 *COCH* Mutations in DFNA9 Families

Origin of families	Exon with mutation[a]	Nucleotide change[b]	Amino acid change[c]	Ref.
Belgium and The Netherlands	4	C207T	P51S	28,29
United States	4	T253G	V66G	2
United States	5	G319A	G88E	2
Australia	5	T382A	I109N	36
United States	5	T405C	W117R	2

[a] For mutation screening of exon 4, the following PCR primers can be used: 5′ cttaaa-tctcacactgtagtc 3′ and 5′ aaaggaaataatcacgtctgc 3′. For mutation screening of exon 5, the following PCR primers can be used: 5′ tctttagatgacttccctgatgag 3′ and 5′ tcacaggtttttccat-caaggtta 3′.

[b] Numbering of nucleotides is according to the human *COCH* cDNA sequence (GenBank Accession No. AF006740), which starts in the 5′ untranslated region, 56 bp upstream of the start ATG.

[c] Numbering of amino acids begins at the start methionine.

may be directly through precipitation and accumulation of the cochlin protein itself, or through abnormal interaction with other extracellular components in the inner ear, required for clearing of these substances or for proper organization of various elements in the inner ear.

V. INNER EAR LOCALIZATION OF *COCH*: CORRELATION WITH DFNA9 HISTOPATHOLOGY

A. Localization of mRNA and Protein Products of *COCH*

Initial in situ hybridization of *Coch* on late embryonic and posthatching chicken cochlear and vestibular labyrinths (2) showed intense *Coch* hybridization in spindle-shaped cells along the pathway of auditory nerve fibers to the habenula perforata, the opening through which neurites extend to innervate hair cells (corresponding to the human osseous spiral lamina), in the area of the cartilaginous plates of the neural limb (corresponding to the human spiral limbus) and the abneural limb (corresponding to human spiral ligament) on medial and lateral edges of the sensory epithelium. No signal was detected in the basilar papilla (sensory epithelium equivalent to the human organ of Corti), the tegmentum vasculosum (equivalent to the human stria vascularis), or spiral ganglion cells. In the vestibular labyrinth, strong *Coch* hybridization was detected in the stroma underlying the sensory epithelium of the crista ampullaris and in the area adjacent to vestibular

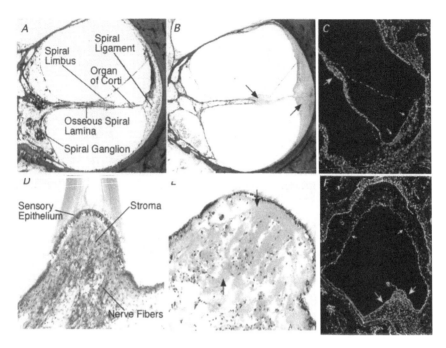

Figure 5 (A and D) Photomicrograph (50×) of (A) the basal turn of the cochlea from an unaffected (control) member of the U.S. DFNA9 family 1W (59-year-old man, postmortem time unknown), and (D) the crista ampullaris of the posterior semicircular canal from a control human temporal bone (81-year-old man, postmortem time 7 h) stained with hematoxylin and eosin. (A) Normal components of the cochlea are indicated. (D) Normal constituents of the crista are shown.

(B and E) Photomicrographs (50×) from two hearing-impaired individuals with DFNA9. (B) The basal turn of the cochlea from an individual with DFNA9 from the U.S. family 1St, with the W117R mutation (71-year-old man, postmortem time unknown) and (E) the crista ampullaris of the posterior semicircular canal from a DFNA9 individual from U.S. family 1W, with the V66G mutation (86-year-old woman, postmortem time 18 h) stained with hematoxylin and eosin. (B) The osseous spiral lamina, spiral limbus, and spiral ligament show loss of cellularity with presence of abundant homogeneous eosinophilic substance (arrows). There is loss of spiral ganglion cells and of their dendrites innervating the organ of Corti and degeneration of the organ of Corti. (E) The stroma of the crista shows abundant eosinophilic deposits (arrows) similar to that found in the cochlea with loss of stromal cells and nerve fibers. The sensory epithelium shows severe degeneration of hair cells, with only supporting cells remaining.

(C and F) In situ hybridization of the *COCH* gene in human fetal inner ear. Silver grains, reflecting hybridization of ^{33}P-labeled *COCH* probe, were captured with bright-field microscopy and pseudocolored red. For tissue morphology, Hoescht 33258 counterstaining of nuclei was visualized by fluorescence microscopy with a DAPI nerve fibers. No signal was detected in the sensory epithelium (hair cells and supporting cells).

Subsequently, in situ hybridization was performed on human fetal and adult mouse inner ears (6), showing strong COCH hybridization in fibrocytes located in the spiral limbus and throughout the spiral ligament (fibrocyte types I, III, and IV), including the suprastriatal zone (Fig. 5C). Because the spiral ligament constitutes a large percentage of the total mass of the membranous cochlea, the abundance of COCH mRNA in this area reflects its overall high-level expression in this organ. In the vestibular labyrinth (Fig. 5F), high levels of COCH mRNA were found in the stromal cells underlying the sensory epithelium in the crista ampullaris of the semicircular canals. These fibrocytic cells surround the Schwann cell bodies and nerve fibers, which do not show COCH expression. Cells in the wall of the semicircular canal also showed presence of COCH mRNA. No hybridization was detected in the sensory epithelia of the cochlea or the vestibule.

The cochlear and vestibular labyrinths have apparent similarities in their structure and function. For example, proteins associated with hair cells, such as the unconventional myosins, have been shown to be important in both systems. However, many of the genes expressed in the cochlea and responsible for deafness have not been studied in the vestibular system. Localization of COCH in mesodermally derived tissues in the support structures underlying and adjacent to the sensory epithelium and surrounding neural fibers of both organs may point toward other common proteins responsible for maintenance of the precise architecture and ionic balance necessary for proper mechanosensory transduction in these analogous systems.

Immunohistochemistry was performed using the anticochlin antibody, developed against the FCH and ivd1 domains of cochlin, on mouse, human adult, and human fetal cochlear sections (6). Immunostaining for cochlin was observed in the area of the fibrocytes of the spiral limbus and spiral ligament (mainly fibrocytes types I and III), in addition to extracellular spaces in these

---

filter and pseudocolored blue. (C) Cross-section of a cochlear duct in human fetal cochlea (19-week developmental age) shows intense COCH hybridization in the fibrocytes of the spiral limbus (large arrow) and throughout the spiral ligament (fibrocyte types I, III, and IV) (small arrows). (F) In the human fetal vestibular system (crista ampullaris of a semicircular canal), strong COCH signal is detected in the stromal cells (fibrocytes) underlying the sensory epithelium (large arrow) and in the surrounding wall of the semicircular canal (small arrows). COCH RNA localization in the inner ear (C and F) correlates well with the sites of abnormal deposits seen in DFNA9 inner ear sections (B and E). Fibrocytes of the cochlear and vestibular labyrinths that express COCH are the same cell types that are markedly absent in DFNA9. (From Refs. 2 and 6.)

structures. The predominant immunostaining pattern obtained with the anticochlin antibody in the spiral limbus and spiral ligament corresponds to *COCH* mRNA expression detected by in situ hybridization.

B. Correlation with DFNA9 Histopathology

A striking feature of the DFNA9 disease phenotype (Fig. 5B,E) is the presence of abundant deposits of a homogeneous acidophilic ground substance that almost completely fills the lateral wall of the cochlear duct in the area of the spiral ligament, the spiral limbus, and osseous spiral lamina, as well as in the stroma of the crista ampullaris and the macula in the vestibular system (24,25,27). These areas closely parallel the sites of the distribution of mRNA and protein products of *COCH* in the cochlea and vestibule.

DFNA9 histopathological findings (Fig. 5B,E) also include marked loss of cellularity in both organs, including loss of the fibrocytes in the spiral limbus, the spiral ligament, and the stromal cells of the crista and macula; these are the very cell types that express *COCH* abundantly in the normal human fetal and mouse inner ears. Neuroepithelial degeneration of the organ of Corti, crista, and macula, and the dendrites and ganglia of the cochlear and vestibular nerves is also seen in some DFNA9 inner ear sections (24,25,27).

The sequence of events leading to deafness and balance dysfunction in DFNA9, the exact composition of the acidophilic material, and the relationship to cellular and neuronal atrophy remain to be elucidated. Previous staining of sections has shown these deposits to contain a mucopolysaccharide-type substance (24). Recent electron microscopic examination of these deposits shows dense, highly branched and disarrayed, nonparallel microfibrils with a granular substance (possibly glycosaminoglycans) scattered among the fibrils (37). There is an apparent degradation and loss of the normal fibrillar type II collagen in the same areas. The spatial correlation of cochlin expression with the abnormal acidophilic deposits in DFNA9 suggests either a direct effect of the mutated protein in these locations or possible altered binding of cochlin with other proteins such as the fibrillar collagens.

Areas of the cochlea that express cochlin also contain a network of gap junctions (38) thought to play an important role in fluid homeostasis by recycling K^+ ions through the spiral limbus and spiral ligament, back into the endolymph of scala media, which bathes the hair cells. Loss of normal fibrocytes and accumulation of the homogeneous acidophilic material in the spiral ligament and spiral limbus caused by *COCH* mutations could interfere with adequate intercellular ion flow through these gap junctions and disrupt the integrity of this system critical for proper cochlear function (6,29).

The late onset and progressive nature of DFNA9 as a result of *COCH* missense mutations may suggest gain of a novel deleterious property of cochlin, affecting the structure and function of this protein, or its interaction with other extracellular components of the inner ear. This in turn could lead to accumulation of the acidophilic deposits and cell death, disrupting the integrity of the support structures, neural elements, and ionic balance necessary for normal functioning of the cochlear and vestibular organs.

VI. FUTURE DIRECTIONS

The prevalence of *COCH* mutations in the population has not been examined systematically, and therefore the true frequency is not known. However, *COCH* may be emerging possibly as a common cause of late-onset deafness and vestibular dysfunction as supported by the finding of *COCH* mutations in geographically distant regions on different continents. Mutation screening for *COCH* worldwide may become more prevalent, as seen in a recent report of a *COCH* mutation identified in Japan (39). A novel missense mutation in exon 5 (FCH domain) of *COCH* (nucletoide G411A, resulting in amino acid substitutions of A119T) was found in a Japanese family with autosomal dominant nonsyndromic sensorineural hearing loss (39, and S. Usami, personal communication, 2002). It will also be of interest to evaluate whether the same mutations in different parts of the world arose independently or from a common ancestor.

In the rare cases of postmortem temporal bone availability, two of the U.S. families were initially identified on the basis of the very unique DFNA9 histopathological findings, in the absence of data from a large number of family members to enable linkage analysis. However, several of the families and individuals found to date to have *COCH* mutations were initially chosen for evaluation on the basis of similarity of symptoms, especially presence of vestibular dysfunction, to the original characterized DFNA9 family in which linkage analysis was performed. This observation further supports the necessity and value of screening sporadic as well as familial cases of late-onset deafness, especially with the presence of balance problems and Meniere-like symptoms, for presence of *COCH* mutations as the etiology. This would be a worthwhile endeavor to provide a more accurate diagnosis and classification of deafness and vestibular problems. In addition, genotype-phenotype correlation studies could reveal possible differences or variations in DFNA9 pathology caused by alternative mutations.

Another important area of investigation will be to elucidate the exact role of cochlin in the cochlear and vestibular labyrinths, and the mechanism of pathogenesis of the *COCH* mutations leading to DFNA9 deafness and perturbations of balance. The deduced amino acid sequence of cochlin is consistent with an extracellular protein with a likely structural or stabilizing role, and binding properties with other proteins, warranting a search for an interaction partner. Because the two types of domains that occur in cochlin are also found in some proteins involved in defense mechanisms, it has been suggested that cochlin may also serve a similar function (18,19).

In light of the fact that all known *COCH* mutations occur in the same domain (the FCH/LCCL module), the function of this domain and the disruptive effects of the single amino acid mutations on the properties and function of cochlin should be investigated. A recent study (19) has shown the folding of the bacterially expressed FCH/LCCL domain of wild-type and mutated cochlin in vitro. Three of the four point mutations tested resulted in misfolding of the domain, causing precipitation of most of the protein during the standard refolding protocol. These results are intriguing with respect to the observation of eosinophilic deposits in DFNA9 inner ear sections. It will be important to test the effects of the *COCH* point mutations within the context of the entire protein in a cellular environment. For example, eukaryotic transfection and expression of wild-type and mutated cochlin can be performed to assess the effects of these mutations on properties such as secretion, subcellular localization, and transport of the protein.

Furthermore, a mouse model can be developed by introduction of the single base pair changes present in DFNA9 leaving the rest of the gene intact. Creating this "knockin" mouse model would most closely duplicate the underlying genetic changes in DFNA9, and would allow for the systematic analysis of clinical, gross, and histological changes and the sequence of events leading to deafness and balance dysfunction in DFNA9.

Future endeavors will provide a better understanding of the role of cochlin in the inner ear and the mechanism of pathogenesis caused by *COCH* mutations, in the hope for better diagnosis, management, counseling, and possibly prevention and treatment of hearing loss and vestibular dysfunction.

REFERENCES

1. Robertson NG, Khetarpal U, Gutiérrez-Espeleta GA, Bieber FR, Morton CC. Isolation of novel and known genes from a human fetal cochlear cDNA library using subtractive hybridization and differential screening. Genomics 1994; 23:42–50.
2. Robertson NG, Lu L, Heller S, Merchant SN, Eavey RD, McKenna M, Nadol JB Jr, Miyamoto RT, Linthicum FH Jr, Lubianca Neto JF, Hudspeth AJ, Seidman CE, Morton CC, Seidman JG. Mutations in a novel cochlear gene cause DFNA9, a human nonsyndromic deafness with vestibular dysfunction. Nat Genet 1998; 20:299–303.

3. Heller S, Sheane CA, Javed Z, Hudspeth AJ. Molecular markers for cell types of the inner ear and candidate genes for hearing disorders. Proc Natl Acad Sci USA 1998; 95:11400–11405.

4. Robertson NG, Skvorak AB, Yin Y, Weremowicz S, Johnson KR, Kovatch KA, Battey JF, Bieber FR, Morton CC. Mapping and characterization of a novel cochlear gene in human and in mouse: a positional candidate gene for a deafness disorder, DFNA9. Genomics 1997; 46:345–354.

5. Ikezono T, Omori A, Ichinose S, Pawankar R, Watanabe A, Yagi T. Identification of the protein product of the *Coch* gene (hereditary deafness gene) as the major component of bovine inner ear protein. Biochim Biophys Acta 2001; 1535:258–265.

6. Robertson NG, Resendes BL, Lin JS, Lee C, Aster JC, Adams JC, Morton CC. Inner ear localization of mRNA and protein products of *COCH*, mutated in the sensorineural deafness and vestibular disorder, DFNA9. Hum Mol Genet 2001; 10:2493–2500.

7. Colombatti A, Bonaldo P. The superfamily of proteins with von Willebrand factor type A–like domains: one theme common to components of extracellular matrix, hemostasis, cellular adhesion, and defense mechanisms. Blood 1991; 77:2305–2315.

8. Colombatti A, Bonaldo P, Doliana R. Type A modules: interacting domains found in several non-fibrillar collagens and in other extracellular matrix proteins. Matrix 1993; 13:297–306.

9. Tuckwell D. Evolution of von Willebrand factor A (VWA) domains. Biochem Soc Trans 1999; 27:835–840.

10. Bonaldo P, Russo V, Bucciotti F, Doliana R, Colombatti A. Structural and functional features of the a3 chain indicate a bridging role for chicken collagen VI in connective tissues. Biochemistry 1990; 29:1245–1254.

11. Roth GJ, Titani K, Hoyer LW, Hickey MJ. Localization of binding sites within human von Willebrand factor for monomeric type III collagen. Biochemistry 1986; 25:8357–8361.

12. Kalafatis M, Takahashi Y, Girma J, Meyer D. Localization of a collagen-interactive domain of human von Willebrand factor between amino acid residues gly 911 and glu 1,365. Blood 1987; 70:1577–1583.

13. Pareti FI, Kenji N, McPherson JM, Ruggeri ZM. Isolation and characterization of two domains of human von Willebrand factor that interact with fibrillar collagen types I and III. J Biol Chem 1987; 262:13835–13841.

14. Lee JO, Rieu P, Arnaout MA, Liddington R. Crystal structure of the A domain from the alpha subunit of integrin CR3 (CD11b/CD18). Cell 1995; 80:631–638.

15. Iwanaga S, Miyata T, Tokunaga F, Muta T. Molecular mechanism of hemolymph clotting system in *Limulus*. Thromb Res 1992; 68:1–32.

16. Muta T, Miyata T, Misumi Y, Tokunaga F, Nakamura T, Toh Y, Ikehara Y, Iwanaga S. *Limulus* factor C: an endotoxin-sensitive serine protease zymogen with a mosaic structure of complement-like, epidermal growth factor-like, and lectin-like domains. J Biol Chem 1991; 266:6554–6561.

17. Nakamura T, Tokunaga F, Morita T, Iwanaga S, Kusumoto S, Shiba T, Kobayashi T, Inoue K. Intracellular serine-protease zymogen, factor C, from

horseshoe crab hemocytes: its activation by synthetic lipid A analogues and acidic phospholipids. Eur J Biochem 1988; 176:89–94.

18. Trexler M, Banyai L, Patthy L. The LCCL module. Eur J Biochem 2000; 267:5751–5757.

19. Liepinsh E, Trexler M, Kaikkonen A, Weigelt J, Banyai L, Patthy L, Otting G. NMR structure of the LCCL domain and implications for DFNA9 deafness disorder. EMBO J 2001; 20:5347–5353.

20. Kaplan F, Ledoux P, Kassamali FQ, Gagnon S, Post M, Koehler D, Deimling J, Sweezey NB. A novel developmentally regulated gene in lung mesenchyme: homology to a tumor-derived trypsin inhibitor. Am J Physiol 1999; 276:L1027–1036.

21. Bork P, Beckmann G. The CUB domain: a widespread module in developmentally regulated proteins. J Mol Biol 1993; 231:539–545.

22. Mayne R, Ren ZX, Liu J, Cook T, Carson M, Narayana S. VIT-1: the second member of a new branch of the von Willebrand factor A domain superfamily. Biochem Soc Trans 1999; 27:832–835.

23. Manolis EN, Yandavi N, Nadol JB Jr, Eavey RD, McKenna M, Rosenbaum S, Khetarpal U, Halpin C, Merchant SN, Duyk GM, MacRae C, Seidman CE, Seidman JG. A gene for non-syndromic autosomal dominant progressive post-lingual sensorineural hearing loss maps to chromosome 14q12-13. Hum Mol Genet 1996; 5:1047–1050.

24. Khetarpal U, Schuknecht HF, Gacek RR, Holmes LB. Autosomal dominant sensorineural hearing loss: pedigrees, audiologic and temporal bone findings in two kindreds. Arch Otolaryngol Head Neck Surg 1991; 117:1032–1042.

25. Khetarpal U. Autosomal dominant sensorineural hearing loss: further temporal bone findings. Arch Otolaryngol Head Neck Surg 1993; 119:106–108.

26. Halpin C, Khetarpal U, McKenna M. Autosomal dominant progressive sensorineural hearing loss in a large North American Family. Am J Audiol 1996; 5:105–111.

27. Merchant SN, Linthicum FH, Nadol JB. Histopathology of the inner ear in DFNA9. Adv Otorhinolaryngol 2000; 56:212–217.

28. deKok YJM, Bom SJH, Brunt TM, Kemperman MH, van Beusekom E, van der Velde-Visser SD, Robertson NG, Morton CC, Huygen PLM, Verhagen WIM, Brunner HG, Cremers CWRJ, Cremers FPM. A Pro51Ser mutation in the COCH gene is associated with late onset autosomal dominant progressive sensorineural hearing loss with vestibular defects. Hum Mol Genet 1999; 8:361–366.

29. Fransen E, Verstreken M, Verhagen WI, Wuyts FL, Huygen PL, D'Haese P, Robertson NG, Morton CC, McGuirt WT, Smith RJ, Declau F, Heyning PH, Camp GV. High prevalence of symptoms of Meniere's disease in three families with a mutation in the COCH gene. Hum Mol Genet 1999; 8:1425–1429.

30. Verhagen WI, Huygen PL, Bles W. A new autosomal dominant syndrome of idiopathic progressive vestibulo-cochlear dysfunction with middle-age onset. Acta Otolaryngol 1992; 112:899–906.

31. Bom SJ, Kemperman MH, De Kok YJ, Huygen PL, Verhagen WI, Cremers

FP, Cremers CW. Progressive cochleovestibular impairment caused by a point mutation in the *COCH* gene at DFNA9. Laryngoscope 1999; 109:1525–1530.

32. Verhagen WI, Huygen PL, Joosten EM. Familial progressive vestibulocochlear dysfunction. Arch Neurol 1988; 45:766–768.

33. Verhagen WI, Huygen PL, Theunissen EJ, Joosten EM. Hereditary vestibulo-cochlear dysfunction and vascular disorders. J Neurol Sci 1989; 92:55–63.

34. Verhagen WI, Huygen PL. Familial progressive vestibulocochlear dysfunction. Arch Neurol 1991; 48:262.

35. Fransen E, Verstreken M, Born SJ, Lemaire F, Kemperman MH, De Kok YJ, Wuyts FL, Verhagen WI, Huygen PL, McGuirt WT, Smith RJ, Van Maldergem LV, Declau F, Cremers CW, Van De Heyning PH, Cremers FP, Van Camp G. A common ancestor for *COCH* related cochleovestibular (DFNA9) patients in Belgium and the Netherlands bearing the P51S mutation. J Med Genet 2001; 38:61–65.

36. Kamarinos M, McGill J, Lynch M, Dahl H. Identification of a novel *COCH* mutation, I109N, highlights the similar clinical features observed in DFNA9 families. Hum Mutat 2001; 17:351.

37. Khetarpal U. DFNA9 is a progressive audiovestibular dysfunction with a microfibrillar deposit in the inner ear. Laryngoscope 2000; 110:1379–1384.

38. Kikuchi T, Kimura RS, Paul DL, Adams JC. Gap junctions in the rat cochlea: immunohistochemical and ultrastructural analysis. Anat Embryol 1995; 191: 101–118.

39. Yuge I, Otsuka A, Harada D, Abe S, Akita J, Kimberling WJ, Usami S. *KCNQ4, TECTA,* and *COCH* are responsible genes for Japanese non-syndromic auto-somal dominant sensorineural hearing loss. The Molecular Biology of Hearing and Deafness Meeting, Bethesda, MD, Oct 4–7, 2001, p 43.

23
Diaphanous

Kelly N. Owens and Mary-Claire King
University of Washington, Seattle, Washington, U.S.A.

I. INTRODUCTION

DFNA1 hearing loss is dominantly inherited, progressive, and nonsyndromic. It is caused by a truncating mutation in the human homolog of *Drosophila* diaphanous, a member of the formin family of proteins. In this chapter we review the clinical features associated with DFNA1, the causative diaphanous mutation, the homologs of diaphanous in humans and other species, and functional roles of diaphanous. Diaphanous is a target of Rho and a binding partner of profilin, which regulates actin polymerization. Diaphanous is required for organization of cytoskeletal structures, including actin stress fibers, focal adhesions, microtubules, and contractile rings, and hence for maintenance of normal cell size, shape, and division.

II. DFNA1 GENETICS

A. DFNA1-Associated Hearing Loss

An extended Costa Rican kindred, Family M, includes more than 150 relatives with dominant, nonsyndromic hearing loss (1). The founding member of this family immigrated to Costa Rica from Jerez de la Frontera, Spain, in about 1600. Written documentation of hearing loss in the family dates from 1745. At onset, affected individuals of Family M exhibit mild to moderate sensorineural hearing loss (SNHL) at low frequencies (250 and 500 Hz) with nearly normal hearing at higher frequencies (Fig. 1). Although age at first detection of hearing loss varies from 5 to 30 years, the majority of affected individuals report initial hearing loss in the first decade of life. Variation in

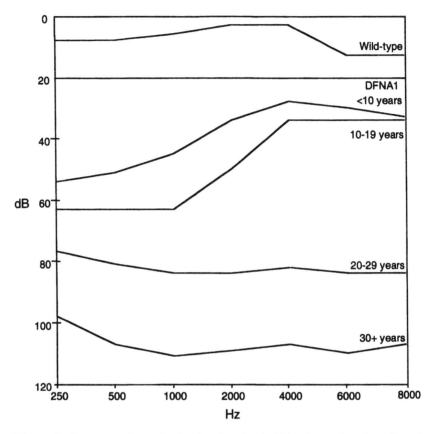

Figure 1 Pure-tone air conduction hearing threshold levels as a function of age for DFNA1 and unaffected members of Family M. Thresholds in decibels (dB) are indicated by age decile for 50 carriers of DFNA1 and for 12 unaffected wild-type adult relatives.

age of onset does not cluster in sibships. Hearing loss of affected individuals is bilateral and severe at all frequencies by age 30 and profound by age 40. Speech reception thresholds of an affected child are slightly lower than normal, with concomitant word recognition scores of 74–78%, in contrast to word recognition scores of affected adults, which were <20% (2). Because hearing loss is postlingual, members of Family M successfully learn speech and lip reading prior to hearing loss. Vocalization often fails as hearing loss becomes severe.

Hearing loss in Family M is sensorineural and appears confined to a cochlear defect. Comprehensive physical examinations and tympanograms indicate normal outer ear structures and middle ear function (1–3). Most affected family members report tonal tinnitus intermittently that disappears with the progression of deafness. Click tinnitus has been reported at the time of onset of hearing loss (2). At onset, family members show positive recruitment tests, negative tone decay tests, and stapedial reflex thresholds consistent with cochlear dysfunction (1). Lynch and Leon commented that some older family members refused to adopt hearing aids with the complaint that high noise levels are uncomfortable and stressful (4). This may reflect positive loudness recruitment. Also, as the vast majority of hearing impairment in the general population is of higher frequency, hearing aids for members of Family M may not be optimized for low-frequency losses. Analysis of residual hearing in a recently diagnosed 7-year-old child revealed the presence of distortion-product-evoked otoacoustic emissions at the higher frequencies and of normal auditory-evoked potentials, indicating that the outer hair cells were functional basally and that the central auditory pathway was intact. Furthermore, high-resolution computed tomography of the temporal bone revealed normal cochlea, semicircular canals, vestibular and cochlear aqueducts, and internal auditory canal, suggesting that the inner ear defect is limited to the membranous labyrinth (2).

Family members do not report any vestibular disturbances or periods of vertigo, and clinical evaluations reveal no nystagmus or balance difficulties. Elevated summating-potential-to-action-potential ratios were observed in one individual, consistent with endolymphatic hydrops (2). Lalwani and colleagues suggested that the presence of cochlear hydrops without vestibular dysfunction may indicate dysfunction of the stria vascularis or endolymphatic sac, leading to dysfunction of fluid homeostasis (2). Further evaluation of young family members at the time of onset is required to determine if this is a consistent or an anomolous feature.

Hearing loss that begins in low frequencies is rare. From a Danish series of nearly 70,000 hearing-impaired individuals, 418 (0.6%) had sensorineural low-frequency hearing loss (LFHL), defined as 20 dB or greater loss at 250 and 500 Hz, at least 15 dB better hearing at higher frequencies, and an air-bone gap of < 15 dB averaged at 500, 1000, and 2000 Hz (5). The hearing loss phenotypes of these individuals with LFHL were heterogeneous, but most frequently included symmetrical loss of hearing at low frequencies with age-related slow deterioration of hearing at 2000–8000 Hz. Of these 418 individuals, 69 reported first- or second-degree relatives with similar low-frequency hearing loss. Based on the size of the Danish population from which the hearing-impaired individuals were ascertained, Parving et al. estimated the population prevalence of inherited LFHL as 1–2 per 10,000 individuals.

In addition to DFNA1, inherited LFHL has been described in families from the United States (DFNA6) (6), Holand (DFNA14) (7), and Newfoundland, Canada (DFNA38) (8). Hearing loss in all these families proved to be due to mutations in the Wolfram syndrome gene WFS1 (8,9). Additional families with hearing loss due to WFS1 have been observed in Japan, Belgium, Germany, and the United Kingdom (10,11). Homozygosity or compound heterozygosity for loss-of-function mutations in WFS1 led to Wolfram syndrome, a severe recessive disorder characterized by diabetes mellitus and optic atrophy but only occasionally including mild-to-moderate high frequency hearing loss (12). In contrast to mutations causing Wolfram syndrome, WFS1 mutations leading to LFHL are dominantly inherited missense substitutions affecting the C-terminus of the wolframin protein. Multiple different WFS1 mutations leading to low-frequency hearing loss have been described, but only one DFNA1 mutation is known. It is possible that only mutations in a restricted region of diaphanous can lead to a hearing loss phenotype.

B. DFNA1 Mutation

DFNA1 was the first autosomal dominant nonsyndromic hearing loss locus mapped in the human genome. Linkage analysis localized hearing loss in Family M to chromosome 5q31 with a lod score of 13.55 at D5S2119 and D5S2010 (13). Positional cloning subsequently revealed a mutation in the human homolog of the *Drosophila melanogaster* diaphanous gene cosegregating with deafness in Family M (3). The human diaphanous gene comprises 27 exons spanning 102 kb of genomic DNA. The wild-type human diaphanous gene encodes a transcript of 4.7 kb and a protein of 1283 amino acids.

The DFNA1 mutation in Family M is $3634(+1)G \rightarrow T$, a nucleotide substitution in the first base of the last intron, immediately 3′ of codon 1211 (3). The DFNA1 mutation abrogates the 5′ splice site of intron 26 so that splicing occurs at a cryptic site between bp $+4$ and $+5$ of the intron. Four additional base pairs are introduced into the mutant transcript, leading to premature truncation of the mutant protein at codon 1233. Mutant diaphanous has 21 aberrant amino acids and lacks 52 amino acids (codon 1212–1263 inclusive) relative to the normal diaphanous protein product. Both normal and mutant alleles are transcribed in lymphoblast cells from affected family members (3). Wild-type diaphanous has no alternative splicing in this region. All carriers of the mutation older than age 20 are affected, suggesting that penetrance of the allele is complete. No gender bias is observed. To date, the Family M mutation has not been observed in several hundred hearing controls or in any other family with hearing loss (3).

Expression of the DFNA1 transcript occurs in all tissues tested including cochlea, brain, heart, lung, placenta, kidney, pancreas, liver, and skeletal muscle (the last of which showed the highest level of expression) (3). RT-PCR of the DFNA1 transcript from cochlear RNA demonstrates that this mRNA is transcribed in the inner ear (3). Expression of diaphanous protein has also been observed in multiple cell lines including fibroblasts (14,15), lymphoblasts (3), kidney cells (16–18), colon epithelial and carcinoma lines (16), fibrosarcomas (18), and several neural carcinoma lines (19).

III. DIAPHANOUS PROTEINS

DFNA1 is a member of the formin gene family. Formins have roles in cytoskeletal organization and cell polarity (20). Proteins encoded by formin genes appear in animals (nematodes, flies, mammals), plants (mustard, tobacco), fungi (yeast, *Aspergillus*), and protozoa (*Entamoeba histolytica*). The first formin gene identified was the mouse limb deformity (ld) gene (21,22). More than 10 members of the extended formin gene family are now known in humans.

Mammalian formins and their *Drosophila* diaphanous homolog share conserved formin homology (FH) domains flanked by coiled-coil domains (CCD) (23) (Fig. 2). Formin homology domain 1 (FH1) is a polyproline rich region of ~ 200 amino acids with multiple repeats of 5–12 consecutive prolines (24). The FH1 region binds both profilin and the SH3 domains of a variety of proteins (25). Formin homology domain 2 (FH2) is highly conserved but its molecular role is less characterized. Sequences of FH1 and FH2 and spacing between them are conserved in formins. The N-terminus contains a third, more loosely conserved domain (FH3) originally defined in the yeast diaphanous homolog Bni1p as essential for protein localization (26). The FH3 domain acts as a binding site and overlaps with a portion of the Rho-binding domain.

Figure 3 illustrates the evolutionary relationships among selected formin family protein sequences. Formin subfamilies include the diaphanous-related genes (DIAPH and Diap), the dishevelled-activator-of-morphogenesis group (DAAM), formin-like homologs (FMNL), formin-homolog-overexpressed-in-spleen (FHOS), and the classic formins. The homologs of *Drosophila* diaphanous include human and mouse diaphanous homologs, *C elegans* cyk-1, *S. cerevisiae* Bni1p, *S. pombe* cdc12, and *E. histolytica* diaphanous.

Three diaphanous homologs exist in humans and mouse. The human and mouse genome informatics groups have adopted *DIAPH1–3* and *Diap1–3* as gene names for human and mouse homologs, respectively (Table 1). Each human *DIAPH* gene is more similar to its mouse counterpart than are the

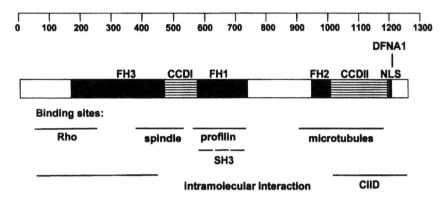

Figure 2 Diaphanous is a member of the formin family defined by conserved formin homology (FH) domains. Protein domains of *Diap1* include FH3 (aa 157–457), polyproline-rich FH1 (aa 570–761), and FH2 (aa 945–1010). Also present are two coiled-coil domains, CCDI and CCDII (aa 457–570 and 1011–1192, respectively), and a putative nuclear localization signal (NLS aa 1196–1202). Rho GTPase binds diaphanous at the N-terminus (aa 63–260). Profilin binds the FH1 domain of diaphanous via polyproline stretches. The SH3 domains of Src, IRSp53, and DIP bind diaphanous via the SH3 binding sites in FH1. The C-terminal portion of the FH3 domain and the first coiled-coil domain (aa 431–603) target diaphanous to the mitotic spindle. The FH2 domain binds stable microtubules in nondividing cells. The diaphanous N-terminus (aa 63–413) and the C-terminal *i*ntramolecular *i*nteraction *d*omain (CIID, aa 1116–1255) interact. The CIID includes a conserved 23-amino-acid region (aa 1177–1199 in *Diap1*) that overlaps the *d*iaphanous *a*utoregulatory *d*omain (DAD) defined in *Diap3*.

DIAPH genes to each other (Fig. 3). DFNA1 is caused by a mutation in human *DIAPH1* on chromosome 5q31. Human and mouse diaphanous1 proteins are 90% identical and 93% similar at the amino acid level. Functional domains are conserved (Fig. 2). The mouse diaphanous1 coding region (1255 amino acids) is nearly identical in size to the human (1263 amino acids) (18). Human *DIAPH2* was initially identified during cloning of DFNA1 and is located at Xq22 (3,27). Disruption of *DIAPH2* is associated with premature ovarian failure in a patient carrying translocation t(X;12)(q21;p2.3) (28,29). Identification of the breakpoint in this and a second patient with premature ovarian failure showed that both breakpoints occur in the last intron of DIAPH2 (28,30). These individuals exhibit mild amenorrhea or premature menopause with associated elevated gonadotropin levels. Neither reports any hearing abnormalities. The association of disruption of *DIAPH2* with ovarian failure is consistent with the observation that mutations in *Drosophila* diaphanous lead to defects in oogenesis. As yet little is known about human *DIAPH3* on chromosome 13. Expression of *DIAPH3* is observed

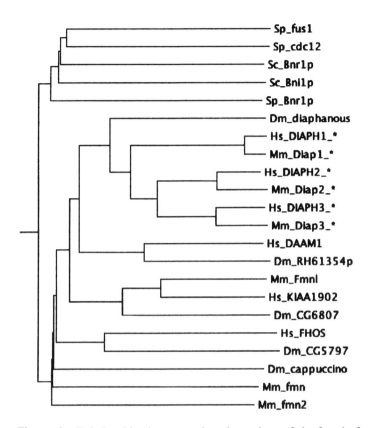

Sp_fus1
Sp_cdc12
Sc_Bnr1p
Sc_Bni1p
Sp_Bnr1p
Dm_diaphanous
Hs_DIAPH1_*
Mm_Diap1_*
Hs_DIAPH2_*
Mm_Diap2_*
Hs_DIAPH3_*
Mm_Diap3_*
Hs_DAAM1
Dm_RH61354p
Mm_Fmnl
Hs_KIAA1902
Dm_CG6807
Hs_FHOS
Dm_CG5797
Dm_cappuccino
Mm_fmn
Mm_fmn2

Figure 3 Relationships between selected members of the formin family are illustrated with an unrooted neighbor-joining tree constructed from comparison of protein sequences using Bonsai software (72). Asterisks indicate the mammalian diaphanous homologs. Two-letter prefixes indicate species: Hs for *Homo sapiens*, Mm for *Mus musculus*, Dm for *Drosophila melanogaster*, Sc for *Saccharomyces cerevisiae*, and Sc for *Schizosaccharomyces pombe*.

Table 1 Diaphanous Homologs in Human and Mouse

Species	Gene	Aliases	Chromosome
Human	*DIAPH1*	DFNA1, Dia, diaph1, hDia1, DRF1	5q31
	DIAPH2	DRF2, dia, diaph2, DIA-156, DIA-12C, POF, POF2	Xq22
	DIAPH3	DRF3, dia3	13q14.3
Mouse	*Diap1*	DRF1, mDIA1, p140Dia	18
	Diap2	DRF2	X
	Diap3	DRF3, Dia2, mdia2, p134mDia2	14

predominantly among hematopoetic lineages and carcinoma cell lines, indicating that *DIAPH3* has a narrower range of expression than *DIAPH1*. No mutations associated with disease have yet been found in *DIAPH3*. Thorough examination of overlap and distinctions between the diaphanous paralogous proteins in vivo remains to be done.

The presence of three diaphanous homologs in humans and mice (Fig. 3) may allow functional redundancy. Diaphanous 1 and 3 can substitute for each other for some functions, such as formation of stress fibers in fibroblasts (16,31). However, there are indications that the diaphanous paralogs have diverged. Not all cell types contain both DIAPH1 and DIAPH3 protein. Also, *Diap3* may be activated in response to broader types of stimuli than *Diap1* (18). The mutation associated with premature ovarian failure in *DIAPH2* is a C-terminal truncation, similar to the Family M mutation in *DIAPH1*, and is likely to be a subtle hypomorphic or dominant negative mutation rather than a null mutation. It remains to be seen what phenotype occurs with a null mutation in any mouse or human diaphanous homolog.

IV. DIAPHANOUS FUNCTION

A. Role of Diaphanous in Regulation of Actin Structures

Diaphanous is a component of a Rho GTPase pathway (Fig. 4) (reviewed in Ref. (32–35)). Rho GTPase pathways are ubiquitous and coordinate external stimuli with internal cellular responses, ultimately regulating organization of the cytoskeleton. Of the 17 members of the Rho family of small GTPase molecules in mammals, the best studied are Rho, Cdc42, and Rac1 (Fig. 4). These related proteins promote different downstream responses by activating various combinations of effectors. Rho is involved in induction of stress fibers and focal contacts, Cdc42 in induction of filopodia, and Rac in induction of membrane ruffing or lamellipodia. Both Rho and Cdc42 are required for cytokinesis. Recent work indicates there may be considerable cross-talk and use of multiple pathways in formation of these cytoskeletal structures. Diaphanous is a target of Rho and performs most, if not all, of its functions via this pathway. When activated by Rho, diaphanous functions in formation and spatial organization of actin-based structures (e.g., stress fibers, focal contacts, contractile rings), organization of microtubules, and transduction of cellular signals.

Rho mediates formation of cytoskeletal structures by binding the diaphanous N-terminus and activating the protein. In the absence of Rho, diaphanous N- and C-termini bind to each other (Fig. 2) and preclude diaphanous activity (Fig. 4) (14,31,36). Activated Rho disrupts this intramolecular

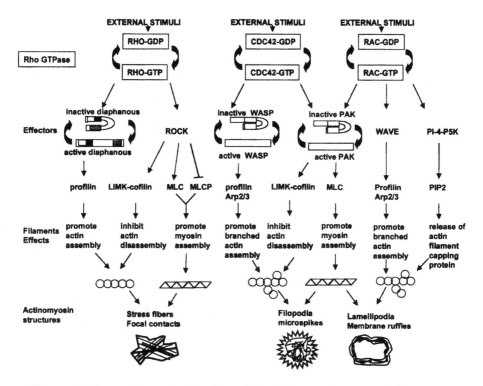

Figure 4 Extracellular stimuli activate Rho GTPase pathways to induce cyto-skeletal reorganization and coordinated cellular events. Rho activates diaphanous. Cdc42 and Rac GTPases Induce different actin structures through activation of other effector molecules.

interaction, apparently leaving diaphanous in an open, active conformation (14). Diaphanous interacts via its FH1 domain with profilin, an actin-binding protein (Fig. 2), thereby regulating actin polymerization (Fig. 4) (18,36). Most of the structures induced by diaphanous are composed of actin-myosin filaments. The *Diap1* Rho-binding domain (RBD) (Fig. 2) is specifically bound by active Rho but not by inactive Rho or by either form of Rac1 or Cdc42 (Fig. 4) (18). In contrast, both Rho and Cdc42 are reported to bind *Diap3* (31). Unlike most Rho targets, diaphanous is not a kinase and contains a distinct Rho binding site (32,35,37). However, Rho often simultaneously activates diaphanous and ROCK, a Rho-associated protein kinase (Fig. 4). Diaphanous and ROCK can act cooperatively, as seen with the induction of stress fibers (14,16,38), or can act antagonistically, as seen with formation of adherens junctions (39).

When activated by Rho, diaphanous regulates formation of stress fibers and focal contacts at the end of stress fibers. Stress fibers are linear, contractile structures of bundled actin and myosin II filaments that influence cell shape and strength. Focal contacts, specialized sites of contact between the plasma membrane and the extracellular matrix, function in adhesion and cell signaling to coordinate cellular response to the extracellular matrix (40). The role of diaphanous in formation of these structures was demonstrated by creating a mutant diaphanous protein lacking the N-terminus. This mutant protein was constitutively active and, when overexpressed, led to formation of parallel stress fibers and focal contacts (14,17). In response to external force, activated diaphanous enables focal contacts to form from focal complexes, smaller integrin-based actin complexes containing distinct proteins (40,41). Riveline et al. noted that focal complexes act as "individual mechanosensors," transducing stimulation by force in a local area into focal contacts (41) if diaphanous is present to mediate their production.

In addition to inducing focal contacts, activated diaphanous regulates formation of other anchoring junctions important for attachment of actin filaments to the plasma membrane: adherens junctions, anchoring sites mediating cell-cell contacts, and fibrillar adhesions, fibronectin-induced sites associated with wound healing and phagocytosis. These anchoring junctions are abundant in tissues subject to mechanical stress and are important for the transmission of force. Diaphanous and actin filaments enable colocalization of E-cadherin and alpha-catenin at adherens junctions (39). Inhibition of diaphanous leads to dynamic instability of the cell periphery, seen as extension and retraction of membrane projections (39). This suggests that diaphanous stabilizes the cell periphery via its effect on cadherins at adherens junctions.

Rho signals both diaphanous and a second effector, Rho-associated kinase or ROCK. ROCK promotes formation of myosin filaments by phosphorylating myosin light chain and myosin light chain phosphatase (Fig. 4) (19). Disassembly and reassembly of stress fibers and focal contacts respectively require inactivation and reactivation of both ROCK and diaphanous (38). Thus, formation of these actinomyosin structures results from cooperative interaction of diaphanous and ROCK. ROCK and diaphanous act antagonistically to determine the spatial organization of these same structures. Overexpression of active diaphanous favors formation of parallel stress fibers and small focal contacts at the cell periphery, whereas overexpression of active ROCK favors formation of radial or stellate stress fibers and large basally located focal contacts. Overexpression of both diaphanous and ROCK yields intermediate stress fiber conformations and moderately sized, evenly distributed focal contacts (14,16,38). Antagonism between diaphanous and ROCK is also seen in the formation of adherens junctions, where diaphanous acts to cluster integrins and stabilize the cell periphery while ROCK destablizes the cell periphery (39).

B. Role of Diaphanous in Cytokinesis

Diaphanous is required for normal cytokinesis. Perturbing interactions of mammalian diaphanous Rho-binding domain disrupts cytokinesis by preventing contractile ring formation and results in binucleated cells (16). Mutations of diaphanous orthologs in *D. melanogaster*, *C. elegans*, *S. cerevisiae*, *S. pombe*, and *A. nidulans* are associated with defects in cytokinesis (23,42–47). Furthermore, diaphanous itself localizes to the midbody and cleavage furrow of dividing fibroblasts (16).

The most comprehensive information about the role of diaphanous in vivo comes from *Drosophila* diaphanous mutants. Null alleles of *Drosophila* diaphanous confer a recessive lethal phenotype in pupae characterized by absence of cleavage furrows and presence of hyperploid cells (23). Weaker alleles allow flies to progress further in development, but these mutants also show defects in cells undergoing rapid division including imaginal discs, ovarian follicle cells, ommatidia of the eye, and neuroblasts.

Absence of diaphanous in flies disrupts both mitosis and meiosis. The mildest *Drosophila* diaphanous allele, dia[1], leads to recessive male sterility. Spermatid production rapidly ceases following an initial burst of division (23,48). Initial rounds of spermatogenesis generate multinucleate spermatids, indicating a failure of cytokinesis following meiosis. Female flies carrying dia[1] and a diaphanous deletion exhibit oogenesis defects as the result of failure of cytokinesis in follicle cells. These gametogenesis defects in flies are reminiscent of the association of *DIAPH2* with premature ovarian failure.

Diaphanous is critical to normal cell division in *Drosophila* embryos (47). It coordinates actin-membrane interactions during cytokinesis. Diaphanous protein is abundant at the leading edge of invaginating cell membranes and appears on the basal surface of each new cell. Diaphanous is essential for proper reorganization of actin during cell division (47). Fly embryos lacking maternal diaphanous have disorganized actin arrays and mislocalize myosin II (47).

Diaphanous functions as a major effector of Rho during cytokinesis. Mutations in *Drosophila* diaphanous act as dominant suppressors of constitutively active mutations of Rho 1 or pebble, a Rho guanine nucleotide exchange factor. Diaphanous mutations dominantly enhance loss of function of pebble (49). The ability of a diaphanous null allele to act dominantly in Rho1 or pebble mutant flies suggests that a precise molecular balance exists.

If the mutation in human DFNA1 results in an unstable protein, decreased levels of diaphanous may cause a similar dominant impact on function of the human Rho pathway.

C. Role of Diaphanous in Regulating Microtubules

Diaphanous is an organizer of microtubules as well as of actin. Diaphanous localizes to spindle microtubules in prophase through telophase and associates with all three types of spindle microtubules: kinetochore, nonkinetochore, and astral microtubules (15). These interactions are independent of Rho activity or the presence of actin structures. A region including part of the diaphanous FH3 and CCDI domains is responsible for microtubule association. However, the FH3-CCDI region of diaphanous does not bind polymerizing microtubules in vitro, indicating that the association of diaphanous with microtubules is indirect (15).

Diaphanous affects organization of spindle microtubules. During *Drosophila* spermatogenesis, diaphanous mutants do not form actin rings and also show defects in the central spindle including fewer microtubules, decreased microtubule interdigitation, and delayed aster positioning. During mitotic divisions, fly embryos lacking maternal diaphanous have disorganized microtubule baskets around nuclei and exhibit abnormal centrosome movements in addition to severe actin defects (47). Signaling from the central spindle is generally required for orienting the contractile ring (50,51). Diaphanous has been proposed to mediate cross-talk between microtubules and actin filaments (47). Such coordinate regulation of microtubules and actin via diaphanous is observed in yeast. In *S. cerevisiae*, Bni1p, the homolog of diaphanous, affects positioning of the central spindle in the bud neck as well as establishment of the contractile ring (52).

In nondividing cells, diaphanous affects the formation and maintenance of microtubules and hence influences cell shape. Overexpression of activated *Diap1* leads to significant elongation of cells (53). Within these elongated cells, actin bundles are aligned in parallel, coordinately oriented with microtubules, and terminate in focal contacts at the cell periphery that contain diaphanous (53). Overexpression of dominant negative mouse Diap1 protein reduces parallel microtubule formation, eliminates formation of focal contacts, and leads to disorganized stress fibers.

Microtubules induced by diaphanous are stable rather than dynamic (54). Stable microtubules have detyrosinated ends and persist for hours in contrast to dynamic, tyrosinated microtubules, which turn over in 5–10 min (55). Mouse diaphanous interacts directly with stable microtubules (54). The action of mouse *Diap1* on microtubules is mediated by the FH2 domain (53). The conservation of the FH1 and FH2 regions among formin homologs may allow coordinate regulation of actin (via FH1) and microtubule processes (via FH2) (53). Similarly, Bni1p, the diaphanous homolog in *S. cerevislae*, is involved in capture and transient capping of microtubules in the cell cortex, thereby positioning the mitotic spindle and moving the yeast nucleus to the budding daughter cell (44,56). Thus diaphanous-induced actin (39) and microtubule structures (54) aid stabilization of the cell periphery.

D. Role of Diaphanous in Transducing Cellular Signals

The role of diaphanous in Rho-mediated transduction of external stimuli involves cellular signaling in addition to cytoskeletal alterations. Accordingly, diaphanous binds several proteins via its SH3 binding sites, which are themselves regulatory molecules: diaphanous interacting protein (DIP) (57), insulin receptor substrate p53 or IRSp53 (58), and Src (16) (Fig. 2). Interaction of IRSp53 and DIP homologs with diaphanous homologs have been conserved from yeast to mammals (45,59). DIP and diaphanous colocalize at the cell periphery and in membrane ruffles in human HeLa cells. Mutant DIP suppresses diaphanous induction of stress fibers (57), suggesting that the interaction of DIP with diaphanous is important for stress fiber formation. In yeast, mutations in DIP or IRSp53 homologs lead to cells with cytokinesis defects akin to mutations in the diaphanous homologs, Bni1p and Bnr1p (60). The phenotypes of these yeast mutants suggest that diaphanous-DIP and diaphanous-IRSp53 interactions are critical both to cell division and to formation of actin structures.

Src interaction with diaphanous is required for some diaphanous-mediated events including cytokinesis and response to serum (16,61). In response to serum, diaphanous activates serum response factor (SRF) via Src (16). SRF is a transcription factor regulating expression of vinculin, β-actin, and sm-α-actin (62,63). Diaphanous-dependent Src activity leads to increased expression of components required for diaphanous-induced structures. Diaphanous is sufficient for SRF activation in fibroblasts (16,39,61) but requires the ROCK target LIMK, in neural cells (61). Src activity is also needed for stress fiber organization (16). Inhibition of Src eliminates cooperative stress fiber formation by diaphanous and ROCK and produces a stellate actin filament pattern reminiscent of activated ROCK alone. Thus the spatial organization of actin by diaphanous requires Src activity (16).

Cross-talk between Rho GTPase pathways can occur via diaphanous. Interaction of Rho and Rac pathways occurs via diaphanous and Src interaction. When ROCK is suppressed, diaphanous activates Rac and induces membrane ruffles via Src (64). When both Rac and ROCK are suppressed, expression of diaphanous leads to filopodia-like protrusions (64) akin to Cdc42-induced filopodia. Cross-talk between the Rho and Cdc42 pathways may occur via DIP and IRSp53, which bind both diaphanous and the Cdc42 effector WASP (60,65,66). Thus, diaphanous provides a point of intersection between the Rho, Cdc42, and Rac pathways.

V. POSSIBLE MOLECULAR MECHANISMS FOR DFNA1 HEARING LOSS

A. Consequences of Loss of the Diaphanous C-Terminus

Complete loss of diaphanous is likely to be devastating to the cytoskeleton and hence lethal. The DFNA1 mutation clearly reflects a more subtle pertubation. Watanabe et al. proposed that the DFNA1 truncation leads to defective diaphanous autoregulation (14). That is, by precluding or reducing the normal intramolecular interaction between diaphanous N- and C-termini, the mutant DFNA1 protein may be open and active even in the absence of activation by Rho (Fig. 4). As a result, the mutant protein may be constitutively active or may interfere with wild-type protein in a dominant negative fashion. However, studies of autoregulation of *Diap3* are not fully consistent with this model. The normal diaphanous autoregulatory domain of *Diap3* ends at residue 1177 corresponding to *DIAPH1* residue 1204. This is the site corresponding to the DFNA1 truncation, suggesting that diaphanous autoregulation may be intact in DFNA1 (31). However, autoregulation of *Diap1* may require a larger region. Although the diaphanous autoregulatory domain is highly conserved between *Diap3* and *Diap1*, the region C-terminal to DFNA1 site is not conserved.

In human HeLa cells, overexpression of diaphanous that is full length except for absence of the C-terminal 63 amino acids (i.e., aa 1–1192 present) induces protruding membranes reminiscent of filopodia or microspikes (14). The same effect is produced by simultaneously inhibiting Rac and ROCK activities (61). That is, these protrusions may be caused by activated diaphanous or by diaphanous uncoupled from ROCK and Rac pathways. Expression of diaphanous constructs missing only the last 39 amino acids (i.e., aa 1–1216 present) do not produce protruding membranes (14). It is not yet known what effect would be seen when 52 amino acids are deleted from the C-terminus, as in Family M.

B. Why Is DFNA1 Nonsyndromic?

Diaphanous induces actin filaments, organizes actin structures and microtubules, and coordinates cell signaling. These functions are central roles within a cell. Why then does Family M exhibit only hearing loss? This may reflect functional redundancy among the DIAPH paralogs in nonauditory cells that is lacking in the inner ear. Alternatively, the DFNA1 mutant phenotype may reflect the prominence in hair cells of cytoskeletal structures such as the actin bundles of the stereocilia or the actin meshwork of the cuticular plate (see Fig. 5) (3,67). Regulation and maintenance of these mechanosensory structures are likely to be extremely sensitive to aberrations in the cytoskeleton. The mechanosensory bristles of flies, which are analogous to vertebrate hair cells (67), are sensitive to cytoskeletal changes that are tolerated in other cell types. For example, viable alleles of *Drosophila* profilin lead to defects in gametogenesis (like *DIAPH2*), roughened eyes

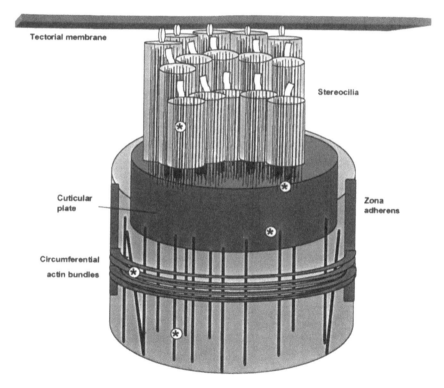

Figure 5 The apical end of an inner hair cell is shown (modified with permission from Ref. 67). Asterisks label potential sites of diaphanous localization and function: parallel actin bundles (thin lines within stereocilia or circumferential bands), parallel microtubules (thick lines), and contact points between the cuticular plate and actin bundles of stereocilia or microtubules. Diaphanous may recruit proteins to actin structures, such as the cuticular plate or zona adherens. Sites of diaphanous localization and function in the hair cell are predicted from experimental results with other cell types.

(indicative of cytokinesis defects), and abnormally formed mechanosensory bristles with disorganized actin bundles (68).

Figure 5 indicates possible hair cell structures that might be perturbed by altered diaphanous activity. These include actin structures with parallel fibers such as hair bundles and the zona adherens, parallel microtubules, or regions of contact between the cuticular plate and actin filaments or microtubules. The function of diaphanous may also be important for maintenance of the zona adherens of the hair cell and for proper localization of E-cadherin and α-catenin, akin to its role in other cell types (39). Furthermore, focal contact formation in response to tension has been observed as a diaphanous-dependent event in fibroblasts. A link between integrins and Rho family GTPases at focal contacts is thought to be a crucial feature in localized control of focal contacts (69). These observations suggest that diaphanous might be important for transduction of signals in response to movement or extracellular matrix signals.

Diaphanous might also have a role in maintenance of hair cells. Development of hair bundles in chick initially involves Rac-dependent, then Cdc42-dependent events (70). Acoustic trauma to chick cochlea leads to an increase in Cdc42, suggesting that induction of a RhoGTPase may be involved in hair cell regeneration of hair bundle repair (71). Perturbation of diaphanous may directly or indirectly inhibit repair of hair bundles, perhaps via interference with Rac or Cdc42 pathways. For example, mutant diaphanous could titrate DIP, which also binds the Cdc42 effector WASP.

In conclusion, DFNA1 is associated with sensorineural hearing loss in the first decade that begins as a low-frequency loss and progresses to profound loss at all frequencies. The protein encoded by the diaphanous gene is a formin family protein that serves as an effector of the small GTPase Rho. Diaphanous regulates formation of actin-based structures (stress fibers, focal contacts, and contractile rings), spatially organizes actin filaments and stable microtubules, and coordinates cytoskeletal changes with cellular signaling. Effects of mutation in DFNA1 in hearing loss are likely to reflect a subtle perturbation of these functions in the cochlea.

ACKNOWLEDGMENTS

We thank the members of Family M, whose generous participation has been essential for work on DFNA1. We thank Karen Avraham, John Kemner, Piri Welsch, and Terry Young for comments during the preparation of this chapter. We thank Jim Thomas for providing the Bonsai software used for creating neighbor-joining trees and multiple alignments of proteins. Research in the laboratory of M.C.K. is supported by the National Institutes of Health (NIDCD Grant RO1 DC01076).

REFERENCES

1. Leon PE, Bonilla JA, Sanchez JR, Vanegas R, Villalobos M, Torres L, Leon F, Howell AL, Rodriguez JA. Low frequency hereditary deafness in man with childhood onset. Am J Hum Genet 1981; 33:209–214.
2. Lalwani AK, Jackler RK, Sweetow RW, Lynch ED, Raventos H, Morrow J, King MC, Leon PE. Further characterization of the DFNA1 audiovestibular phenotype. Arch Otolaryngol Head Neck Surg 1998; 124:699–702.
3. Lynch ED, Lee MK, Morrow JE, Welcsh PL, Leon PE, King MC. Non-syndromic deafness DFNA1 associated with mutation of a human homolog of the *Drosophila* gene diaphanous. Science 1997; 278:1315–1318.
4. Lynch ED, Leon PE. Non-syndromic dominant DFNA1. Adv Otorhinolaryngol 2000; 56:60–67.
5. Parving A, Sakihara Y, Christensen B. Inherited sensorineural low-frequency hearing impairment: some aspects of phenotype and epidemiology. Audiology 2000; 39:50–60.
6. Lesperance MM, Helfert RH, Altschuler RA. Deafness induced cell size changes in rostral AVCN of the guinea pig. Hearing Res 1995; 86:77–81.
7. Van Camp G, Kunst H, Flothmann K, McGuirt W, Wauters J, Marres H, Verstreken M, Bespalova IN, Burmeister M, Van de Heyning PH, Smith RJ, Willems PJ, Cremers CW, Lesperance MM. A gene for autosomal dominant hearing impairment (DFNA14) maps to a region on chromosome 4p16.3 that does not overlap the DFNA6 locus. J Med Genet 1999; 36:532–536.
8. Young TL, Ives E, Lynch E, Person R, Snook S, MacLaren L, Cater T, Griffin A, Fernandez B, Lee MK, King MC, Cator T. Non-syndromic progressive hearing loss DFNA38 is caused by heterozygous missense mutation in the Wolfram syndrome gene *WFS1*. Hum Mol Genet 2001; 10:2509–2514.
9. Bespalova IN, Van Camp G, Bom SJ, Brown DJ, Cryns K, DeWan AT, Erson AE, Flothmann K, Kunst HP, Kumool P, Sivakumaran TA, Cremens CW, Leal SM, Burmeister M, Lesperance MM. Mutations in the Wolfram syndrome 1 gene (*WFS1*) are a common cause of low frequency sensorineural hearing loss. Hum Mol Genet 2001; 10:2501–2508.
10. Komatsu K, Nakamura N, Ghadami M, Matsumoto N, Kishino T, Ohta T, Niikawa N, Yoshiura K. Confirmation of genetic homogeneity of nonsyndromic low-frequency sensorineural hearing loss by linkage analysis and a DFNA6/14 mutation in a Japanese family. J Hum Genet 2002; 47:395–399.
11. Cryns K, Pfister M, Pennings RJ, Bom SJ, Flothmann K, Caethoven G, Kremer H, Schatteman I, Koln KA, Toth T, Kupka S, Blin N, Nurnberg P, Thiele H, van de Heyning PH, Reardon W, Stephens D, Cremers CW, Smith RJ, Van Camp G. Mutations in the WFS1 gene that cause low-frequency

sensorineural hearing loss are small non-inactivating mutations. Hum Genet 2002; 110:389–394.

12. Khanim F, Kirk J, Latif F, Barrett TG. *WFS1*/wolframin mutations, Wolfram syndrome, and associated diseases. Hum Mutat 2001; 17:357–367.

13. Leon PE, Raventos H, Lynch E, Morrow J, King MC. The gene for an inherited form of deafness maps to chromosome 5q31. Proc Natl Acad Sci USA 1992; 89:5181–5184.

14. Watanabe N, Kato T, Fujita A, Ishizaki T, Narumiya S. Cooperation between mDia1 and ROCK in Rho-induced actin reorganization. Nat Cell Biol 1999; 1:136–143.

15. Kato T, Watanabe N, Morishima Y, Fujita A, Ishizaki T, Narumiya S. Localization of a mammalian homolog of diaphanous, mDia1, to the mitotic spindle in HeLa cells. J Cell Sci 2001; 114:775–784.

16. Tominaga T, Sahai E, Chardin P, McCormick F, Courtneidge SA, Alberts AS. Diaphanous-related formins bridge Rho GTPase and Src tyrosine kinase signaling. Mol Cell 2000; 5:13–25.

17. Takaishi K, Mino A, Ikeda W, Nakano K, Takai Y. Mechanisms of activation and action of mDia1 in the formation of parallel stress fibers in MDCK cells. Biochem Biophys Res Commun 2000; 274:68–72.

18. Watanabe N, Madaule P, Reid T, Ishizaki T, Watanabe G, Kakizuka A, Saito Y, Nakao K, Jockusch BM, Narumiya S. p140mDia, a mammalian homolog of *Drosophila* diaphanous, is a target protein for Rho small GTPase and is a ligand for profilin. EMBO J 1997; 16:3044–3056.

19. Kosako H, Yoshida T, Matsumura F, Ishizaki T, Narumiya S, Inagaki M. Rho-kinase/ROCK is involved in cytokinesis through the phosphorylation of myosin light chain and not ezrin/radixin/moesin proteins at the cleavage furrow. Oncogene 2000; 19:6059–6064.

20. Zeller R, Haramis AG, Zuniga A, McGuigan C, Dono R, Davidson G, Chabanis S, Gibson T. Formin defines a large family of morphoregulatory genes and functions in establishment of the polarising region. Cell Tissue Res 1999; 296:85–93.

21. Woychik RP, Generoso WM, Russell LB, Cain KT, Cacheiro NL, Bultman SJ, Selby PB, Dickinson ME, Hogan BL, Rutledge JC. Molecular and genetic characterization of a radiation-induced structural rearrangement in mouse chromosome 2 causing mutations at the limb deformity and agouti loci. Proc Natl Acad Sci USA 1990; 87:2588–2592.

22. Woychik RP, Stewart TA, Davis LG, D'Eustachio P, Leder P. An inherited limb deformity created by insertional mutagenesis in a transgenic mouse. Nature 1985; 318:36–40.

23. Castrillon DH, Wasserman SA. Diaphanous is required for cytokinesis in *Drosophila* and shares domains of similarity with the products of the limb deformity gene. Development 1994; 120:3367–3377.

24. Frazier JA, Field CM. Actin cytoskeleton: are FH proteins local organizers? Curr Biol 1997; 7:R414–R417.

25. Ren R, Mayer BJ, Cicchetti P, Baltimore D. Identification of a ten-amino acid proline-rich SH3 binding site. Science 1993; 259:1157–1161.

26. Petersen J, Nielsen O, Egel R, Hagan IM. FH3, a domain found in formins,

targets the fission yeast formin Fus1 to the projection tip during conjugation. J Cell Biol 1998; 141:1217–1228.

27. Banfi S, Borsani G, Bulfone A, Ballabio A. *Drosophila*-related expressed sequences. Hum Mol Genet 1997; 6:1745–1753.

28. Bione S, Sala C, Manzini C, Arrigo G, Zuffardi O, Banfi S, Borsani G, Jonveaux P, Philippe C, Zuccotti M, Ballabio A, Toniolo D. A human homologue of the *Drosophila melanogaster* diaphanous gene is disrupted in a patient with premature ovarian failure: evidence for conserved function in oogenesis and implications for human sterility. Am J Hum Genet 1998; 62:533–541.

29. Sala C, Arrigo G, Torri G, Martinazzi F, Riva P, Larizza L, Philippe C, Jonveaux P, Sloan F, Labella T, Toniolo D. Eleven X chromosome breakpoints associated with premature ovarian failure (POF) map to a 15-Mb YAC contig spanning Xq21. Genomics 1997; 40:123–131.

30. Marozzi A, Manfredini E, Tibiletti MG, Furlan D, Villa N, Vegetti W, Crosignani PG, Ginelli E, Meneveri R, Dalpra L. Molecular definition of Xq common-deleted region in patients affected by premature ovarian failure. Hum Genet 2000; 107:304–311.

31. Alberts AS. Identification of a carboxy-terminal diaphanous-related formin homology protein autoregulatory domain. J Biol Chem 2001; 276:2824–2830.

32. Wherlock M, Mellor H. The Rho GTPase family: a Racs to Wrchs story. J Cell Sci 2002; 115:239–240.

33. Ridley AJ. Rho family proteins: coordinating cell responses. Trends Cell Biol 2001; 11:471–477.

34. Weed SA, Parsons JT. Cortactin: coupling membrane dynamics to cortical actin assembly. Oncogene 2001; 20:6418–6434.

35. Bishop AL, Hall A. Rho GTPases and their effector proteins. Biochem J 2000; 348:348(Pt 2):241–255.

36. Krebs A, Rothkegel M, Klar M, Jockusch BM. Characterization of functional domains of mDia1, a link between the small GTPase Rho and the actin cytoskeleton. J Cell Sci 2001; 114:3663–3672.

37. Fujisawa K, Madaule P, Ishizaki T, Watanabe G, Bito H, Saito Y, Hall A, Narumiya S. Different regions of Rho determine Rho-selective binding of different classes of Rho target molecules. J Biol Chem 1998; 273:18943–18949.

38. Nakano K, Takaishi K, Kodama A, Mammoto A, Shiozaki H, Monden M, Takai Y. Distinct actions and cooperative roles of ROCK and mDia in Rho small G protein-induced reorganization of the actin cytoskeleton in Madin-Darby canine kidney cells. Mol Biol Cell 1999; 10:2481–2491.

39. Sahai E, Marshall CJ. ROCK and Dia have opposing effects on adherens junctions downstream of Rho. Nat Cell Biol 2002; 4:408–415.

40. Geiger B, Bershadsky A. Assembly and mechanosensory function of focal contacts. Curr Opln Cell Biol 2001; 13:584–592.

41. Riveline D, Zamir E, Balaban NQ, Schwarz US, Ishizaki T, Narumiya S, Kam Z, Geiger B, Bershadsky AD. Focal contacts as mechanosensors: externally applied local mechanical force induces growth of focal contacts by an mDia1-dependent and ROCK-independent mechanism. J Cell Biol 2001; 153:1175–1186.

42. Swan KA, Severson AF, Carter JC, Martin PR, Schnabel H, Schnabel R, Bowerman B. cyk-1: a *C. elegans* FH gene required for a late step in embryonic cytokiness. J Cell Sci 1998; 111:2017–2027.

43. Chang F, Drubin D, Nurse P. cdc12p, a protein required for cytokinesis in fission yeast, is a component of the cell division ring and interacts with profilin. J Cell Biol 1997; 137:169–182.

44. Fujiwara T, Tanaka K, Inoue E, Kikyo M, Takai Y. Bni1p regulates microtubule-dependent nuclear migration through the actin cytoskeleton in *Saccharomyces cerevisiae*. Mol Cell Biol 1999; 19:8016–8027.

45. Kamei T, Tanaka K, Hihara T, Umikawa M, Imamura H, Kikyo M, Ozaki K, Takai Y. Interaction of Bnr1p with a novel Src homology 3 domain-containing Hof1p. Implication in cytokinesis in *Saccharomyces cerevisiae*. J Biol Chem 1998; 273:28341–28345.

46. Kohno H, Tanaka K, Mino A, Umikawa M, Imamura H, Fujiwara T, Fujita Y, Hotta K, Qadota H, Watanabe T, Ohya Y, Takai Y. Bni1p implicated in cytoskeletal control is a putative target of Rho1p small GTP binding protein in *Saccharomyces cerevisiae*. EMBO J 1996; 15:6060–6068.

47. Afshar K, Stuart B, Wasserman SA. Functional analysis of the *Drosophila* diaphanous FH protein in early embryonic development. Development 2000; 127:1887–1897.

48. Gonczy P, DiNardo S. The germ line regulates somatic cyst cell proliferation and fate during *Drosophila* spermatogenesis. Development 1996; 122:2437–2447.

49. Prokopenko SN, Brumby A, O'Keefe L, Prior L, He Y, Saint R, Bellen HJ. A putative exchange factor for Rho1 GTPase is required for initiation of cytokinesis in *Drosophila*. Genes Dev 1999; 13:2301–2314.

50. Severson AF, Bowerman B. Cytokinesis: closing in on the central spindle. Dev Cell 2002; 2:4–6.

51. Glotzer M. Animal cell cytokinesis. Annu Rev Cell Dev Biol 2001; 17:351–386.

52. Lee L, Klee SK, Evangelista M, Boone C, Pellman D. Control of mitotic spindle position by the *Saccharomyces cerevisiae* formin Bni1p. J Cell Biol 1999; 144: 947–961.

53. Ishizaki T, Morishima Y, Okamoto M, Furuyashiki T, Kato T, Narumiya S. Coordination of microtubules and the actin cytoskeleton by the Rho effector mDia1. Nat Cell Biol 2001; 3:8–14.

54. Palazzo AF, Cook TA, Alberts AS, Gundersen GG. mDia mediates Rho-regulated formation and orientation of stable microtubules. Nat Cell Biol 2001; 3:723–729.

55. Webster DR, Gundersen GG, Bulinski JC, Borisy GG. Differential turnover of tyrosinated and detyrosinated microtubules. Proc Natl Acad Sci USA 1987; 84:9040–9044.

56. Gundersen GG. Evolutionary conservation of microtubule-capture mechanisms. Nat Rev Mol Cell Biol 2002; 3:296–304.

57. Satoh S, Tominaga T. mDia-interacting protein acts downstream of Rho-mDia and modifies Src activation and stress fiber formation. J Biol Chem 2001; 276:39290–39294.

58. Fujiwara T, Mammoto A, Kim Y, Takai Y. Rho small G-protein-dependent

binding of mDia to an Src homology 3 domain-containing IRSp53/BAIAP2. Biochem Biophys Res Commun 2000; 271:626–629.

59. Vallen EA, Caviston J, Bi E. Roles of Hof1p, Bni1p, Bnr1p, and myo1p in cytokinesis in *Saccharomyces cerevisiae*. Mol Biol Cell 2000; 11:593–611.

60. Naqvi SN, Feng Q, Boulton VJ, Zahn R, Munn AL. Vrp1p functions in both actomyosin ring-dependent and Hof1p-dependent pathways of cytokinesis. Traffic 2001; 2:189–201.

61. Geneste O, Copeland JW, Treisman R. LIM kinase and diaphanous cooperate to regulate serum response factor and actin dynamics. J Cell Biol 2002; 157:831–838.

62. Sotiropoulos A, Gineitis D, Copeland J, Treisman R. Signal-regulated activation of serum response factor is mediated by changes in actin dynamics. Cell 1999; 98:159–169.

63. Gineitis D, Treisman R. Differential usage of signal transduction pathways defines two types of serum response factor target gene. J Biol Chem 2001; 276:24531–24539.

64. Tsuji T, Ishizaki T, Okamoto M, Higashida C, Kimura K, Furuyashiki T, Arakawa Y, Birge RB, Nakamoto T, Hirai H, Narumiya S. ROCK and mDia1 antagonize in Rho-dependent Rac activation in Swiss 3T3 fibroblasts. J Cell Biol 2002; 157:819–830.

65. Martinez-Quiles N, Rohatgi R, Anton IM, Medina M, Saville SP, Miki H, Yamaguchi H, Takenawa T, Hartwig JH, Geha RS, Ramesh N. WIP regulates N-WASP-mediated actin polymerization and filopodium formation. Nat Cell Biol 2001; 3:484–491.

66. Ramesh N, Anton IM, Hartwig JH, Geha RS. WIP, a protein associated with Wiskott-Aldrich syndrome protein, induces actin polymerization and redistribution in lymphoid cells. Proc Natl Acad Sci USA 1997; 94:14671–14676.

67. Muller U, Littlewood-Evans A. Mechanisms that regulate mechanosensory hair cell differentiation. Trends Cell Biol 2001; 11:334–342.

68. Verheyen EM, Cooley L. Profilin mutations disrupt multiple actin-dependent processes during *Drosophila* development. Development 1994; 120:717–728.

69. Juliano RL. Signal transduction by cell adhesion receptors and the cytoskeleton: functions of integrins, cadherins, selectins, and immunoglobulin-superfamily members. Annu Rev Pharmacol Toxicol 2002; 42:283–323.

70. Kollmar R. Who does the hair cell's 'do? Rho GTPases and hair-bundle morphogenesis. Curr Opin Neurobiol 1999; 9:394–398.

71. Gong TW, Hegeman AD, Shin JJ, Adler HJ, Raphael Y, Lomax MI. Identification of genes expressed after noise exposure in the chick basilar papilla. Hearing Res 1996; 96:20–32.

72. Thomas JH, Bonsai. Beta. (Dept. of Genome Sciences, University of Washington, Seattle, WA, 2002). http://calliope.gs.washington.edu/software/index.html.

24
Claudin 14

Tamar Ben-Yosef, Edward R. Wilcox, and Thomas B. Friedman
National Institute on Deafness and Other Communication Disorders,
National Institutes of Health, Rockville, Maryland, U.S.A.

I. TIGHT JUNCTIONS

A. Background

A hallmark in the development of multicellular organisms is the assembly of cellular sheets that separate compartments of different compositions. For example, in the cochlea of the inner ear the perilymph of the scala vestibuli and scala tympani has very different ionic composition as compared to the endolymph of the scala media (1,2). Maintenance of different compartments is performed by epithelial or endothelial cells, which adhere to each other by forming different types of intercellular junctions (3), including desmosomes (4), adherens junctions (5), gap junctions (6), and tight junctions (7,8) (Fig. 1A). Epithelial cells execute a variety of vectorial functions in transport and secretion. To accomplish this they are organized in a polarized fashion with structurally and functionally distinct apical and basolateral plasma membrane domains (reviewed in Ref. 9). The movement of solutes, ions, and water through epithelia occurs both across and between individual cells, and is referred to as the transcellular and the paracellular routes, respectively (Fig. 1B). Both routes display cell-specific and tissue-specific variations in permeability, and together account for the distinct transport properties of each tissue. The basis for transcellular transport, through specific membrane pumps and channels that actively generate the unique electroosmotic gradients and secretory fluids characteristic of each epithelium, is well known. In contrast, our understanding of the epithelial paracellular pathway, which is responsible for maintenance of gradients by restricting back diffusion between cells,

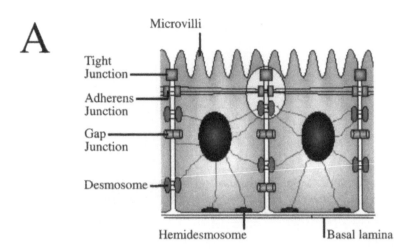

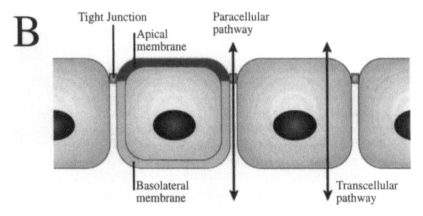

Figure 1   Intercellular junctions and pathways across cellular sheets. (A) Schematic drawing of intestinal epithelial cells. Different types of intercellular junctions, including desmosomes, adherens junctions, gap junctions, and tight junctions (TJs), are illustrated. The junctional complex, which is located at the most apical region of lateral membranes, is circled. (B) Distinct pathways across cellular sheets: a schematic representation of the transcellular versus the paracellular route. (Reprinted by permission from *Nature Reviews Molecular Cell Biology* (8), copyright 2001, Macmillan Magazines Ltd.).

and of the mechanisms that establish and maintain epithelial cell polarity, is more limited.

The major barrier in the paracellular pathway is created by the tight junction (TJ), also known as zonula occludens (ZO; "occluding belt"). TJs can be found in various epithelial tissues, in which they form regions of intimate contact between the plasma membranes of adjacent cells (3). In freeze-fracture replicas of epithelial cells prefixed with glutaraldehyde, TJs usually appear either as a continuous band-like network of branching and interconnecting thin ridges on P faces (the cytoplasmic leaflet of plasma membranes), or as a corresponding pattern of grooves on E faces (the extracytoplasmic leaflet of plasma membranes) (10) (Fig. 2). A closer examination of these structures suggested that each of the interconnected lines of attachment of TJ regions consists of two adhering rows, one in each membrane, of closely spaced adhesion particles (11). These particles are proteins that bridge the width of the adjoining membranes and are linked together in the plane of the intercellular space. There is some evidence that TJs form an intramembrane diffusion barrier that restricts the lateral diffusion of apical and basolateral membrane components, thus maintaining cellular polarity ("fence function") (12–15). TJs also close or seal the space between

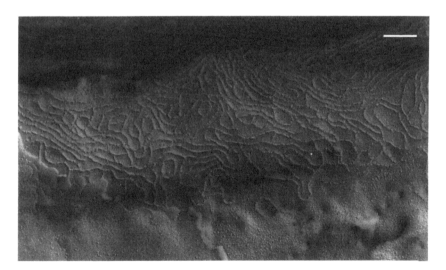

Figure 2 Freeze-fracture electron microscopy image of the apical membrane and the TJ region of marginal cells in the stria vascularis. TJs appear as a continuous band-like network of branching and interconnecting thin ridges on the P face. Scale bar = 200 nm. (Courtesy of A. Forge, Institute of Laryngology and Otology, University College London Medical School, London.)

cells and thus set up a semipermeable barrier that prevents or reduces paracellular diffusion ("barrier function") (16). The actual barrier capacity of TJs can be determined by measurements of the electrical resistance across the epithelium (17). Barrier function of TJs was demonstrated for relatively large molecules, such as hemoglobin (3), as well as for smaller molecules, such as the colloidal tracer lanthanum hydroxide (18). TJs partly block the paracellular transport of water and small electrolytes. Depending on the functional requirements of an epithelium, there may be small or large amounts of water and small solutes flowing passively through the TJ (17). The paracellular permeability of different epithelia was found to correlate with the number of TJ strands along the apical-basal axis (19). The morphological pattern of the strands also varies among tissues; however, the physiological correlate of these ultrastructural differences is yet unknown.

B. Tight Junction Proteins

TJ strands are composed of at least three types of membrane-spanning proteins: occludin (20), different members of the claudin family (21), and junction adhesion molecule (JAM) (22,23). These strand-associated membrane proteins interact with the actin-based cytoskeleton (24), as well as with membrane-associated proteins that function as adapters and signaling proteins (reviewed in Refs. 25,26).

1. Occludin

Occludin was the first identified TJ protein (20). It is exclusively localized to TJs of both epithelial and endothelial cells (20). It spans the membrane four times with cytoplasmic amino and carboxy termini and forms two extracellular loops that are composed mostly of glycine and tyrosine (20). Initially occludin was thought to be the main TJ sealing protein. Several lines of evidence supported this hypothesis: Occludin expression induced adhesion in suspended cell assays (27); disruption of occludin interactions by the addition of peptides corresponding to its extracellular loops resulted in a drop in transepithelial electrical resistance (28,29); mutation or overexpression of occludin in cultured cells affected permeability properties (30–32). However, several studies suggested that occludin might not be absolutely required for TJ formation. Some cell types have TJs although they express only low levels of occludin (33,34). Expression of a carboxy terminus truncated occludin or addition of peptides corresponding to occludin extracellular loops disrupted occludin localization in TJs in cultured cells, but did not affect gross TJ morphology (29,30). Moreover, occludin-null embryonic stem cells differentiated into epithelial cells and formed well-developed TJ structures (35).

Occludin-null mice demonstrated a wide variety of histological abnormalities, including the gut, brain, testis, salivary glands, and bone, but TJs appeared unaffected and the epithelial barrier function was normal. This phenotype suggested that TJs and occludin have a more complex function than previously assumed (36).

2. The Claudin Family

The claudins are a family of more than 20 genes encoding TJ proteins. Claudin 1 and 2 were discovered first, based on their cofractionation with occludin from isolated chicken liver junctions (37). Both of these 22-kD proteins have no sequence similarity to occludin, but they share the same topology of four transmembrane domains with two extracellular loops, and cytoplasmic amino and carboxy termini (37). Immunofluorescence and immunoelectron microscopy revealed that claudin 1 and 2 were both targeted to and incorporated into the TJ strand itself (37). When each of these proteins was transfected into cells that lack TJs, they were highly concentrated at cell-cell contact sites. In freeze-fracture replicas of these contact sites, well-developed networks of strands were identified that were similar to TJ strand networks in vivo (38). Although occludin was also concentrated at cell contact sites when transfected into cells, it created only a small number of short strands. However, when cotransfected with claudin 1, occludin was incorporated into well-developed claudin 1–based strands (38). These findings suggested that claudins are mainly responsible for TJ strand formation, and that occludin is an accessory protein in the TJ, although it might have additional functions that are not yet understood (38).

After the discovery of claudin 1 and 2, additional family members were identified through amino acid sequence similarity searches (39), and to date more than 20 known claudin paralogs have been identified in humans (Table 1). All members of the claudin family share the same membrane topology and other structural features, as indicated by the observation that eight different claudins can bind to the three submembrane proteins ZO-1, -2, and -3 through their carboxy terminus cytosolic domain (40). Similar to claudin 1 and 2, other claudins are also concentrated at preexisting TJs when transfected into MDCK cells (39). Northern blotting showed that the tissue distribution pattern varies significantly among different claudin family members, and that many tissues express multiple claudin species (39). These findings suggested that multiple claudin family members are involved in the formation of TJ strands in a tissue-dependent manner. When claudin 1, 2, and 3 were coexpressed in mouse L fibroblasts in different combinations, different claudins were copolymerized into individual TJ strands (heteropolymers) (Fig. 3A), and when two transfected clones of mouse L fibroblasts singly

Table 1 The Claudin Family

Protein name	Synonymous names	Gene name	Human chromosome	GenBank Accession Number		Related phenotype	Ref.
				Gene	cDNA		
Claudin 1	SEMP1 (senescence-associated epithelial membrane protein 1)	*CLDN1*	3q28–29	AH010563	NM_021101	*Cldn1*-null mice die postnatally due to dysfunction of the epidermal permeability barrier	37,64,71
Claudin 2		*CLDN2*	Xq22.3–23	AL158821	NM_020384		37
Claudin 3	RVP1 (rat ventral prostate 1 protein), CPETR2 (*Clostridium perfringens* enterotoxin receptor 2)	*CLDN3*	7q11	AF007189	NM_001306		39,65
Claudin 4	CPE-R (*Clostridium perfringens* enterotoxin receptor)	*CLDN4*	7q11.23		NM_001305		39,66
Claudin 5	TMVCF (transmembrane protein deleted in velo-cardio-facial syndrome), MBEC (mouse brain endothelial cell 1)	*CLDN5*	22q11.2	NT_011519	NM_003277	Within the region of 22q11 that is commonly deleted in patients with velocardiofacial syndrome (VCFS) (MIM 192430)	39,67,68
Claudin 6		*CLDN6*	16p13.2–13.3	NM_021195	XM_012518	Transgenic mice overexpressing *Cldn6* die postnatally due to dysfunction of the epidermal permeability barrier	39,72
Claudin 7		*CLDN7*	17p12	NT_010692	NM_001307		39
Claudin 8		*CLDN8*	21q22.1	AJ250711	NM_012132		39

	Symbol	Location			Other name	Notes	Ref.
Claudin 9	CLDN9	16p13.2–13.3	AJ130941	NM_020982			
Claudin 10	CLDN10	13q21.2–22		NM_006984			
Claudin 11	CLDN11	3q26.2–26.3	NT_025667	NM_005602	OSP (oligodendrocyte-specific protein)	*Cldn11*-null mice exhibit both neurological and reproductive deficits, including slowed CNS nerve conduction, conspicuous hindlimb weakness, and male sterility	45,69
Claudin 12	CLDN12	7q21	AJ250713	NM_012129			
Claudin 13[a]	Cldn13		NT_039314	NM_020504			
Claudin 14	CLDN14	21q22.1	AJ132445	NM_012130		Mutated in humans with profound, congenital, recessive deafness *DFNB29* (MIM 605608)	46
Claudin 15	CLDN15	7q21.3–22.1		NM_138429			
Claudin 16	CLDN16	3q		NM_006580	Paracellin-1	Mutated in humans with primary hypomagnesemia (MIM 603959); mutated in bovine chronic interstitial nephritis	43,44
Claudin 17	CLDN17	21q22.1	AJ250712	NM_012131			
Claudin 18	CLDN18	3q21–23	NT_005832	NM_016369			
Claudin 19	CLDN19	1p33–34.2		NM_148960			
Claudin 20	CLDN20	6q25	P56880 (protein)				70
Claudin 21[b]	CLDN21	4pter-qter					
Claudin 22[b]	CLDN22	4pter-qter					

[a] Found in the mouse, no human ortholog found yet.
[b] Symbol and cytogenetic location reserved on the human gene nomenclature database (http://www.gene.ucl.ac.uk/nomenclature). No sequence information available.

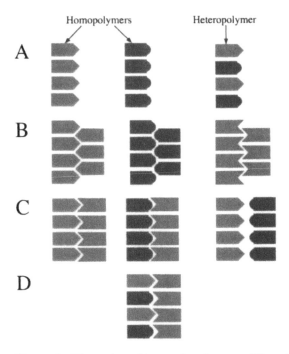

Figure 3 Illustration of interactions between different claudins within and between TJ strands. Claudins can form homopolymers or heteropolymers (A), which can interact with other homo- and heteropolymers (B–D) (18,38). Various claudin combinations increase both the structural and the functional diversity of TJs in different tissues, and might explain the difference in transepithelial resistance found between "tight" and "leaky" epithelia. (Based on Ref. 21.)

expressing claudin 1, 2, or 3 were cocultured it was found that claudin 1- or claudin 2–based strands (homopolymers) laterally associated with claudin 3–based strands but not with each other (Fig. 3C) (41). When L fibroblasts transfectants singly expressing claudin 1 were cocultured with transfectants coexpressing claudin 1 and 2, claudin 1 homopolymers laterally associated with claudin 1 and 2 heteropolymers to form paired strands (Fig. 3D) (21). Since the claudin family includes more than 20 members, a very large number of combinations are possible within and between TJ strands in different tissues (Fig. 3). This mode of assembly of claudins increases both the structural and the functional diversity of TJs in different tissues (41), and might explain the 100,000-fold difference in transepithelial resistance found between "tight" and "leaky" epithelia (19).

Convincing support for the function of the claudins in creating the TJ physiological barrier came from several sources. *Clostridium perfringens* enterotoxin removes specific claudins from TJ strands, causing TJ disintegration and reduction of the TJ barrier function (42). Additional evidence came from the phenotypes of humans and animals with mutations in specific claudin genes (Table 1). Mutations in human *CLDN16* cause renal hypomagnesemia with hypercalciuria and nephrocalcinosis, due to a defect in paracellular resorption of Mg^{2+} in the thick ascending limb of Henle in the kidney (43). A null mutation in bovine *Cldn16* causes chronic interstitial nephritis, which is characterized by failures in selective filtration and absorption in surface renal epithelium, due to dysfunction of paracellular renal transport systems (44). In addition, *Cldn11*-null mice demonstrate both neurological and reproductive deficits, due to the absence of TJs in the central nervous system myelin and between Sertoli cells (45). Finally, we demonstrated that mutations of *CLDN14* in humans cause profound, congenital, recessive deafness *DFNB29*, and hypothesized a failure to maintain the electrochemical gradient between the endolymph and its surrounding tissues in the inner ear's organ of Corti (46).

Taken together, the evidence strongly suggests that claudins are the primary proteins responsible for the physiological and structural paracellular barrier function of TJs (21). Yet the discovery that at least one of the family members, claudin 1, is not restricted to TJs in the rat epididymis raises the possibility that claudins might have additional roles, such as cell-cell adhesion (47). Claudins were also suggested to participate in morphogenesis, based on their strong and specific expression in vertebrate primordia (48).

II. CLAUDIN 14

A. Mutations in the Human *CLDN14* Gene Cause Autosomal Recessive Deafness *DFNB29*

The *DFNB29* locus on chromosome 21q22.1 was defined by two large consanguineous Pakistani families segregating profound, congenital, recessive deafness (46). *DFNB29*-affected individuals in these families show no signs of vestibular dysfunction or any other symptoms beside deafness. The *DFNB29* 2.3-Mb interval included three genes: *CLDN14* (claudin 14), *KIAA0136*, a gene of unknown function, and *CHAF1B* (chromatin assembly factor 1B-p60 subunit) (49), and excluded the *DFNB10* locus, which was later found to encode a novel serine protease, *TMPRSS3* (50,51). Mutations of gap junction proteins encoded by *GJB2* (*Cx26*) and *GJB3* (*Cx31*) are significant causes of deafness (52–55). It was thus hypothesized that other proteins with functions important for inner ear intercellular junctions might be essential for hearing. This hypothesis made *CLDN14*, encoding a member of the claudin family of TJ proteins, an excellent candidate gene for *DFNB29*.

Comparison of *CLDN14* cDNA sequence to the genomic sequence of human chromosome 21 indicated that the *CLDN14* gene has three exons, with the entire protein of 239 amino acid residues encoded in exon 3 (46). Sequencing of exon 3 led to the identification of two *CLDN14* mutations that cosegregated with deafness in both *DFNB29* families (46). One of the families cosegregated 398delT, a single nucleotide deletion within codon Met133, located in the third transmembrane domain. This frameshift mutation is predicted to cause premature translation termination 69 nucleotides later, after the incorporation of 23 incorrect amino acids and the loss of almost half of the predicted claudin 14 protein (46). The second family cosegregated a missense mutation, V85D (aspartic acid substituted for valine), due to a transversion of T to A at position 254. Valine 85 is conserved among 12 of 20 claudins, while isoleucine is present among five claudins, and the remaining three claudins have either a cysteine or a proline at this position (46). Aspartic acid at position 85 is predicted to affect hydrophobicity and disrupt the predicted secondary structure in the second transmembrane domain (46). Neither one of the two *CLDN14* mutations was detected in 300 normal control chromosomes from Pakistani individuals, indicating that these two variants are not common polymorphisms in the Pakistani population (46). Among 100 Pakistani families that could support statistically significant linkage of recessive nonsyndromic deafness (56), only these two families segregated deafness that was linked to *CLDN14* (46). Therefore, mutations of *CLDN14* probably account for a small portion of recessive nonsyndromic deafness in Pakistan. Finding two mutant alleles of *CLDN14* cosegregating with recessive deafness in two consanguineous families demonstrates the significant role of claudin 14 in the cochlea and its importance in the hearing process.

B. *Cldn14* Knockout Mice Are Deaf: A Mouse Model for Autosomal Recessive Deafness *DFNB29*

To explore the role of claudin 14 in the inner ear and in other organs and tissues a targeted deletion of *Cldn14* was used to create *Cldn14*-null mice, on a C57BL6/129SVj mixed background. *Cldn14*-null homozygous mice are viable, healthy, and fertile. To evaluate their hearing, *Cldn14*-null homozygous and heterozygous mice and their wild-type (WT) littermates underwent auditory brainstem response (ABR) analyses at 4 weeks of age. Responses to 50-μs duration clicks, and 8-, 16-, and 32-kHz tone bursts were recorded. Thresholds were determined in 5-dB steps of decreasing stimulus intensity, until waveforms lost reproducible morphology. *Cldn14*-null homozygous mice were found to be deaf, while thresholds of their heterozygous and homozygous WT littermates were indistinguishable (T. Ben-Yosef, personal communication, 2003). *Cldn14* knockout mice are therefore a valuable model for studying the pathophysiology of autosomal recessive deafness *DFNB29*.

C. *CLDN14* Expression

Northern blot analysis demonstrated *CLDN14* expression in human kidney and liver (46). *CLDN14* is probably expressed in much lower levels in additional human and mouse tissues, including brain, pancreas, spleen, skin, colon, and testis, as indicated by RT-PCR (46) and by the presence of several *CLDN14/Cldn14* expressed sequence tags (ESTs) in the NCBI EST database (http://www.ncbi.nlm.nih.gov/dbEST/index.html), but the physiological significance of these findings is not clear. The *CLDN14* transcript is alternatively spliced, as indicated by the finding of two splicing isoforms in human liver cDNA, with and without exon 2, and by Northern blot analysis showing a shorter transcript in human kidney (46). Although RNA stability or rate of translation may differ, these splice isoforms do not alter the amino acid sequence of claudin 14, which is encoded entirely by exon 3. The functional distinctions, if any, between these splice isoforms remain to be explored.

The developmental profile and cell-specific expression pattern of *Cldn14* in the mouse inner ear was investigated using in situ hybridization and immunocytochemistry to detect *Cldn14* mRNA and protein, respectively. In the inner ear no expression was detected by in situ hybridization at embryonic days 15 or 17, but it was detected at postnatal days 4 and 8 (46). At postnatal day 4, *Cldn14* expression was apically located in the inner and outer hair cell region of the entire organ of Corti. At postnatal day 8, the highest *Cldn14* expression was detected in the supporting cells of the organ of Corti, including the pillar, Deiters', and inner sulcus cells (46).

The cochlea of the inner ear has two compartments with different ionic compositions. The perilymph of the scala vestibuli and scala tympani has low K^+ and high Na^+ concentrations, similar to cerebrospinal fluid (2). The ionic composition of the endolymph of the scala media is similar to that of an intracellular microenvironment, which has high K^+ and low Na^+ concentrations (reviewed in Ref. 1). This large K^+ gradient contributes to an 80–100-mV endocochlear potential, attributed in part to Na^+ - K^+-ATPase activity in the stria vascularis (57–61). This electrochemical gradient is critical for the depolarization of sensory hair cells, increasing the sensitivity of the mechanically activated transduction channels located at the top of stereocilia (62,63). The postnatal onset and rise of the endocochlear potential is presumably dependent upon the development of the paracellular barrier between the basal cells of the stria vascularis by TJs (60). The onset of claudin 14 in the inner ear is temporally correlated with the appearance of the endocochlear potential (60), suggesting that claudin 14 is important for sealing the scala media. An alternative or additional role for claudin 14 in the organ of Corti might be related to its hypothesized TJ fence function in developing and maintaining the polarity of inner and outer hair cells. These two hypotheses can be tested by measuring endocochlear potential and by examining hair cell structure and integrity in *Cldn14*-null mice.

III. SUMMARY

Claudin 14 is required for hearing, as demonstrated by profound congenital deafness caused by homozygosity for recessive *CLDN14* mutations in humans and mice. In addition to the inner ear, claudin 14 is expressed in kidney and liver, yet no obvious kidney or liver pathophysiology was observed in deaf individuals homozygous for *CLDN14* mutations, or in *Cldn14*-null mice. This indicates that in kidney and liver claudin 14 is not necessary for normal function under regular conditions. It remains to be determined if the role of claudin 14 in the auditory system is important for paracellular transport or epithelial cell polarity and/or hair cell development. Further characterization of *Cldn14*-null mice will lead to a better understanding of the role of tight junctions in the development and maintenance of the processes necessary for sound transduction in the ear.

REFERENCES

1. Ferrary E, Sterkers O. Mechanisms of endolymph secretion. Kidney Int Suppl 1998; 65:S98–103.
2. Ryan AF, Wickham MG, Bone RC. Element content of intracochlear fluids, outer hair cells, and stria vascularis as determined by energy-dispersive roentgen ray analysis. Otolaryngol Head Neck Surg 1979; 87:659–665.
3. Farquhar MG, Palade GE. Junctional complexes in various epithelia. J Cell Biol 1963; 17:375–412.
4. Kowalczyk AP, Bornslaeger EA, Norvell SM, Palka HL, Green KJ. Desmosomes: intercellular adhesive junctions specialized for attachment of intermediate filaments. Int Rev Cytol 1999; 185:237–302.
5. Nagafuchi A. Molecular architecture of adherens junctions. Curr Opin Cell Biol 2001; 13:600–603.
6. Goodenough DA, Goliger JA, Paul DL. Connexins, connexons, and intercellular communication. Annu Rev Biochem 1996; 65:475–502.

7. Anderson JM. Molecular structure of tight junctions and their role in epithelial transport. News Physiol Sci 2001; 16:126–130.

8. Tsukita S, Furuse M, Itoh M. Multifunctional strands in tight junctions. Nat Rev Mol Cell Biol 2001; 2:285–293.

9. Yeaman C, Grindstaff KK, Nelson WJ. New perspectives on mechanisms involved in generating epithelial cell polarity. Physiol Rev 1999; 79:73–98.

10. Staehelin LA. Structure and function of intercellular junctions. Int Rev Cytol 1974; 39:191–283.

11. Staehelin LA. Further observations on the fine structure of freeze-cleaved tight junctions. J Cell Sci 1973; 13:763–786.

12. Cereijido M, Valdes J, Shoshani L, Contreras RG. Role of tight junctions in establishing and maintaining cell polarity. Annu Rev Physiol 1998; 60:161–177.

13. Dragsten PR, Blumenthal R, Handler JS. Membrane asymmetry in epithelia: is the tight junction a barrier to diffusion in the plasma membrane? Nature 1981; 294:718–722.

14. van Meer G, Simons K. The function of tight junctions in maintaining differences in lipid composition between the apical and the basolateral cell surface domains of MDCK cells. EMBO J 1986; 5:1455–1464.

15. van Meer G, Gumbiner B, Simons K. The tight junction does not allow lipid molecules to diffuse from one epithelial cell to the next. Nature 1986; 322:639–641.

16. Madara JL. Regulation of the movement of solutes across tight junctions. Annu Rev Physiol 1998; 60:143–159.

17. Fromter E, Diamond J. Route of passive ion permeation in epithelia. Nat New Biol 1972; 235:9–13.

18. Reese TS, Karnovsky MJ. Fine structural localization of a blood-brain barrier to exogenous peroxidase. J Cell Biol 1967; 34:207–217.

19. Claude P, Goodenough DA. Fracture faces of zonulae occludentes from "tight" and "leaky" epithelia. J Cell Biol 1973; 58:390–400.

20. Furuse M, Hirase T, Itoh M, Nagafuchi A, Yonemura S, Tsukita S. Occludin: a novel integral membrane protein localizing at tight junctions. J Cell Biol 1993; 123:1777–1788.

21. Tsukita S, Furuse M. Pores in the wall: claudins constitute tight junction strands containing aqueous pores. J Cell Biol 2000; 149:13–16.

22. Martin-Padura I, Lostaglio S, Schneemann M, Williams L, Romano M, Fruscella P, Panzeri C, Stoppacciaro A, Ruco L, Villa A, Simmons D, Dejana E. Junctional adhesion molecule, a novel member of the immunoglobulin superfamily that distributes at intercellular junctions and modulates monocyte transmigration. J Cell Biol 1998; 142:117–127.

23. Williams LA, Martin-Padura I, Dejana E, Hogg N, Simmons DL. Identification and characterisation of human junctional adhesion molecule (JAM). Mol Immunol 1999; 36:1175–1188.

24. Turner JR. "Putting the squeeze" on the tight junction: understanding cytoskeletal regulation. Semin Cell Dev Biol 2000; 11:301–308.

25. Gonzalez-Mariscal L, Betanzos A, Avila-Flores A. MAGUK proteins: structure and role in the tight junction. Semin Cell Dev Biol 2000; 11:315–324.

26. Mitic LL, Van Itallie CM, Anderson JM. Molecular physiology and pathophysiology of tight junctions I. Tight junction structure and function: lessons from mutant animals and proteins. Am J Physiol Gastrointest Liver Physiol 2000; 279:G250–254.

27. Van Itallie CM, Anderson JM. Occludin confers adhesiveness when expressed in fibroblasts. J Cell Sci 1997; 110:1113–1121.

28. Lacaz-Vieira F, Jaeger MM, Farshori P, Kachar B. Small synthetic peptides homologous to segments of the first external loop of occludin impair tight junction resealing. J Membr Biol 1999; 168:289–297.

29. Wong V, Gumbiner BM. A synthetic peptide corresponding to the extracellular domain of occludin perturbs the tight junction permeability barrier. J Cell Biol 1997; 136:399–409.

30. Balda MS, Whitney JA, Flores C, Gonzalez S, Cereijido M, Matter K. Functional dissociation of paracellular permeability and transepithelial electrical resistance and disruption of the apical-basolateral intramembrane diffusion barrier by expression of a mutant tight junction membrane protein. J Cell Biol 1996; 134:1031–1049.

31. Chen Y, Merzdorf C, Paul DL, Goodenough DA. COOH terminus of occludin is required for tight junction barrier function in early *Xenopus* embryos. J Cell Biol 1997; 138:891–899.

32. McCarthy KM, Skare IB, Stankewich MC, Furuse M, Tsukita S, Rogers RA, Lynch RD, Schneeberger EE. Occludin is a functional component of the tight junction. J Cell Sci 1996; 109:2287–2298.

33. Hirase T, Staddon JM, Saitou M, Ando-Akatsuka Y, Itoh M, Furuse M, Fujimoto K, Tsukita S, Rubin LL. Occludin as a possible determinant of tight junction permeability in endothelial cells. J Cell Sci 1997; 110:1603–1613.

34. Moroi S, Saitou M, Fujimoto K, Sakakibara A, Furuse M, Yoshida O, Tsukita S. Occludin is concentrated at tight junctions of mouse/rat but not human/guinea pig Sertoli cells in testes. Am J Physiol 1998; 274:C1708–1717.

35. Saitou M, Fujimoto K, Doi Y, Itoh M, Fujimoto T, Furuse M, Takano H, Noda T, Tsukita S. Occludin-deficient embryonic stem cells can differentiate into polarized epithelial cells bearing tight junctions. J Cell Biol 1998; 141:397–408.

36. Saitou M, Furuse M, Sasaki H, Schulzke JD, Fromm M, Takano H, Noda T, Tsukita S. Complex phenotype of mice lacking occludin, a component of tight junction strands. Mol Biol Cell 2000; 11:4131–4142.

37. Furuse M, Fujita K, Hiiragi T, Fujimoto K, Tsukita S. Claudin-1 and -2: novel integral membrane proteins localizing at tight junctions with no sequence similarity to occludin. J Cell Biol 1998; 141:1539–1550.

38. Furuse M, Sasaki H, Fujimoto K, Tsukita S. A single gene product, claudin-1 or -2, reconstitutes tight junction strands and recruits occludin in fibroblasts. J Cell Biol 1998; 143:391–401.

39. Morita K, Furuse M, Fujimoto K, Tsukita S. Claudin multigene family encoding four-transmembrane domain protein components of tight junction strands. Proc Natl Acad Sci USA 1999; 96:511–516.

40. Itoh M, Furuse M, Morita K, Kubota K, Saitou M, Tsukita S. Direct binding of three tight junction-associated MAGUKs, ZO-1, ZO-2, and ZO-3, with the COOH termini of claudins. J Cell Biol 1999; 147:1351–1363.

41. Furuse M, Sasaki H, Tsukita S. Manner of interaction of heterogeneous claudin species within and between tight junction strands. J Cell Biol 1999; 147:891–903.

42. Sonoda N, Furuse M, Sasaki H, Yonemura S, Katahira J, Horiguchi Y, Tsukita S. *Clostridium perfringens* enterotoxin fragment removes specific claudins from tight junction strands: evidence for direct involvement of claudins in tight junction barrier. J Cell Biol 1999; 147:195–204.

43. Simon DB, Lu Y, Choate KA, Velazquez H, Al-Sabban E, Praga M, Casari G, Bettinelli A, Colussi G, Rodriguez-Soriano J, McCredie D, Milford D, Sanjad S, Lifton RP. Paracellin-1, a renal tight junction protein required for paracellular Mg2+ resorption. Science 1999; 285:103–106.

44. Hirano T, Kobayashi N, Itoh T, Takasuga A, Nakamaru T, Hirotsune S, Sugimoto Y. Null mutation of PCLN-1/Claudin-16 results in bovine chronic interstitial nephritis. Genome Res 2000; 10:659–663.

45. Gow A, Southwood CM, Li JS, Pariali M, Riordan GP, Brodie SE, Danias J, Bronstein JM, Kachar B, Lazzarini RA. CNS myelin and sertoli cell tight junction strands are absent in Osp/claudin-11 null mice. Cell 1999; 99:649–659.

46. Wilcox ER, Burton QL, Naz S, Riazuddin S, Smith TN, Ploplis B, Belyantseva I, Ben-Yosef T, Liburd NA, Morell RJ, Kachar B, Wu DK, Griffith AJ, Friedman TB. Mutations in the gene encoding tight junction claudin-14 cause autosomal recessive deafness DFNB29. Cell 2001; 104:165–172.

47. Gregory M, Dufresne J, Hermo L, Cyr D. Claudin-1 is not restricted to tight junctions in the rat epididymis. Endocrinology 2001; 142:854–863.

48. Kollmar R, Nakamura SK, Kappler JA, Hudspeth AJ. Expression and phylogeny of claudins in vertebrate primordia. Proc Natl Acad Sci USA 2001; 98:10196–10201.

49. Hattori M, Fujiyama A, Taylor TD, et al. The DNA sequence of human chromosome 21. Nature 2000; 405:311–319.

50. Scott HS, Kudoh J, Wattenhofer M, Shibuya K, Berry A, Chrast R, Guipponi M, Wang J, Kawasaki K, Asakawa S, Minoshima S, Younus F, Mehdi SQ, Radhakrishna U, Papasavvas MP, Gehrig C, Rossier C, Korostishevsky M, Gal A, Shimizu N, Bonne-Tamir B, Antonarakis SE. Insertion of beta-satellite repeats identifies a transmembrane protease causing both congenital and childhood onset autosomal recessive deafness. Nat Genet 2001; 27:59–63.

51. Ben-Yosef T, Wattenhofer M, Riazuddin S, Ahmed ZM, Scott HS, Kudoh J, Shibuya K, Antonarakis SE, Bonne-Tamir B, Radhakrishna U, Naz S, Ahmed Z, Pandya A, Nance WE, Wilcox ER, Friedman TB, Morell RJ. Novel mutations of TMPRSS3 in four DFNB8/B10 families segregating congenital autosomal recessive deafness. J Med Genet 2001; 38:396–400.

52. Kelsell DP, Dunlop J, Stevens HP, Lench NJ, Liang JN, Parry G, Mueller RF, Leigh IM. Connexin 26 mutations in hereditary non-syndromic sensorineural deafness. Nature 1997; 387:80–83.

53. Liu XZ, Xia XJ, Xu LR, Pandya A, Liang CY, Blanton SH, Brown SD, Steel

KP, Nance WE. Mutations in connexin 31 underlie recessive as well as dominant non-syndromic hearing loss. Hum Mol Genet 2000; 9:63–67.

54. Morell RJ, Kim HJ, Hood LJ, Goforth L, Friderici K, Fisher R, Van Camp G, Berlin CI, Oddoux C, Ostrer H, Keats B, Friedman TB. Mutations in the connexin 26 gene (GJB2) among Ashkenazi Jews with nonsyndromic recessive deafness. N Engl J Med 1998; 339:1500–1505.

55. Xia JH, Liu CY, Tang BS, Pan Q, Huang L, Dai HP, Zhang BR, Xie W, Hu DX, Zheng D, Shi XL, Wang DA, Xia K, Yu KP, Liao XD, Feng Y, Yang YF, Xiao JY, Xie DH, Huang JZ. Mutations in the gene encoding gap junction protein beta-3 associated with autosomal dominant hearing impairment. Nat Genet 1998; 20:370–373.

56. Friedman T, Battey J, Kachar B, Riazuddin S, Noben-Trauth K, Griffith A, Wilcox E. Modifier genes of hereditary hearing loss. Curr Opin Neurobiol 2000; 10:487–493.

57. Johnstone BM, Sellick PM. The peripheral auditory apparatus. Q Rev Biophys 1972; 5:1–57.

58. Gratton MA, Smyth BJ, Lam CF, Boettcher FA, Schmiedt RA. Decline in the endocochlear potential corresponds to decreased Na,K-ATPase activity in the lateral wall of quiet-aged gerbils. Hearing Res 1997; 108:9–16.

59. Marcus DC, Chiba T. K^+ and Na^+ absorption by outer sulcus epithelial cells. Hearing Res 1999; 134:48–56.

60. Souter M, Forge A. Intercellular junctional maturation in the stria vascularis: possible association with onset and rise of endocochlear potential. Hearing Res 1998; 119:81–95.

61. Stankovic KM, Brown D, Alper SL, Adams JC. Localization of pH regulating proteins H^+ ATPase and Cl-/HCO3- exchanger in the guinea pig inner ear. Hearing Res 1997; 114:21–34.

62. Hudspeth AJ. How the ear's works work. Nature 1989; 341:397–404.

63. Milhaud PG, Nicolas MT, Bartolami S, Cabanis MT, Sans A. Vestibular semicircular canal epithelium of the rat in culture on filter support: polarity and barrier properties. Pflugers Arch 1999; 437:823–830.

64. Swisshelm K, Machl A, Planitzer S, Robertson R, Kubbies M, Hosier S. SEMP1, a senescence-associated cDNA isolated from human mammary epithelial cells, is a member of an epithelial membrane protein superfamily. Gene 1999; 226:285–295.

65. Peacock RE, Keen TJ, Inglehearn CF. Analysis of a human gene homologous to rat ventral prostate. 1. Protein. Genomics 1997; 46:443–449.

66. Paperna T, Peoples R, Wang YK, Kaplan P, Francke U. Genes for the CPE receptor (CPETR1) and the human homolog of RVP1 (CPETR2) are localized within the Williams-Beuren syndrome deletion. Genomics 1998; 54:453–459.

67. Sirotkin H, Morrow B, Saint-Jore B, Puech A, Das Gupta RPatanjali SR, Skoultchi A, Weissman SM, Kucherlapati R. Identification, characterization, and precise mapping of a human gene encoding a novel membrane-spanning protein from the 22q11 region deleted in velo-cardio-facial syndrome. Genomics 1997; 42:245–251.

68. Chen Z, Zandonatti M, Jakubowski D, Fox HS. Brain capillary endothelial cells express MBEC1, a protein that is related to the *Clostridium perfringens* enterotoxin receptors. Lab Invest 1998; 78:353–363.
69. Morita K, Sasaki H, Fujimoto K, Furuse M, Tsukita S. Claudin-11/OSP-based tight junctions of myelin sheaths in brain and Sertoli cells in testis. J Cell Biol 1999; 145:579–588.
70. Niimi T, Nagashima K, Ward JM, Minoo P, Zimonjic DBPopescu NC, Kimura S. Claudin-18, a novel downstream target gene for the T/EBP/NKX2.1 homeodomain transcription factor, encodes lung- and stomach-specific isoforms through alternative splicing. Mol Cell Biol 2001; 21:7380–7390.
71. Furuse M, Hata M, Furuse K, Yoshida Y, Haratake A, Sugitani Y, Noda T, Kubo A, Tsukita S. Claudin-based tight junctions are crucial for the mammalian epidermal barrier: a lesson from claudin-1-deficient mice. J Cell Biol 2002; 156: 1099–1111.
72. Turksen K, Troy TC. Permeability barrier dysfunction in transgenic mice overexpressing claudin 6. Development 2002; 129:1775–1784.

25
CDH23

Julie M. Schultz, Robert J. Morell, Andrew J. Griffith, and Thomas B. Friedman
National Institute on Deafness and Other Communication Disorders, National Institutes of Health, Rockville, Maryland, U.S.A.

I. CELLULAR ADHESION

Adhesion molecules mediate cell-to-cell contact, and participate in the regulation of the development of tissues. Cell adhesion molecules can be classified into four families: immunoglobin-like proteins, integrins, selectins, and cadherins (1). In general, cadherins are membrane-bound glycoprotein receptors that function in cell-to-cell adhesion at adherens junctions, where cytoskeleton components are assembled intracellularly (2). The cadherin superfamily members are grouped as a family of proteins by virtue of tandem repeats of an extracellular cadherin-specific motif referred to as the EC domain, and are distinguished from each other by their unique structural features (3). The cadherin superfamily includes the classical cadherins, desmosomal cadherins, protocadherins, and cadherin-related proteins (3,4). They are classified into these specific subgroups based on the motifs of their cytoplasmic domain, the number of membrane-spanning regions, or the number of EC domains (5). The majority of cadherins have a single membrane-spanning domain, and a cytoplasmic domain involved in linkage to the cytoskeleton (1,6,7). Each extracellular EC domain is approximately 110 amino acids in length and contains highly conserved amino acid motifs (DXD, LDRE, and DXNDNXPXF), which are involved in Ca^{2+}-mediated intermolecular association among cadherins on the same cell as well as adjacent cells (1,3).

The classical cadherins have five EC domains, whereas other cadherins may have more than 30 EC domains. E-cadherin, N-cadherin, and P-cadherin are classical cadherins that have been extensively studied in the context of intercellular adhesion. The high-resolution structure of E-cadherin shows that the first EC domain binds Ca^{2+} and has an exposed protein surface that may provide homophilic binding specificity (8). X-ray crystallographic studies of N-cadherin show that the EC domains are involved in higher-order protein organization through the formation of dimers with cadherin EC domains on the same cell surface that interact with cadherin dimers on adjacent cells (9). Cells transfected with E-cadherin or P-cadherin preferentially aggregate with cells expressing the same cadherins during cell-sorting experiments (10).

Some cadherin proteins are necessary for the integrity of the retinal photoreceptor sensory cells and the cochlear neurosensory cells. A photoreceptor-specific cadherin (prCAD) was identified by subtractive hybridization of a bovine retina cDNA library and was shown to be localized at the base of the outer segment (11). Mice with a presumptive null mutation of prCAD initially develop normal retinae. However, from 1 to 5 months after birth there is a progressive loss of photoreceptor cells.

Immunocytochemistry experiments suggest that E-cadherin is involved in reticular lamina maintenance in the organ of Corti before the development of fluid spaces in the cochlea (12). In humans, Usher syndrome type 1F (deafness and progressive blindness) is caused by mutations of *PCDH15*, encoding protocadherin 15 (13,14). Finally, mutations of the cadherin-related 23 gene, *CDH23*, cause Usher syndrome type 1D, as well as nonsyndromic hearing loss *DFNB12*, which are the topics of this chapter.

II. *CDH23*

CDH23 spans more than 250 kb of genomic DNA, with 69 exons encoding a 9–10-kb transcript; three of the exons are alternatively spliced (15,16). The largest *CDH23* isoform encodes a deduced 3354-amino-acid protein that is predicted, by TMpred and TMHMM, to have one membrane-spanning region that divides cadherin 23 into a large extracellular domain with 27 EC domains and a cytoplasmic domain of 268 amino acids (15). The extracellular domain contains two alternatively spliced miniexons (16), and the cytoplasmic domain contains one alternatively spliced exon encoding 35 amino acids (15). The cytoplasmic domain of *CDH23* is highly conserved among the human, mouse, rat, bovine, and pufferfish homologs, but is unique from the cytoplasmic domains of other cadherin proteins.

III. *DFNB12*

Affected individuals with nonsyndromic hereditary hearing loss are often clinically indistinguishable. However, genetic linkage studies provide the information necessary to distinguish between different hereditary hearing loss loci. In 1996, a new locus for nonsyndromic recessive deafness, *DFNB12*, was mapped to chromosome 10q21–q22 (17). Affected individuals from families with nonsyndromic deafness, linked to *DFNB12*, present with prelingual, bilateral, moderate to profound sensorineural hearing loss (SNHL) in the absence of any extra-auditory features (15,17,17a). Clinical evaluations of balance, the attainment of motor developmental milestones, and, when tested, electronystagmography (ENG) with caloric testing are all within normal limits for *DFNB12* patients, suggesting normal vestibular function. Affected *DFNB12* individuals lack a clinically significant vestibular dysfunction, although partial vestibular deficits may be overlooked without a comprehensive vestibular evaluation. Ocular funduscopy or electroretinography (ERG) of affected *DFNB12* individuals confirms the absence of retinitis pigmentosa (RP).

IV. *USH1D*

Three clinical subtypes of Usher syndrome (USH) are distinguished on the basis of the auditory, visual, and vestibular phenotypes (18–20). Type 1 USH (*USH1*) is the most severe subtype and is characterized by congenital profound hearing loss, vestibular areflexia, and onset of RP by age 10. The loci for *USH1* (designated *USH1A–USH1G*) are distinguishable only on the basis of their genetic map location (21). Five *USH1* genes have been identified (*USH1B, USH1C, USH1D, USH1F,* and *USH1G*) (13–16,22–24,24a).

The *USH1D* locus was mapped in 1996 to chromosome 10q (25), overlapping the *DFNB12* locus. Affected individuals with *USH1D* have profound SNHL and vestibular areflexia, which is demonstrated by pure-tone audiometry and a lack of responses to caloric irrigation, respectively. If calorics cannot be performed, a history of delayed motor developmental milestones and abnormal performance in tandem gait and Romberg evaluations are consistent with vestibular areflexia. The onset of retinal degeneration typically presents as nyctalopia during the first decade of life, with progressive loss of peripheral vision, and, in some cases, leads to complete blindness. RP is confirmed by ERG or ocular funduscopy in patients.

V. POSITIONAL CLONING OF *DFNB12*

We used a positional cloning strategy to identify the *DFNB12* gene. Consanguineous families segregating SNHL were used to refine the linked interval of *DFNB12* on chromosome 10q21–q22 (15). One *DFNB12* family, PKSR46a, had recombinations in two individuals that reduced the *DFNB12* interval to 0.5 cM. The gene for *DFNB12* was positionally cloned based on an evaluation of genomic DNA sequence of 18 genes from the critical chromosomal interval, and missense mutations of *CDH23* were identified in five *DFNB12* families (15). Since the *DFNB12* and *USH1D* loci overlapped and might be allelic, we also sequenced the *CDH23* gene in six *USH1D* families. We identified nonsense and splice-site mutations cosegregating with the Usher syndrome phenotype, demonstrating allelism. Simultaneously and independently, mutations in the mouse ortholog (*Cdh23*) were identified in *waltzer* mice (26), which led to the identification of *CDH23* mutations in *USH1D* patients (16). *CDH23* is one of three known examples of a gene in which mutations can cause nonsyndromic deafness or Usher syndrome. Mutations of *MYO7A* are associated with *DFNA11*, *DFNB2*, and *USH1B* (22,27–29), and mutations in *USH1C* are associated with both *USH1C* and *DFNB18* (23,24,30).

VI. *CDH23* MUTANT ALLELES

CDH23 homozygous missense mutations were identified in children of consanguineous marriages segregating hearing loss and exhibiting linkage to the *DFNB12* locus (15). *CDH23* nonsense, splice-site, frameshift, and missense mutations were identified in *USH1D* families (15,16). We proposed a genotype-phenotype correlation where some amino acid replacements in cadherin 23 were presumed to cause partial loss of function and nonsyndromic deafness while more disabling mutations and functional null alleles of *CDH23* cause RP and vestibular dysfunction in addition to deafness (15). This genotype-phenotype correlation was further examined in a larger cohort of nonsyndromic deafness and Usher syndrome type I patients. More than 100 probands with nonsyndromic deafness or *USH1* were screened for *CDH23* mutations (31) and the type of mutant alleles of *CDH23* characterized was consistent with the genotype-phenotype correlation.

The 19 *CDH23* mutations identified in *DFNB12* families are homozygous missense mutations or compound heterozygous missense mutations in the putative extracellular domain of cadherin 23. Many of the nonsyndromic deafness families have missense mutations that occur in the conserved calcium-binding motifs of the extracellular EC domains (15,31,31a). This suggests that Ca^{2+} chelation by the EC domains of cadherin 23 is required in the organ of Corti but may not be necessary in the retina. However, we do know that some "nonsyndromic deafness families" have presymptomatic signs of RP revealed by ERG and fundus examinations (31), suggesting that even missense mutations of *CDH23* may have a subclinical effect on the retina.

Nonsense mutations, insertions, deletions, splicing variants, and missense mutations have all been identified in *USH1* probands, many of whom have a typical USH1 phenotype. Not surprisingly, some families with *CDH23* mutations exhibit an atypical *USH1* phenotype. Affected members of family PKSR7a were found to be homozygous for the IVS66 + 1G > A mutation at the splice donor site of an exon-intron boundary encoding the putative cytoplasmic domain of cadherin 23. This Pakistani family was originally diagnosed with nonsyndromic deafness, but reevaluation of the two oldest affected individuals (27 and 28 years old) by an ophthalmologist revealed early-stage RP (15).

The identification of late-onset RP demonstrates the importance of monitoring *DFNB12*-affected individuals for presymptomatic development of RP. Likewise, three branches of a Cuban family were reported to have variable degrees and ages of onset of retinal degeneration depending on their *CDH23* genotypes; homozygous R1746Q, homozygous Q1496H (a putative splice-site mutation), or compound heterozygous R1746Q/Q1496H (16). Moreover, additional affected individuals have been diagnosed with atypical Usher syndrome by virtue of an absent, mild, and/or late-onset phenotype (31).

To date, 27 missense, five nonsense, two insertions, seven deletions, and 10 splice-site mutations of *CDH23* have been identified and are associated with a range of hearing and retinal phenotypes (summarized in Ref. (31)). All reported *CDH23* alleles identified in nonsyndromic deafness patients have been missense mutations (15,31), with the exception of one profoundly deaf individual. She is compound heterozygous for a *DFNB12* missense mutation and a truncating mutation in the region of *CDH23* encoding the extracellular domain, and has normal vestibular and visual function at age 26 (JM Schultz and AJ Griffith, unpublished data, 2003). This suggests that a single hypomorphic missense allele is sufficient for a normal retinal phenotype. However, until we understand the function of cadherin 23 in the retina and auditory system, and the role of modifier genes, we cannot accurately predict the phenotype of an individual who is compound heterozygous for a hypomorphic and a more severe mutant allele of *CDH23*.

VII. *CDH23* EXPRESSION ANALYSIS

Northern blot analysis of human RNA, from dissected ocular tissues and brain, probed with the portion of *CDH23* encoding the unique cytoplasmic domain, demonstrates a ~9.5–10 kb mRNA expressed in the retina, but not in the ciliary body, retinal pigmented epithelium-choroid, lens, iris, or occipital cortex (15). The 488-bp probe of our Northern blot was derived from a portion of exons 66–69 and could be amplified from a human cochlear cDNA library, demonstrating its expression in the cochlea. No Northern hybridization signal was observed for human RNA from heart, brain, placenta, lung, liver, skeletal muscle, or kidney using the same probe derived from the cytoplasmic domain. However, a 1.35-kb mRNA was detected in human pancreas but has not been further characterized (15). *CDH23* message was detected in RNA from human retina, brain, kidney, skeletal muscle, and blood by RT-PCR analysis using primers that hybridize to the region of the gene encoding the twenty-second and twenty-third EC domains (16).

Using RT-PCR, *Cdh23* expression in the mouse was found in the brain, heart, kidney, eye, and ear (26). In the auditory system, in situ hybridization experiments demonstrate *Cdh23* expression in the mouse cochlear neuroepithelium with specific staining of neurosensory cells (26,32). Using embryonic day 18 tissue, Wilson and co-workers reported a more extensive in situ expression analysis with a *Cdh23* probe showing hybridization in the hair cells of the vestibular sensory epithelium and cells comprising Reissner's membrane, as well as the cochlear inner and outer hair cells (32). *Cdh23* expression was also observed in the tongue and olfactory bulbs (32). For both of these studies, it would be interesting to know whether their in situ probes would fail to detect *Cdh23* message in a *Cdh23*-null mouse.

The localization of the *CDH23/Cdh23* mRNA expression is not consistent among these studies and appears to be dependent upon the assay used to detect the message. The probes for RT-PCR and in situ hybridization were derived from regions of the extracellular domain that also encode EC repeats, which may not be specific for *CDH23/Cdh23*, while the probe for our Northern blot analysis was directed against the novel cytoplasmic domain. RT-PCR is a more sensitive method of detecting low levels of message in comparison to Northern blot hybridization analyses. However, the physiological relevance of these potentially low mRNA levels in tissues other than the inner ear and retina has not been determined.

VIII. MOUSE MODEL FOR STUDYING
CADHERIN 23 FUNCTION

Nonsense, splice-site, and frameshift mutations of *Cdh23* have been identified in 10 strains of *waltzer* mice, which have sensorineural deafness and vestibular defects (26,32–34). Each mutant allele is predicted to be a functional null. *Cdh23* mRNA localizes to the cochlear hair cells by in situ hybridization (26,32). Scanning electron microscopy of the cochlear inner and outer hair cells of mice with *Cdh23* mutations reveals disorganized stereocilia (26,33,35). Unlike humans with *CDH23*-null alleles, no retinal phenotype was observed for *waltzer* mice with *Cdh23*-null mutations. Species-specific variations may account for the differences in the retinal phenotype of humans and mice. The mouse retina may express another cadherin that is able to compensate for the loss of cadherin 23, or the retinal phenotype may be late-onset or subtle. Alternatively, since the 10 *Cdh23* alleles are not on the same genetic background, some *waltzer* strains may harbor a modifier gene that suppresses retinal degeneration but not hearing loss.

IX. FUNCTION OF CADHERIN 23

Although there is no published supporting data, perhaps cadherin 23 is involved in the organization of hair cell stereocilia through homophilic interactions on adjacent stereocilia. The stereocilia of hair cells are arranged in rows of decreasing height and are interconnected by tip links, shaft connectors, side links, and ankle links that have been identified in ultrastructural studies (36,37). Perhaps cadherin 23 is a molecular correlate of one or more of these structures.

In other tissues, some cadherins are bound to β-catenin or plakoglobin, which in turn binds to other proteins such as α-catenin, vinculin, and Z0–1 (2). Cadherin 23 likely does not bind any of these proteins since the cytoplasmic domain does not contain these protein-binding motifs. *CDH23* has an alternatively spliced exon in the region encoding the cytoplasmic domain. Mutations in this alternate exon 68 have not yet been identified in *DFNB12* or *USH1D* probands. RT-PCR experiments conducted with RNA from adult mice show that the cadherin 23 isoform containing exon 68 is expressed in the inner ear but not in the retina (38). Yeast two-hybrid and biochemical assays demonstrate an interaction of the cytoplasmic domain of cadherin 23 with the PDZ domains of harmonin, the *USH1C* gene product (38,39).

In summary, missense mutations of *CDH23* with presumed subtle functional disablements of cadherin 23 are associated with nonsyndromic deafness, while mutant alleles of *CDH23* with a more severe effect cause deafness accompanied by vestibular and progressive retinal dysfunction. Studies of the phenotypic variation caused by different mutations of *CDH23* coupled with the assignment of functions to cadherin 23 within the inner ear and retina may eventually permit the rational design of therapies.

REFERENCES

1. Nollet F, Kools P, van Roy F. Phylogenetic analysis of the cadherin superfamily allows identification of six major subfamilies besides several solitary members. J Mol Biol 2000; 299:551–572.
2. Nagafuchi A. Molecular architecture of adherens junctions. Curr Opin Cell Biol 2001; 13:600–603.
3. Suzuki ST. Structural and functional diversity of cadherin superfamily: are new members of cadherin superfamily involved in signal transduction pathway? J Cell Biochem 1996; 61:531–542.
4. Ivanov DB, Philippova MP, Tkachuk VA. Structure and functions of classical cadherins. Biochemistry 2001; 66:1450–1464.
5. Yagi T, Takeichi M. Cadherin superfamily genes: functions, genomic organization, and neurologic diversity. Genes Dev 2000; 14:1169–1180.
6. Gumbiner BM. Cell adhesion: the molecular basis of tissue architecture and morphogenesis. Cell 1996; 84:345–357.
7. Kemler R. From cadherins to catenins: cytoplasmic protein interactions and regulation of cell adhesion. Trends Genet 1993; 9:317–321.
8. Overduin M, Harvey TS, Bagby S, Tong KI, Yau P, Takeichi M, Ikura M. Solution structure of the epithelial cadherin domain responsible for selective cell adhesion. Science 1995; 267:386–389.
9. Shapiro L, Fannon AM, Kwong PD, Thompson A, Lehmann MS, Grubel G, Legrand J-F, Als-Nielsen J, Colman DR, Hendrickson WA. Structural basis of cell-cell adhesion by cadherins. Nature 1995; 374:327–337.
10. Nose A, Nagafuchi A, Takeichi M. Expressed recombinant cadherins mediate cell sorting in model systems. Cell 1988; 54:993–1001.
11. Rattner A, Smallwood PM, Williams J, Cooke C, Savchenko A, Lyubarsky A, Pugh ENJ, Nathans J. A photoreceptor-specific cadherin is essential for the structural integrity of the outer segment and for photoreceptor survival. Neuron 2001; 32:775–786.
12. Whitlon DS. E-cadherin in the mature and developing organ of Corti of the mouse. J Neurocytol 1993; 22:1030–1038.
13. Ahmed ZM, Riazuddin S, Bernstein SL, Ahmed Z, Khan S, Griffith AJ, Morell RJ, Friedman TB, Wilcox ER. Mutations of the protocadherin gene PCDH15 cause Usher syndrome type 1F. Am J Hum Genet 2001; 69:25–34.
14. Alagramam KN, Yuan B, Kuehn MH, Murcia CL, Wayne S, Srisailapathy CR, Lowry RB, Knaus R, Laer LV, Bernier FP, Schwartz S, Lee C, Morton CC, Mullins RF, Ramesh A, Van Camp G, Hagemen GS, Woychik RP, Smith RJH. Mutations in the novel protocadherin PDCH15 cause Usher syndrome type 1F. Hum Mol Genet 2001; 10:1709–1718.
15. Bork JM, Peters LM, Riazuddin S, et al. Usher syndrome 1D and non-syndromic autosomal recessive deafness DFNB12 are caused by allelic mutations of the novel cadherin-like gene CDH23. Am J Hum Genet 2001; 68:26–37.
16. Bolz H, von Brederlow B, Ramirez A, Bryda EC, Kutsche K, Nothwang HG,

Seeliger M, Cabrera MdC-S, Vila MC, Molina OP, Gal A, Kubisch C. Mutation of *CDH23*, encoding a new member of the cadherin gene family, causes Usher syndrome type 1D. Nat Genet 2001; 27:108–112.

17. Chaib H, Place C, Salem N, Dode C, Chardenoux S, Weissenbach J, El Zir E, Loiselet J, Petit C. Mapping of *DFNB12*, a gene for a non-syndromal autosomal recessive deafness, to chromosome 10q21–22. Hum Mol Genet 1996; 5:1061–1064.

17a. Bork JM, Morell RJ, Khan S, Riazuddin S, Wilcox ER, Friedman TB, Griffith AJ. Clinical presentation of DFNB12 and Usher syndrome type 1D. Adv Oto-Rhino-Laryngol 2002; 61:145–152.

18. Smith RJ, Berlin CI, Hejtmancik JF, Keats BJ, Kimberling WJ, Lewis RA, Moller CG, Pelias MZ, Tranebjaerg L. Clinical diagnosis of the Usher syndromes. Usher Syndrome Consortium. Am J Med Genet 1994; 50:32–38.

19. Kimberling WJ, Moller C. Clinical and molecular genetics of Usher syndrome. J Am Acad Audiol 1995; 6:63–72.

20. Otterstedde CR, Spandau U, Blankenagel A, Kimberling WJ, Reisser C. A new clinical classification for Usher's syndrome based on a new subtype of Usher's syndrome type I. Laryngoscope 2001; 111:84–86.

21. Van Camp G, Smith RJH. Hereditary hearing loss homepage. http://dnalab-www.uia.ac.be/dnalab/hhh/.

22. Weil D, Blanchard S, Kaplan J, Guilford P, Gibson F, Walsh J, Mburu P, Varela A, Levilliers J, Weston MD, Kelley PM, Kimberling WJ, Wagenaar M, Levi-Acobas F, Larget-Piet D, Munnich A, Steel KP, Brown SDM, Petit C. Defective myosin VIIA gene responsible for Usher syndrome type 1B. Nature 1995; 374:60–61.

23. Bitner-Glindzicz M, Lindley KJ, Rutland P, Blaydon D, Smith VV, Milla PJ, Hussain K, Furth-Lavi J, Cosgrove KE, Shepherd RM, Barnes PD, O'Brien RE, Farndon PA, Sowden J, Liu X-Z, Scanlan MJ, Malcolm S, Dunne MJ, Aynsley-Green A, Glaser B. A recessive contiguous gene deletion causing infantile hyperinsulinism, enteropathy and deafness identifies the Usher type 1C gene. Nat Genet 2000; 26:56–60.

24. Verpy E, Leibovici M, Zwaenepoel I, Liu X-Z, Gal A, Salem N, Mansour A, Blanchard S, Kobayashi I, Keats BJ, Slim R, Petit C. A defect in harmonin, a PDZ domain-containing protein expressed in the inner ear sensory hair cells, underlies Usher syndrome type 1C. Nat Genet 2000; 26:51–55.

24a. Weil D, El-Amraoui A, Masmoudi S, Mustapha M, Kikkawa Y, Laine S, Delmaghani S, Adato A, Nadifi S, Zina ZB, Hamel C, Gal A, Ayadi H, Yonekawa H, Petit C. Usher syndrome type 1G (USH1G) is caused by mutations in the gene encoding SANS, a protein that associates with the USH1C protein, harmonin. Hum Mol Genet 2003; 12:463–471.

25. Wayne S, Der Kaloustian VM, Schloss M, Polomeno R, Scott DA, Hejtmancik JF, Sheffield VC, Smith RJ. Localization of the Usher syndrome type ID gene (*Ush1D*) to chromosome 10. Hum Mol Genet 1996; 5:1689–1692.

26. Di Palma F, Holme RH, Bryda EC, Belyantseva IA, Pellegrino R, Kachar B, Steel KP, Noben-Trauth K. Mutations in *Cdh23*, encoding a new type of

cadherin, cause stereocilia disorganization in *waltzer*, the mouse model for Usher syndrome type 1D. Nat Genet 2001; 27:103–107.

27. Liu XZ, Walsh J, Mburu P, Kendrick-Jones J, Cope MJ, Steel KP, Brown SD. Mutations in the myosin VIIA gene cause non-syndromic recessive deafness. Nat Genet 1997; 16:188–190.

28. Liu XZ, Walsh J, Tamagawa Y, Kitamura K, Nishizawa M, Steel KP, Brown SD. Autosomal dominant non-syndromic deafness caused by a mutation in the myosin VIIA gene [letter]. Nat Genet 1997; 17:268–269.

29. Weil D, Kussel P, Blanchard S, Levy G, Levi-Acobas F, Drira M, Ayadi H, Petit C. The autosomal recessive isolated deafness, *DFNB2*, and the Usher 1B syndrome are allelic defects of the myosin-VIIA gene. Nat Genet 1997; 16:191–193.

30. Ahmed ZM, Smith TN, Riazuddin S, Makishima T, Ghosh M, Bokhari S, Puthezhath SN, Menon PSN, Deshmukh D, Griffith AJ, Riazuddin S, Friedman TB, Wilcox ER. Nonsyndromic recessive deafness *DFNB18* and Usher syndrome type 1C are allelic mutations of *USH1C*. Hum Genet 2002; 110:527–531.

31. Astuto LM, Bork JM, Weston MD, Askew JW, Fields RR, Orten DJ, Ohliger SJ, Riazuddin S, Morell RJ, Khan S, Riazuddin S, Kremer H, Van Hauwe P, Moller C, Cremers CWRJ, Ayuso C, Heckenlively JR, Rohrschneider K, Spandau U, Greenberg J, Ramesar R, Reardon W, Bitoun P, Millan J, Legge R, Friedman TB, Kimberling WJ. *CDH23* mutation and phenotype heterogeneity: profile of 107 diverse families with Usher syndrome and non-syndromic deafness. Am J Hum Genet 2002; 71:262–275.

31a. de Brouwer AP, Pennings RJ, Roeters M, Van Hauwe P, Astuto LM, Hoefsloot LH, Huygen PL, van den Helm B, Deutman AF, Bork JM, Kimberling WJ, Cremers FP, Cremers CW, Kremer H. Mutations in the calcium-binding motifs of *CDH23* and the 35delG mutation in *GJB2* cause hearing loss in one family. Hum Genet 2003; 112:156–163.

32. Wilson SM, Householder DB, Coppola V, Tessarollo L, Fritzsch B, Lee E-C, Goss D, Carlson GA, Copeland NG, Jenkins NA. Mutations in *Cdh23* cause nonsyndromic hearing loss in *waltzer* mice. Genomics 2001; 74:228–233.

33. Wada T, Wakabayashi Y, Takahashi S, Ushiki T, Kikkawa Y, Yonekawa H, Kominami R. A point mutation in a cadherin gene, *Cdh23*, causes deafness in a novel mutant, *watlzer mouse niigata*. Biochem Biophys Res Commun 2001; 283:113–117.

34. Di Palma F, Pellegrino R, Noben-Trauth K. Genomic structure, alternative splice forms and normal and mutant alleles of cadherin 23 (*Cdh23*). Gene 2001; 281:31–41.

35. Holme RH, Steel KP. Stereocilia defects in *waltzer* (*Cdh23*), *shaker1* (*Myo7a*) and *double waltzer/shaker1* mutant mice. Hearing Res 2002; 3862:1–11.

36. Corwin JT, Warchol ME. Auditory hair cells: structure, function, development, and regeneration. Annu Rev Neurosci 1991; 14:301–333.

37. Muller U, Littlewood-Evans A. Mechanisms that regulate mechanosensory hair cell differentiation. Trends Cell Biol 2001; 11:334–342.

38. Siemens J, Kazmierczak P, Reynolds A, Sticker M, Littlewood-Evans A, Muller U. The Usher syndrome proteins cadherin 23 and harmonin form a complex by means of PDZ-domain interactions. Proc Natl Acad Sci 2002; 99:14946–14951.

39. Boeda B, El-Amraoui A, Bahloul A, Goodyear R, Daviet L, Blanchard S, Perfettini I, Fath KR, Shorte S, Reiners J, Houdusse A, Legrain P, Wolfrum U, Richardson G, Petit C. Myosin VIIa, harmonin and cadherin 23, three Usher I gene products that cooperate to shape the sensory hair cell bundle. EMBO J 2002; 21:6689–6699.

26
TMPRSS3

Stylianos E. Antonarakis
University of Geneva Medical School and University Hospitals, Geneva, Switzerland

Hamish S. Scott
The Walter and Eliza Hall Institute of Medical Research, Parkville, Victoria, Australia

I. INTRODUCTION

Mutant alleles in the *TMPRSS3 (ECHOS1)* gene on chromosome 21 have been identified in two forms of hereditary nonsyndromic recessive deafness, DFNB10 and DFNB8. A novel mutation mechanism, insertion of β-satellites, has been found in one of these families. *TMPRSS3* encodes for a transmembrane serine protease that also contains LDLRA and SRCR domains. Missense mutations in all of these domains have been identified in patients with deafness. Although *TMPRSS3* mutations are not a common cause of hereditary deafness, the elucidation of their pathogenetic mechanisms is important for the understanding of the hearing process, and may provide targets for therapeutic interventions.

II. LOCI FOR DEAFNESS *DFNB10* AND *DFNB8* ON CHROMOSOME 21

Among the numerous genetic loci of nonsyndromic autosomal recessive deafness, three map to chromosome 21, namely *DFNB8*, *DFNB10*, and *DFNB29* (http://dnalab-www.uia.ac.be/dnalab/hhh). In this chapter we summarize the molecular genetics aspects of the first two phenotypes that are due to defects of the same gene, *TMPRSS3*, or *ECHOS1*.

A large Palestinian family from a small town in Israel (BT117) was described with more than 40 deaf individuals segregating an autosomal recessive form of nonsyndromic deafness (1). This kindred showed extensive consanguinity over the last seven generations. Hearing evaluation of affected and nonaffected members by pure-tone audiometric tests showed severe deafness in the affected individuals, without any hearing remnants at a level of 75–80 dB. The same level of hearing loss was evident in all affected individuals, ruling out progressive deafness. The diagnosis of sensorineural deafness was confirmed in two 1-week-old girls by a brainstem-evoked potential test. None of the deaf individuals showed any signs of vestibular involvement, defects in ear morphology, mental retardation, or any other aberrations that could indicate that the deafness was part of a syndrome. A genome-wide linkage analysis using short sequence repeat (SSR) polymorphic markers resulted in mapping of the locus to chromosome 21q22.3 between markers *D21S1Z60* and 21qter, a region of 12 cM. Homozygosity of only the most telomeric marker, *D21S1259*, was observed (1). This family defined *DFNB10*, an autosomal recessive, nonsyndromic, congenital deafness.

A large consanguineous Pakistani family (1DF) was described that segregated a recessive, nonsyndromic childhood-onset deafness (2). The age of onset of deafness was 10–12 years and hearing was completely lost within 4–5 years. Pure-tone audiometric tests, between 125 and 8000 Hz up to 120 dB, revealed a maximum audio threshold in both ears of affected individuals of 105 dB at 1000 Hz. Linkage analysis using SSR markers mapped this disease locus telomeric to *D21S212* on chromosome 21q22.3, a large region of more that 15 cM (2). This family defined *DFNB8*, an autosomal recessive, nonsyndromic childhood-onset deafness.

As the description of these two families occurred independently in the same year, two different locus numbers were attributed to them. From various linkage and physical maps of distal chromosome 21q22.3 in 1996, it was clear that the two large genomic regions of linkage on chromosome 21 were overlapping. However, as the phenotypes of these two pedigrees were not identical, childhood onset in *DFNB8* versus congenital deafness in *DFNB10*, it was thought they were likely to define two different loci as opposed to allelic variants (3).

III. POSITIONAL CLONING OF THE *TMPRSS3* GENE

A. A *TMPRSS3* Mutation Causes *DFNB10*

The group of Shimizu and Kudoh at Keio University in Japan was active in physical and transcription mapping of 21q22.3 as a preliminary to compiling the complete genomic sequence of the region. The advances of the physical map and preliminary genomic sequence of chromosome 21 allowed identification and ordering of a total of 50 SSR markers in 21q22.3, comprising 16 published and 34 new markers, precisely mapped and ordered on BAC/cosmid contigs. The use of these markers in linkage analysis on previously analyzed and additional members of the Palestinian family revealed informative recombinants that narrowed down the genomic mapping of the *DFNB10* locus to between markers *1016E7.CA60* and *1151C12.GT45*, a critical region (CR) of approximately 1 Mb (Fig. 1) (4).

With the available DNA samples from members of the Pakistani family, it was only possible to further refine the *DFNB8* locus as being telomeric to *D21S1225* (itself only approximately 500 kb telomeric to *D21S212*). By assuming *DFNB8* and *DFNB10* were in fact caused by the same gene, the CR could be refined to approximately 740 kb between *D21S1225* and *1151C12. GT45*.

Initially, there were six known genes/transcripts in the *DFNB10* CR and all these genes (*ABCG1, TFF3, TFF2, TFF1, PDE9A, NDUVF3*) were excluded as being responsible for *DFNB10* (4). By a combination of techniques, ending with detailed analysis of the complete genomic sequence of the CR, seven novel genes were defined (*WDR4, SLC37A1, UBASH3A, ZNF295, UMODL1, TMPRSS3,* and *TSGA2*). As transcript mapping and mutation analyses (by direct sequencing) were being performed at the same time, several predicted exons were analyzed for mutations that did not end up being part of the 13 defined genes in the CR. Mutation analysis was

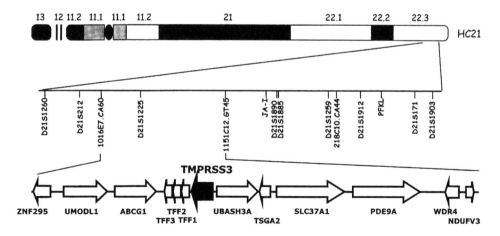

Figure 1 Schematic representation of the critical region of *DFNB10* and *DFNB8* om chromosome 21q22.3. The genes and their transcription orientation within the critical region are depicted as arrows.

performed in affected members of the BT117 Palestinian family for a total of 166 exons, 48 from the six known genes, 93 from the seven novel genes, and 25 orphan exons.

After the mutation analysis of 163 exons was completed with negative results, an amplicon that had been refractory using DNA from affected, but not normal, individuals finally yielded a product. However, instead of the normal 476 nts the amplified product was abnormally large at 1702 nts and was present in homozygosity and heterozygosity in all affected individuals and obligate heterozygotes, respectively, of family BT117. This amplicon was exon 11 of the *TMPRSS3* gene. Sequence of the abnormal DNA fragment in the patients revealed a deletion of 8 bp and the insertion of 18 complete β-satellite repeat monomers (~68 bp) in addition to 10 and two nucleotides derived from β-satellite repeats at the 5' and 3' end of the rearrangment, respectively. This would result in a frameshift mutation from G393 within the protease domain of *TMPRSS3* and termination at 404 amino acids after the addition of 11 unrelated amino acids. We concluded that this mutation in *TMPRSS3* causes *DFNB10* (5).

The sequences of the 18 inserted β-satellite monomers, although highly conserved, were also variable (52–93% divergence between repeats). The basic repetitive unit of β-satellites (or Sau3A repeats) is a monomer of ~68 bp that has been detected on the short arms of all human acrocentric chromosomes (13, 14, 15, 21, 22) in addition to chromosomes 1, 9 (centromeric) 19p, and Y (6–8). Shiels et al. (9) showed that in a 1.5-Mb domain on the short-arm chromosome 22, α-satellites were interspersed between satellite 3 and satellite 1 sequences, between α-satellite repeats and rRNA. At least four families of β-satellites have been defined to date, mainly by their mapping position and the restriction enzyme used to define a higher-order repeat (HOR). pβ4 (AccI HOR) and p21β2 (no HOR) satellites have been detected both distal and proximal to the rRNA genes on the acrocentric chromosomes while the p21β7 (AvaI HOR) satellites have only been detected distal to the rRNA genes. pβ3 satellites are defined by a 2.5-kb EcoRI HOR. In the 1234-bp insertion of β-satellites into exon 11 of *TMPRSS3*, there are no AvaI or EcoRI sites and two AccI. While the length of the β-satellite insertion does not allow definitive identification of the subfamily, it seems likely to be derived from either p21β2 or p21β7 repeats.

The mobile nature of repetitive sequences on the short arms of acrocentric chromosomes is well documented with frequent exchanges between the short arms of the different acrocentric chromosomes (e.g., Ref. 10). Small polydisperse circular DNAs (spcDNA) produced by unequal homologous recombination between or within repetitive sequences are a heterogeneous population of extrachromosomal circular molecules present in a large variety of eukaryotic cells. They contain repetitive sequences including β-satellite repeats (11,12), and many of the other repeats present on the short arms of

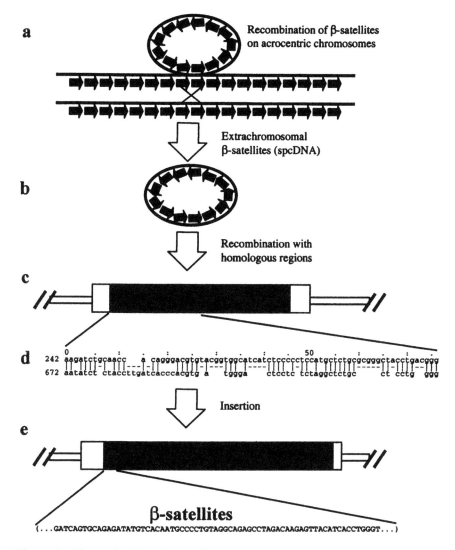

Figure 2 The mechanism of β-satellite insertion. The proposed mechanism for the insertion of β-satellite repeats into the *TMPRSS3* gene in the BT117 Palestinian DFNB10 family is shown with unequal crossing over (a) producing circular extrachromosomal DNA fragments containing β -satellite repeats (shaded gray, b). Homologous recombination within exon 11 of *TMPRSS3* (c and d) results in the insertion of 18 β-satellite repeats (e).

human acrocentric chromosomes (reviewed in Ref. 13). The β-satellites inserted into *TMPRSS3* in the *DFNB10* family may be derived from recombination of spcDNA containing β-satellite repeats with a region of minimal homology spanning exon 11 of the *TMPRSS3* gene (Fig. 2). While more classic chromosomal rearrangements involving β-satellites, such as Robertsonian translocations and inversions, have been described (14,15), this was the first description of β-satellite insertion into an active gene resulting in a pathogenic state. Our model of insertion of a repeat sequence into an area of a gene with minimal homology implies that other repetitive units may also be involved in similar mutagenic events, and it may be possible to predict potential sites of insertion. Insertions of nonretrotransposon repetitive elements into genes may not previously have been described as it may occur mainly in sporadic cases and may also happen during mitosis resulting in somatic mutation.

B.   A *TMPRSS3* Mutation Also Causes *DFNB8*

We subsequently tested for *TMPRSS3* mutations in the DNA of the patients of the Pakistani family 1DF with *DFNB8*, since the *DFNB8* CR overlapped with the *DFNB10* CR on chromosome 21q22.3. A mutation G to A in position -6 of IVS4, possibly creating a novel acceptor splice site, was found in homozygosity in the affected members of this family. In vitro splicing analyses of normal and mutant genomic fragments containing exons 4 and 5 of *TMPRSS3* revealed a 4-bp insertion between exons 4 and 5, consistent with the use of the putative splice acceptor site created by IVS4-6G > A. The 4-bp insertion would result in a frameshift from C107, and termination at 132 amino acids after the addition of 25 unrelated amino acids. Thus IVS4-6G > A can be considered a pathogenic mutation.

Splice acceptor site mutations allowing the production of small amounts of normal splicing and thus protein resulting in comparatively mild phenotypes compared to other mutations in the same gene have been described (e.g., Ref. (17)). Despite the fact that no normally spliced transcript could be detected in the in vitro system, it is likely that IVS4-6G > A allows the production of small amounts of normal splicing and thus TMPRSS3 protein, accounting for the phenotypic difference between the *DFNB8* and 10 families having childhood onset and congenital deafness, respectively (3).

IV.   THE *TMPRSS3* GENE, TRANSCRIPTS AND EXPRESSION

TMPRSS3 stands for transmembrane protease, serine 3, and is the name approved by the human gene nomenclature committee (http://www.gene.

ucl.ac.uk/nomenclature/). We also named the gene *ECHOS1*, from the Greek work *echos* for sound. The *TMPRSS3* gene has 13 exons spanning 24 kb (Fig. 3a). Four alternative transcripts, *TMPRSS3a–d* encoding putative polypeptides of 454, 327, 327, and 344 amino acids, respectively, were detected (b and c code for the same peptides). The *TMPRSS3a* transcript contains all 13 exons with the initiating methionine in exon 2. The *TMPRSS3b* and *c* transcripts start in introns 2 and 3, respectively, with putative initiating methlonines in exon 5. The 3'-end of *TMPRSS3d* continues into intron 9 (Fig. 3b).

Detection of *TMPRSS3* transcripts by Northern blot analysis was difficult showing that the gene is expressed at low levels in the 23 gross organs/tissues/cells analyzed. Semiquantitative RT-PCR specific to the four *TMPRSS3* transcripts on a multiple-tissue cDNA panel from 27 human tissues and human fetal cochlea cDNA showed that all four transcripts show distinct patterns of expression but *TMPRSS3a*, containing all 13 exons, is the most highly and widely expressed transcript. Both *TMPRSS3a* and *TMPRSS3d* expression were detected in fetal cochlea.

V. THE TMPRSS3 PROTEIN

The *TMPRSS3a* transcript encodes a putative 454-amino-acid peptide that contains in order a transmembrane (TM), a low-density lipoprotein receptor A (LDLRA), a scavenger receptor cysteine-rich (SRCR) domain, and a serine protease domain (Fig. 3c). This domain structure has been observed in other proteases including the human transmembrane serine protease *TMPRSS2*, which shows the highest homology to *TMPRSS3*. *TMPRSS2* also maps on 21q just centromeric of the *DFNB10* critical region (18). The domain structure of the TMPRSS3 protein is reflected in the gene structure with the TM domain encoded by exon 3, the LDLRA domain by exon 4, and the SRCR domain by exons 5 and 6.

The serine protease domain of *TMPRSS3* (residues 217–444) shows between 45 and 38% identity with other transmembrane serine proteases (Fig. 3f). The *TMPRSS3* protease domain is compatible with the S1 family of the SA clan of serine-type peptidases for which the prototype is chymotrypsin (19) (http://www.merops.co.uk/). The serine protease active-site residues (H257, D304, and S401) are conserved and *TMPRSS3* is predicted to cleave after K or R residues as it contains D395 at the base of the specificity pocket (S1 subsite) that binds to the substrate. The N-terminus of the protease domain is immediately preceded by the peptide sequence, RIVGG. Proteolytic cleavage between R and I would result in protease activation similar to other serine protease zymogens (19), converting *TMPRSS3* to a noncatalytic and catalytic subunit linked by a disulfide bond (probably C207 to C324). The

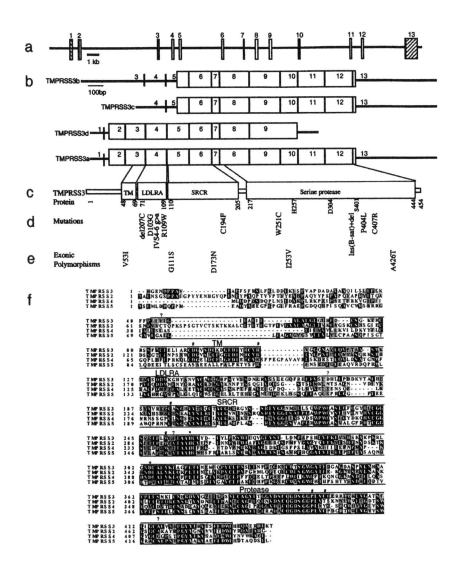

TMPRSS3 serine protease domain contains six conserved cysteine residues, which, by homology to other proteases and 3D modeling, are likely to form the following intrasubunit disulfide bonds: C242–C258, C370–C386, C397–C425.

As no recognizable leader sequence precedes the predicted hydrophobic TM domain (residues 48–69), *TMPRSS3* is likely to be a type II integral membrane protein. Eleven human type II transmembrane serine proteases (TTSPs) have been described to date (many are reviewed in Ref. 20). Where the subcellular localization is described, the TTSPs are anchored to the plasma membrane with a cytosolic N-terminus and extracellular protease domain (e.g., Ref. 21,22). Similarly, *TMPRSS3* is predicted to have its N-terminus on the inside of a membrane and the protease domain on the outside of a membrane.

The ~40-amino-acid-long LDLRA domain, which contains six disulfide-bound cysteines (C72, C79, C85, C92, C98, C107), was originally found in the low-density lipoprotein receptor as the binding sites for LDL (23) and calcium (24,25), and has subsequently been described in numerous extracellular and membrane proteins (PDOC00929; http://www.expasy.ch/cgi-bin/get-prodoc-entry?PDOC00929).

An ~100-residue-long putative adhesive extracellula SRCR domain was also identified in TMPRSS3. SRCR domains linked to serine protease domains have been reported in secreted or membrane-bound molecules with diverse biological roles in development and immunity (26) (PDOC00929; http://www.expasy.ch/cgi-bin/get-prodoc-entry?PDOC00348). The LDLRA and SRCR domains of *TMPRSS3* are potentially involved in binding with extracellular molecules and/or the cell surface.

Figure 3 The *TMPRSS3* gene, transcripts, protein, and mutations. (a) *TMPRSS3* contains 13 exons (boxes) spanning 24kb. (b) There are four different transcripts *TMPRSS3a–d* (coding regions in boxes, noncoding regions indicated by lines). (c) A schematic of the TMPRSS3 protein showing the transmembrane (TM), LDLRA, SRCR, and protease domains and their position in the 454-amino-acid peptide. The active site-residues His257, Asp304, and Ser401 are indicated. (d) The position of the nine *TMPRSS3* mutations relative to the protein is indicated. (e) Exonic polymorphisms that change amino acids are indicated. (f) Representative protein homologies with other human transmembrane proteases are shown. They are *TMPRSS2* (015393), *TMPRSS4* (AAF74526), and *TMPRSS5* (AB028140). Domains, as detected in *TMPRSS3*, are boxed according to their position in *TMPRSS3* and labeled underneath with the active-site residues His257, Asp304, and Ser401 indicated by asterisks (*) above the alignment. Mutations are indicated above the sequence alignment with a number sign (#) while polymorhisms that change amino acids are indicated with a question mark (?). *TMPRSS2* and *4* share exactly the same domain structure as *TMPRSS3* while *TMPRSS5* lacks an LDLRA domain.

The putative peptides encoded by the *TMPRSS3b* and *c* transcripts would contain only half the SRCR domain while *TMPRSS3d* would contain only half the protease domain. The TMPRSS3b and c transcripts may be experimental artifacts or, alternatively, produce soluble forms of the protease as has been observed for the archetypal transmembrane protease, hepsin or *TMPRSS1* (27) and other TTSPs (20).

VI. *TMPRSS3* MUTATION SPECTRUM IN DEAFNESS

Subsequent to the discovery that *TMPRSS3* was mutated in the nonsyndromic autosomal recessive deafness *DNFB10*, and *DFNB8*, we and other investigators examined the DNA of additional patients in both familial and sporadic cases of deafness. The nine pathogenic changes detected to date are summarized in Table 1 and Figure 3d. In addition to the evidence detailed below, all pathogenic changes were excluded as polymorphisms after examination of a large number of control chromosomes from relevant populations.

A. Familial Mutations

Supportive evidence for linkage to the *DFNB8/10* locus was found in 5/159 additional consanguineous Pakistani families segregating profound congenital autosomal recessive deafness.

A missense mutation, R109W, was found in homozygosity in Pakistani family PKSR51a31. This substitution is in the last amino acid of the LDLRA domain, which is potentially involved in binding of *TMPRSS3* with extracellular molecules and/or the cell surface. Two of the other three most closely

Table 1   Pathogenic Mutations in *TMPRSS3*

	Exon/intron	Nucleotide change	AA level	Origin/ref
1	Exon 4	del207C	Frameshift + STOP	Spanish, Greek (30)
2	Exon 4	308A	D103G	Greek (30)
3	Intron 4	IVS4-6 G > A	Frameshift + STOP	Pakistani (5)
4	Exon 5	325C > T	R109W	Pakistani (31)
5	Exon 7	581G > T	C194F	Pakistani (31)
6	Exon 8	753G > C	W251C	Tunisian (28)
7	Exon 11	Ins (β-sat) + del	Frameshift + STOP	Palestinian (5)
8	Exon 12	1211C > T	P404L	Tunisian (28)
9	Exon 12	1219T > C	C407R	Pakistani (31)

TTSPs have either Arg or the similar positively charged Lys at this position (Fig. 3f).

A second missense mutation, C194F, was detected in homozygosity in affected members of the Pakistani PKB16 pedigree (31). The mutation is within the SRCR domain and affects a highly conserved Cys residue.

A third missense mutation, C407R, was found in homozygosity in two Pakistani pedigrees, PKSN37 and PKSN18b. This substitution is within the serine protease domain only a few amino acids from the active-site residue S401 within the substrate pocket. Although C407 is not highly conserved, the nonconservative substitution of a small polar uncharged Cys to a large positively charged Arg so close to the S401 active-site residue is expected to alter the geometry of the active-site loop and therefore affect the serine protease activity (31).

Supportive evidence for linkage to the *DFNB8/B10* locus was also found in 2/39 Tunisian families segregating profound congenital autosomal recessive deafness.

The W251C missense mutation was found in homozygosity in a consanguineous Tunisian family Z with profound nonsyndromic congenital recessive deafness. This mutation lies in the serine protease domain and affects a Trp residue that is highly conserved among serine proteases of the S1 type (Fig. 3f). Examination of the predicted 3D-structure suggests that the W251C mutation might lead to a destabilization of *TMPRSS3* as the large side chain of the Trp residue occupies a large hydrophobic pocket on the exterior of the protein, and structural rearrangements caused by substituting the smaller Cys would likely affect the nearby active-site H257 residue and thus the activity of the enzyme (28).

The P404L missense mutation was observed in homozygosity in a consanguineous Tunisian family R with profound, nonsyndromic deafness. This mutation is located within the sequence signature characteristic of serine proteases active sites, separated from the catalytic Ser by two Gly residues (-Ser-Gly-Gly-Pro-Leu-). P404 is well conserved among the members of the S1 chymotrypsin family of proteases (Fig. 3f). For an exchange of Pro with Leu at position 404 we would expect a significant alteration of the geometry of the active-site loop affecting the catalytic activity (28).

B. *TMPRSS3* Mutations in Sporadic Deafness Cases

A total of 512 sporadic cases of deafness negative for the common 35delG GJB2 mutation (Cx26 gene) (29) have been analyzed for *TMPRSS3* mutations. These include 86 Greek, 99 Spanish, 198 Italian, 65 Australian, and 64 North American patients. Definitive mutations were detected in only 2/512 patients (30).

A deletion of one nucleotide (207delC) was found in homogygosity in a Spanish family SDP26, resulting in a frameshift after amino acid I69 just after the transmembrane domain, addition of 18 novel amino acids, and premature termination of *TMPRSS3* (30).

The D103G missense mutation was found in heterozygosity in a Greek pedigree K208. The other mutant allele in this family was 207delC. The D103G mutation affects an Asp residue of the LDLRA domains that is well conserved. 3D modeling of the mutation suggested that this substitution impairs the Ca^{2+}-binding site of the LDLRA domain (30).

From the large number of patients now screened for *TMPRSS3* mutations, 28 polymorphisms or rare sequence variants were also identified and are shown in Table 2. These include the five amino acid substitutions: V53I, G111S, D173N, I253V, A426T (30). Two of the missense variants, D173N and A426T, were observed only once in heterozygosity in different patients (1/896 Caucasian chromosomes). By direct sequencing, no other changes were found in the patients heterozygous for D173N and A426T. These sequence variants cannot formally be ruled out as mutations without a functional assay. However, D173 is not well conserved between SRCR domains, within SRCR domains of TTSPs (Fig. 3f), and the mouse Tmprss3 has an N at this position. While A426 is relatively well conserved in TTSPs, it is not well conserved in serine protease domains in general and 3D modeling of the conservative substitution of A426 by threonine in *TMPRSS3* does not have any obvious deleterious effect (30).

Thus the analysis of *TMPRSS3* to date indicates that the frequency of *TMPRSS3* mutations in a European childhood deaf population is approximately 0.4% (4 in 1024 deaf alleles) after exclusion of the common 35delG GJB2 mutation. However, the estimate in the Pakistani and Indian Muslim population is approximately 3% (5/160), and 5% (2/39) in Tunisian families. In both these populations, GJB2 mutations were not excluded and thus *TMPRSS3* mutations are still a significant cause of deafness. This is supported by the fact that the IVS4-6G > A (*DFI/DFNB8*) and C407R (PKSN37 and PKSN18b) mutations were found in 1 of 160 and 1 of 200 Muslim Indian control chromosomes, respectively (5,31).

VII. FUTURE INVESTIGATIONS

The following studies will enhance our understanding of the molecular pathophysiology of *TMPRSS3*-related deafness, and may allow the introduction of new therapeutic possibilities.

1. Cloning of the mouse homolog of *TMPRSS3* and determining its temporal and spacial expression pattern, particularly in the ear.

Table 2 Nonpathogenic Sequence Variants in *TMPRSS3*

	Exon/intron	Intronic SNP	Exonic SNP	AA level	First ref.
1	Exon 2		21T > G	P7P	30
2	Exon 3		157G > A	V53I	5
3	Intron 3	IVS3-23C > A			30
4	Intron 4	IVS4 + 70 T > A			30
5	Intron 4	IVS4 + 74 A > T			30
6	Exon 5		331G > A	G111S	31
7	Exon 5		339G > A	Q113Q	30
8	Exon 5		378G > A	K126K	30
9	Intron 5	IVS5 + 91 G > A			30
10	Intron 5	IVS5-13 A > G			31
11	Exon 6		453G > A	V151V	5
12	Exon 6		517G > A	D173N	30
134	Intron 6	IVS6 + 13 A > G			30
14	Intron 7	IVS7 + 85 A > G			30
15	Intron 7	IVS7 + 129 T > A			30
16	Intron 7	IVS7 + 145 C > G			30
17	Intron 7	IVS7-105 A > G			30
18	Intron 7	IVS7-3 Ins (TA)			5
19	Exon 8		757A > G	I253V	5
20	Exon 9		789C > T	Y263Y	30
21	Intron 10	IVS10-120			30
22	Intron 10	IVS10-118			30
23	Exon 11		1128C > T	Y376Y	31
24	Exon 12		1275C > T	C425C	30
25	Exon 12		1276G > A	A426T	30
26	Exon 13		1367G > A	3'-UTR	5
27	Exon 13		1451T > A	3'-UTR	31
28	Exon 13		1571A > G	3'-UTR	5

The generation of a targeted disruption of *Tmprss3* in mice will provide an outstanding animal model to study the molecular pathology of this particular recessive deafness.

2. Functional analysis of TMPRSS3 protein and its different domains. Identifying the substrates for the *TMPRSS3*, its interacting proteins, and the pathways of its involvement. Furthermore, determining the intracellular localization of the protein and its biosynthetic pathways. This knowledge may provide targets for therapeutic interventions.

3. Examining the involvement of different alleles of *TMPRSS3* in hearing loss in older adults.

4. Determining the physiological role of TMPRSS3 protein outside the ear.

5. Evaluating the involvement of other TTSPs in hereditary deafness.

The study described above provides another example of the utility of results of exploration of the human genome in terms of DNA markers and nucleotide sequences that, when coupled with excellent clinical material and careful phenotyping, result in the determination of disease-related genes. Functional analysis of the predicted proteins adds to our understanding of complex processes such hearing.

ACKNOWLEDGMENTS

We are grateful to the patients and their family members for their participation in the described studies. We thank all clinicians who collected patients' samples and performed clinical and audiological laboratory investigations. We also thank our collaborators N. Shimizu, J. Kudoh, B. Bonne-Tamir, A. Gal, and members of our laboratories particularly M.L. Guipponi and M. Wattenhofer. The laboratory of SEA is supported by grants 31.57149.99 from the Swiss FNRS, 98-3039 from the OFES/EU, the Foundation Child Care, and funds from the University and Cantonal Hospital of Geneva. The laboratory of HSS is supported by the National Health and Medical Research Council of Australia (project grant 215305 and fellowship 171601), by the Nossal Leadership award from the Walter and Eliza Hall Institute of Medical Research, and a grant from the Rebecca L. Cooper Foundation.

REFERENCES

1. Bonne-Tamir B, DeStefano AL, Briggs CE, Adair R, Franklyn B, Weiss S, Korostishevsky M, Frydman M, Baldwin CT, Farrer LA. Linkage of congenital recessive deafness (gene *DFNB10*) to chromosome 21q22.3. Am J Hum Genet 1996; 58:1254–1259.

2. Veske A, Oehlmann R, Younus F, Mohyuddin A, Muller-Myhsok B, Mehdi SQ, Gal A. Autosomal recessive non-syndromic deafness locus (*DFNB8*) maps on chromosome 21q22 in a large consanguineous kindred from Pakistan. Hum Mol Genet 1996; 5:165–168.

3. Scott HS, Antonarakis SE, Mittaz L, Lalioti MD, Younus F, Mohyuddin A, Mehdi SQ, Gal A. Refined genetic mapping of the autosomal recessive non-syndromic deafness locus *DFNB8* on human chromosome 21q22.3. Adv Otorhinolaryngol 2000; 56:158–163.

4. Berry A, Scott HS, Kudoh J, Talior I, Korostishevsky M, Wattenhofer M,

Guipponi M, Barras C, Rossier C, Shibuya K, Wang J, Kawasaki K, Asakawa S, Minoshima S, Shimizu N, Antonarakis S, Bonne-Tamir B. Refined localization of autosomal recessive nonsyndromic deafness *DFNB10* locus using 34 novel microsatellite markers, genomic structure, and exclusion of six known genes in the region. Genomics 2000; 68:22–29.

5. Scott HS, Kudoh J, Wattenhofer M, Shibuya K, Berry A, Chrast R, Guipponi M, Wang J, Kawasaki K, Asakawa S, Minoshima S, Younus F, Mehdi SQ, Radhakrishna U, Papasavvas MP, Gehrig C, Rossier C, Korostishevsky M, Gal A, Shimizu N, Bonne-Tamir B, Antonarakis SE. Insertion of beta-satellite repeats identifies a transmembrane protease causing both congenital and childhood onset autosomal recessive deafness. Nat Genet 2001; 27:59–63.

6. Waye JS, Willard HF. Human beta satellite DNA: genomic organization and sequence definition of a class of highly repetitive tandem DNA. Proc Natl Acad Sci USA 1989; 86:6250–6254.

7. Greig GM, Willard HF. Beta satellite DNA: characterization and localization of two subfamilies from the distal and proximal short arms of the human acrocentric chromosomes. Genomics 1992; 12:573–580.

8. Eichler EE, Hoffman SM, Adamson AA, Gordon LA, McCready P, Lamerdin JE, Mohrenweiser HW. Complex beta-satellite repeat structures and the expansion of the zinc finger gene cluster in 19p12. Genome Res 1998; 8:791–808.

9. Shiels C, Coutelle C, Huxley C. Contiguous arrays of satellites 1, 3, and beta form a 1.5-Mb domain on chromosome 22p. Genomics 1997; 44:35–44.

10. Farrell SA, Winsor EJ, Markovic VD. Moving satellites and unstable chromosome translocations: clinical and cytogenetic implications. Am J Med Genet 1993; 46:715–720.

11. Hollis M, Hindley J. Human Sau3A repeated DNA is enriched in small polydisperse circular DNA from normal lymphocytes. Gene 1986; 46:153–160.

12. Assum G, Fink T, Steinbeisser T, Fisel KJ. Analysis of human extrachromosomal DNA elements originating from different beta-satellite subfamilies. Hum Genet 1993; 91:489–495.

13. Gaubatz JW. Extrachromosomal circular DNAs and genomic sequence plasticity in eukaryotic cells. Mutat Res 1990; 237:271–292.

14. Wolff DJ, Schwartz S. Characterization of Robertsonian translocations by using fluorescence in situ hybridization. Am J Hum Genet 1992; 50:174–181.

15. Samonte RV, Conte RA, Ramesh KH, Verma RS. Molecular cytogenetic characterization of breakpoints involving pericentric inversions of human chromosome 9. Hum Genet 1996; 98:576–580.

16. Kazazian HH Jr. Mobile elements and disease. Curr Opin Genet Dev 1998; 8: 343–350.

17. Scott HS, Litjens T, Nelson PV, Thompson PR, Brooks DA, Hopwood JJ, Morris CP. Identification of mutations in the alpha-L-iduronidase gene (IDUA) that cause Hurler and Scheie syndromes. Am J Hum Genet 1993; 53:973–986.

18. Paoloni-Giacobino A, Chen H, Peitsch MC, Rossier C, Antonarakis SE. Cloning of the *TMPRSS2* gene, which encodes a novel serine protease with transmembrane, LDLRA, and SRCR domains and maps to 21q22.3. Genomics 1997; 44:309–320.

19. Rawlings ND, Barrett AJ. Families of serine peptidases. Meth Enzymol 1994; 244:19–61.

20. Hooper JD, Clements JA, Quigley JP, Antalis TM. Type II transmembrane serine proteases: insights into an emerging class of cell surface proteolytic enzymes. J Biol Chem 2001; 276:857–860.

21. Leytus SP, Loeb KR, Hagen FS, Kurachi K, Davie EW. A novel trypsin-like serine protease (hepsin) with a putative transmembrane domain expressed by human liver and hepatoma cells. Biochemistry 1988; 27:1067–1074.

22. Tsuji A, Torres-Rosado A, Arai T, Le Beau MM, Lemons RS, Chou SH, Kurachi K. Hepsin, a cell membrane-associated protease: characterization, tissue distribution, and gene localization. J Biol Chem 1991; 266:16948–16953.

23. Sudhof TC, Goldstein JL, Brown MS, Russell DW. The LDL receptor gene: a mosaic of exons shared with different proteins. Science 1985; 228:815–822.

24. van Driel IR, Goldstein JL, Sudhof TC, Brown MS. First cysteine-rich repeat in ligand-binding domain of low density lipoprotein receptor binds Ca^{2+} and monoclonal antibodies, but not lipoproteins. J Biol Chem 1987; 262:17443–17449.

25. Mahley RW. Apolipoprotein E: cholesterol transport protein with expanding role in cell biology. Science 1988; 240:622–630.

26. Resnick D, Pearson A, Krieger M. The SRCR superfamily: a family reminiscent of the Ig superfamily. Trends Biochem Sci 1994; 19:5–8.

27. Kawamura S, Kurachi S, Deyashiki Y, Kurachi K. Complete nucleotide sequence, origin of isoform and functional characterization of the mouse hepsin gene. Eur J Biochem 1999; 262:755–764.

28. Masmoudi S, Antonarakis SE, Schwede T, Ghorbel AM, Gratri M, Pappasavas MP, Drira M, Elgaied-Boulila A, Wattenhofer M, Rossier C, Scott HS, Ayadi H, Guipponi M. Novel missense mutations of *TMPRSS3* in two consanguineous Tunisian families with non-syndromic autosomal recessive deafness. Hum Mutat 2001; 18:101–108.

29. Gasparini P, Rabionet R, Barbujani G, Melchionda S, Petersen M, Brondum-Nielsen K, Metspalu A, Oitmaa E, Pisano M, Fortina P, Zelante L, Estivill X. High carrier frequency of the 35delG deafness mutation in European populations. Genetic Analysis Consortium of GJB2 35delG. Eur J Hum Genet 2000; 8:19–23.

30. Wattenhofer M, Di Iorio V, Rabionet R, Dougherty L, Pampanos A, Schwede T, Montserrat-Sentis B, Arbones L, Iliades T, Pasquadibisceglie A, D'Amelio M, Alwan S, Rossier C, Dahl HH, Petersen MB, Estivill X, Gasparini P, Scott HS, Antonarakis SE. Mutations in the *TMPRSS3* gene are a rare cause of childhood nonsyndromic deafness in Caucasian patients. J Mol Med 2002; 80:124–131.

31. Ben-Yosef T, Wattenhofer M, Riazuddin S, Ahmed ZM, Scott HS, Kudoh J, Shibuya K, Antonarakis SE, Bonne-Tamir B, Radhakrishna U, Naz S, Ahmed Z, Pandya A, Nance WE, Wilcox ER, Friedman TB, Morell RJ. Novel mutations of *TMPRSS3* in four *DFNB8/B10* families segregating congenital autosomal recessive deafness. J Med Genet 2001; 38:396–400.

27
Otosclerosis

Kris Van Den Bogaert and Guy Van Camp
University of Antwerp, Antwerp, Belgium

Richard J. H. Smith
University of Iowa, Iowa City, Iowa, U.S.A.

I. INTRODUCTION

Among white adults, otosclerosis is the single most common cause of hearing impairment. The disease is caused by abnormal bone homeostasis of the otic capsule, which usually results in a conductive hearing loss due to fixation of the stapes footplate, although sensorineural hearing loss also may occur. The etiology of otosclerosis is unknown, and both genetic and environmental factors have been implicated. Epidemiological studies support autosomal dominant inheritance with reduced penetrance, although viral involvement also has been suggested. Otosclerosis is one of the last important types of hearing impairment for which any genetic cause remains to be elucidated. At the moment, only three loci for otosclerosis have been localized, although additional studies provide significant evidence for the involvement of at least one other locus; none of the responsible genes has been identified. Because the etiology of otosclerosis remains poorly characterized, effective medical therapy to prevent or stabilize the disease has not been developed.

II. CLINICAL SIGNIFICANCE

Clinical otosclerosis (MIM 166800) has a prevalence of 0.3–0.4% among white adults, making it the single most common cause of hearing impairment in this group (1). The disease is characterized by isolated endochondral bone sclerosis of the labyrinthine capsule leading to hearing loss. Auditory impairment is heralded by the appearance of otosclerotic foci that invade the stapediovestibular joint (oval window) and interfere with free motion of the stapes (2). Mean age-of-onset is in the third decade, and 90% of affected persons are under 50 years of age at the time of diagnosis (3,4). In approximately 10% of persons with clinically significant otosclerosis, a profound sensorineural hearing loss develops across all frequencies (3,5), reflecting either mechanical or toxic damage to the inner ear as otosclerotic foci invade the cochlear endosteum and encroach on the membranous labyrinth. While the sensorineural component of the hearing loss cannot be corrected, stapes microsurgery has proven to be a highly successful means to restore the normal conduction mechanism and can improve hearing thresholds by as much as 50 dB (5).

III. A POSSIBLE VIRAL ETIOLOGY?

Retroviral infections are believed to play a role in several bone diseases (6,7) and consistent with this hypothesis are several studies that suggest a viral etiology in the pathogenesis of otosclerosis. By immunofluorescence with polyclonal and monoclonal antibodies against mumps, rubella, and measles viruses, the presence of viral antigen, most commonly measles, has been found in otosclerotic foci (8). PCR amplification of the measles nucleocapsid gene also has been used to confirm the presence of retroviral RNA in temporal bone specimens from persons with otosclerosis but not in histologically negative controls. These results suggest that a viral insult, most likely measles, triggers the development of otosclerotic foci in susceptible individuals. Several investigators believe that after the middle ear mucosa becomes infected, viral particles invade the bone of the labyrinth via lymphatic or pericapillary spaces with otosclerosis developing as a consequence of the induced inflammation (9,10).

A causal role for measles in otosclerosis, however, has not been proven. Grayeli et al. (11) could not detect measles virus in any bone samples or primary bone cultures in 35 persons with otosclerosis, and the disparate ethnic-based epidemiological data for otosclerosis and measles suggest that the detection of measles in otosclerotic foci may represent a secondary, unrelated event. Measles is a highly infectious disease and a major cause of morbidity and mortality in all ethnic groups worldwide (12,13). In contrast, otosclerosis shows a racial bias. Histological evidence of otosclerosis is found in approximately 2.5% of whites (1) but in only 1% of blacks (14). Among the Japanese, its prevalence is approximately one-half that in whites (15), and among South American Indians, its prevalence drops to only 0.04% (16).

IV. THE GENETICS OF OTOSCLEROSIS

The etiology of otosclerosis is unknown and its genetics is poorly understood. Reports of an inherited disease that probably represents otosclerosis date to the mid-nineteenth century when Toynbee described a familial pattern of conductive hearing loss (17). In his catalogue of 1837, he noted that thickening of the anterior two-thirds of the stapedial footplate resembled ivory and originated from the vestibular surface of the labyrinth. In 1876, Magnus documented a family in which the father and seven of 13 children had conductive hearing impairment, verified in one child to be due to ankylosis of the stapes (18). Eighteen years later, Politzer coined the term "otosclerosis," in reference to a "disease that has its seat in the labyrinthine capsule [and] leads, through new formation and growth of osseous tissue, to ankylosis of the stapes in the fenestra ovalis" (19).

Although the genetics of otosclerosis is controversial, the majority of studies indicate autosomal dominant inheritance, a conclusion first reached by Albrecht (20). This observation was supported by Larsson's analyses of 262 probands in which he also recognized that penetrance is incomplete (21,22). In a detailed study of 150 probands, Morrison calculated the fractions of affected first-, second-, and third-degree relatives, and noted that the observed ratios were consistent with autosomal dominant inheritance with 40% penetrance (23). Other studies have confirmed these findings (24–26). Detailed mathematical calculations by Larsson (22) and Gapany-Gapanavicius (27) suggest that other modes of transmission are unlikely, but Baurer and Stein have postulated digenic recessive inheritance based on a study of 94 families (24). Hernandez-Orozco and Courtney also favor digenic inheritance, but of a dominant X-linked gene and an autosomal recessive gene (25).

Lack of a positive family history in 40–50% of cases has added to the heritability controversy (28–30). These cases have been hypothesized by some to represent an autosomal recessive form of otosclerosis in which the heterozygote is identifiable only by histological examination of the temporal bones (31).

In the 1960s and 1970s it was often tried to explain complex genetic characteristics with monogenic concepts. As described higher, this has also been done for otosclerosis. However, little further understanding was gained from these studies. Nowadays, complex diseases are looked upon differently, and analyzed without prior assumption on the mode of inheritance.

V. MONOGENIC AND COMPLEX DISEASES

The spectrum of human diseases forms a continuum between purely genetic and purely environmental conditions (Fig. 1). At one extreme are purely genetic conditions typified by the monogenic diseases showing autosomal dominant, recessive, or X-linked inheritance. Although complicating factors such as reduced penetrance can be present, a disease is not considered truly complex unless different genes or environmental factors also impact phenotype. At the other extreme are purely environmental diseases, including many types of infectious illnesses.

With respect to hearing, while most cases of congenital deafness have a single cause that is either monogenic (e.g., a *GJB2* mutation) or environmental (prematurity, infections), the etiology in late-onset deafness, such as age-related hearing impairment, otosclerosis, or Menière's disease, is complex. In many of these cases, there is thought to be an interaction between several genes and different environmental triggers.

Large autosomal dominant families segregating otosclerosis are very rare—in the majority of cases there are only a few, if any, other affected family members. While this presentation may reflect reduced penetrance, it is more consistent with the interaction of other complicating factors. Otosclerosis can therefore be considered a complex disease with rare monogenic autosomal dominant families. Much can be learned from the analysis of monogenic otosclerosis that may be applicable to otosclerosis as a complex

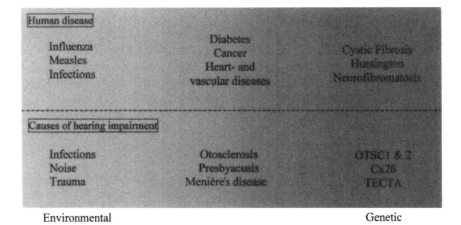

Figure 1 The spectrum of human diseases forms a continuum between purely genetic and purely environmental conditions.

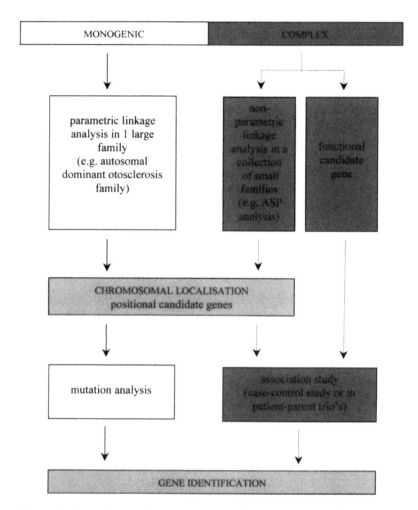

Figure 2 Strategies used to study monogenic versus complex diseases.

disease, but in general, the analysis of these two types of otosclerosis will require different research strategies (Fig. 2).

A. Monogenic Forms of Otosclerosis

Genes responsible for monogenic forms of otosclerosis can be identified by a positional cloning strategy in large families segregating autosomal dominant otosclerosis (12 or more persons). Initially, a genome-wide scan is completed to identify a genomic region that segregates with the otosclerosis phenotype. A computer algorithm then is used to calculate the likelihood that the genome segregation pattern and the clinical status are linked and not chance events. If a "linked" interval is found, it will contain the disease-causing gene. To minimize the size of the linked interval and thereby reduce the number of genes that must be considered, additional family members can be studied and additional markers can be used. Mutation screening of the genes in the candidate interval is used to find the disease-causing gene.

To date, only three otosclerosis-causing genes have been localized using three large families showing an autosomal dominant inheritance pattern. In 1998, we localized the first otosclerosis-causing gene, *OTSCI*, to a 14.5-cM interval on chromosome 15q between FES and D15S657 (32). An additional family originating from Tunisia also has been reported to be linked to this locus (33). In 2001, we mapped a second locus, *OTSC2*, flanked by two markers on chromosome 7q, D7S495 and D7S2426, that define a 16-cM interval (34). Recently, OTSC3 was mapped to chromosome 6p21-22 (35). None of the responsible genes has been cloned. Furthermore, the analysis of additional families segregating otosclerosis has provided evidence for further genetic heterogeneity; in addition to the three known loci, at least one additional otosclerosis locus must exist (36).

B. Complex Forms of Otosclerosis

Genome scans for complex diseases are carried out using a large collection of small families. Instead of the standard parametric linkage analysis used for monogenic conditions—where parameters such as inheritance pattern and penetrance need to be defined—nonparametric methods are used. The most frequently used nonparametric linkage method, affected sib-pair (ASP) analysis, has been applied to many complex diseases besides otosclerosis. Examples include schizophrenia, bipolar disorder, diabetes, autism, multiple sclerosis, and lupus. For many of these diseases, significant linkage has been detected. A genome search by ASP analysis identifies the chromosomal regions that are likely to be shared between affected sibs. Chromosomal regions resulting from the genome searches are large and contain a large number of genes.

Another tool for the analysis of complex diseases are association studies in a large number of affected individuals and controls (case-control study) or in patient-parent trios. An allele is associated with a disease in a population if patients have this allele more often than the controls. The disease-associated allele may be the direct cause of the disease (causative effect) or it may be very close to the disease-causing mutation so that the two are coinherited. This latter situation holds if the mutation occurred only once in the population (founder effect). An advantage of association studies is that they are more powerful to detect weak effects. A major difference with linkage is that association can be detected only over very small genetic distances (less than 1 cM). A total genome scan by association would require 10,000 markers and is not possible with current technology. Association studies are therefore limited to candidate genes. These genes can be selected on the basis of functional information or can be located in candidate regions from genome scans.

Results of nonparametric linkage analysis for otosclerosis have not yet been published. A single candidate-gene-based association study has been performed by McKenna et al. (37). Because of the clinical and histopathological similarities between otosclerosis and type I osteogenesis imperfecta, they investigated a possible association between otosclerosis and three collagen genes. Because mutations of type I collagen genes underlie the milder forms of osteogenesis imperfecta (38), the *COL1A1*, *COL1A2*, and *COL2A1* genes were studied. The investigators found a statistically significant association between otosclerosis and *COL1A1*, while differences in allele frequencies could not be detected between the otosclerosis group and controls for *COL1A2* and *COL2A1*. This result indicates that the *COL1A1* gene may play a role in the etiology of otosclerosis; however, further elucidation of a role for *COL1A1* in the development of otosclerosis has not been reported.

VI. CONCLUSION

Based on available data, we hypothesize that most cases of otosclerosis represent a complex disease with a genetic basis acting on a complex genetic background and requiring an environmental trigger to become activated. Less frequent are the monogenic forms of otosclerosis. Currently, three autosomal dominant otosclerosis loci are mapped, but none of the genes has yet been cloned. The genes responsible for otosclerosis are likely to have specific roles in bone homeostasis in the otic capsule. Little is known about this process at the molecular level and the identification of these genes is the first step in the elucidation of mechanisms of bone turnover of the otic capsule. Elucidating the genetics of otosclerosis will have a significant impact on our understanding of this disease and may enable us to prevent a leading cause of hearing loss in the white adult population.

ACKNOWLEDGMENTS

This study was supported in part by grants from the University of Antwerp and from the Vlaams Fonds voor Wetenschappelijk Onderzoek (FWO) to

GVC and by NIH grant R01DC05218 to GVC and RJHS. KVDB holds a predoctoral research position with the Instituut voor de aanmoediging van Innovatie door Wetenschap en Technologie in Vlaanderen (IWT-Vlaanderen), and GVC holds a research position with the FWO.

REFERENCES

1. Declau F, Qiu JP, Timmermans JP, Van Spaendonck M, Michaels L, Van de Heyning P. Prevalence of otosclerosis in a non-selected series of temporal bones. Otol Neurotol 2001; 22(5):596–602.
2. Hueb MM, Goycoolea MV, Paparella MM, Oliveira JA. Otosclerosis: the University of Minnesota temporal bone collection. Otolaryngol Head Neck Surg 1991; 105:396–405.
3. Browning GG, Gatehouse S. Sensorineural hearing loss in stapedial otosclerosis. Ann Otol Rhinol Laryngol 1984; 93:13–16.
4. Gordon MA. The genetics of otosclerosis: a review. Am J Otol 1989; 10:426–438.
5. Ramsay HAW, Linthicum FH. Mixed hearing loss in otosclerosis: indication for long-term follow-up. Am J Otol 1994; 15:536–539.
6. Mills BG, Frausto A, Singer FR, Ohsaki Y, Demulder A, Roodman GD. Multinucleated cells formed in vitro from Paget's bone marrow express viral antigens. Bone 1994; 15:443–448.
7. Labat ML. Retroviruses and bone diseases. Clin Orthop 1996; 326:287–309.
8. Arnold W, Friedmann I. Immunohistochemistry of otosclerosis. Acta Otolaryngol Suppl 1990; 470:124–129.
9. Arnold W, Niedermeyer HP, Lehn N, Neubert W, Höfler H. Measles virus in otosclerosis and the specific immune response of the inner ear. Acta Otolaryngol 1996; 116:705–709.
10. McKenna MJ, Kristiansen AG, Haines J. Polymerase chain reaction amplification of a measles virus sequence from human temporal bone sections with active otosclerosis. Am J Otol 1996; 17:827–830.
11. Grayeli AB, Palmer P, Huy PTB, Soudant J, Sterkers O, Lebon P, Ferrary E. No evidence of measles virus in stapes samples from patients with otosclerosis. J Clin Microbiol 2000; 38:2655–2660.
12. Clements CJ, Cutts FT. The epidemiology of measles: thirty years of vaccination. Curr Top Microbiol Immunol 1995; 191:13–33.
13. Nokes DJ, Williams JR, Butler AR. Towards eradication of measles virus: global progress and strategy evaluation. Vet Microbiol 1995; 44(2–4):333–350.
14. Guild SR. Histologic otosclerosis. Ann Otol Rhinol Laryngol 1944; 53:246–267.
15. Joseph RB, Frazer JP. Otosclerosis incidence in Caucasians and Japanese. Arch Otolaryngol 1964; 80:256–257.
16. Tato JM, Tato JM. Otosclerosis and races. Ann Otol Rhinol Laryngol 1967; 76:1018–1025.

17. Toynbee J. Pathological and surgical observations on the diseases of the ear. Med Chir Trans 1861; 24:190–205.

18. Magnus A. Über Verlauf and Sectionsbefund eines Falles von hochgradiger and eigenthumlicher Gehörstörung. Arch Ohrenheilk 1876; 11:244–251.

19. Politzer A. Über premare Erkrankung der knockernen Labrynthkapsel. Z Ohrenheilk 1894; 25:309–327.

20. Albrecht W. Über der Vererbung der hereditären Labyrinthschwerkörigkeit und der Otosclerose. Arch Ohr Nas Kehlkopfheilk 1922; 110:15–48.

21. Larsson A. Otosclerosis: a genetic and clinical study. Acta Otolaryngol Suppl 1960; 154:1–86.

22. Larsson A. Genetic problems in otosclerosis. In: Schuknecht HF, ed. Otosclerosis. Boston: Little Brown, 1962:109–117.

23. Morrison AW. Genetic factors in otosclerosis. Ann R Coll Surg Engl 1967; 41:202–237.

24. Bauer J, Stein C. Vererbung and Konstitution bei Ohrenkrankheiten. Seitschrift fur die gesamte Anatomie, Part II. Ztschr Konstitut 1925; 10:483–545.

25. Hernandez-Orozco F, Courtney GT. Genetic aspects of clinical otosclerosis. Ann Otol Rhinol Laryngol 1964; 73:632–644.

26. Causse JR, Causse JP. Otospongiosis as a genetic disease. Am J Otol 1984; 5:211–223.

27. Gapany-Gapanavicius B. Otosclerosis: Genetics and Surgical Rehabilitation. Jerusalem: Keter, 1975.

28. Nager FR. Zur klinik und pathologischen Anatomie der Otosklerose. Acta Otolaryngol 1939; 27:542–551.

29. Cawthorn T. Otosclerosis. J Laryngol Otol 1955; 69:437–456.

30. Shambaugh GE. Otosclerosis. In: Coates GM, Schenk HP, Miller MV, eds. Otolaryngology. Vol 2. Hagerstown, MD: WF Prior, 1956:1–17.

31. Morrison AW, Bundey SE. The inheritance of otosclerosis. J Laryngol Otol 1970; 84:921–932.

32. Tomek MS, Brown MR, Mani SR, Ramesh A, Srisailapathy CRS, Coucke P, Zbar RIZ, Bell AM, McGuirt WT, Fukushima K, Willems PJ, Van Camp G, Smith RJH. Localization of a gene for otosclerosis to chromosome 15q25–q26. Hum Mol Genet 1998; 7:285–290.

33. Drira M, Ghorbel A, Chakroun A, Charfeddine L, Fakhfakh M, Bouguecha M, Sakka M, Ayadi H, Habib C. Étude génètique et localisation d'un gene de l'otospongiose chez familles Tunisiennes. 106th Congrès Français d'Oto-Rhino-Laryngologie et de Chirurgie de la Face et du Cou, Paris, Oct 3–5, 1999

34. Van Den Bogaert K, Govaerts PJ, Schatteman I, Brown MR, Caethoven G, Offeciers FE, Somers T, Declau F, Coucke P, Van de Heyning P, Smith RJH, Van Camp G. A second gene for otosclerosis (*OTSC2*) maps to chromosome 7q34–36. Am J Hum Genet 2001; 68:495–500.

35. Chen W, Campbell C, Green V, Van Den Bogaert K, Komodikis C, Manolidis LS, Economou E, Kyamides Y, Christodoulou K, Faghel C, Giguere C, Alford RL, Manolidis S, Van Camp G, Smith RJH. Linkage of otosclerosis to a third locus on human chromosome 6p21.2-22.3. J Med Genet 2002; 39:473–477.

36. Van Den Bogaert K, Govaerts PJ, De Leenheer EMR, Schatteman I, Declau F, Smith RJH, Cremers CWRJ, Van de Heyning PH, Offeciers FE, Somers T, Van Camp G. Otosclerosis—a genetically heterogeneous disease involving at least 3 different genes. Bone 2002; 30(4):624–630.

37. McKenna MJ, Kristiansen AG, Bartley ML, Rogus JJ, Haines JL. Association of *COL1A1* and otosclerosis: evidence for a shared genetic etiology with mild osteogenesis imperfecta. Am J Otol 1998; 19:604–610.

38. Willing MC, Pruchno CJ, Atkinson M, Byers PH. Osteogenesis imperfecta type I is commonly due to a *COL1A1* null allele of type I collagen. Am J Hum Genet 1992; 51(3):508–515.

28

Mechanisms that Regulate Hair Cell Differentiation and Regeneration

Brigitte Malgrange, Ingrid Breuskin, Gustave Moonen, and Philippe P. Lefebvre
University of Liège, Liège, Belgium

I. INTRODUCTION

Hair cells (HCs) are the mechanoreceptors, i.e., biological devices converting mechanical energy (e.g., sound pressure or acceleration) into electrochemical energy (i.e., neurotransmission), that are involved in the detection of sound, balance, orientation, and movements. HCs are present in the lateral lines and inner ears of fish and amphibians, in the basilar papilla and vestibule of birds, and in the cochlea and vestibule of mammals. Disease, aging, infection, and exposure to noise or ototoxic drugs cause HC loss. Age and trauma-induced susceptibility is a major health problem because a significant proportion of humans suffer from deafness or balance disorders directly resulting from HC loss. In contrast, HC production is an ongoing phenomenon in the sensory maculae of fishes (1–4), amphibians (5), and in the vestibular epithelium of birds (2,6–8). In the auditory and vestibular epithelia of the mammalian inner ear and the auditory epithelium of birds, i.e., the basilar papilla, the production of HCs occurs over only a brief period during the early stages of development (9–12). However, in the basilar papilla, lost HCs following drug or noise-induced damage are replaced through a regenerative process (reviewed in Ref. 13).

In mammals, embryonic HCs and supporting cells (SCs) proliferation within the sensory epithelia culminates between embryonic day 13 (E13) and 15 (E15) in mice (9) and HC production never occurs at later stages in normal conditions. Increasing experimental evidence suggests, however, that new HCs can be produced in adult mammalian vestibular organs following ototoxic damage (14–17). In the embryonic mammalian cochlea, laser-ablated HCs in cultured organs of Corti can be replaced by new HCs (18) and at the neonatal stage, there is some evidence that HCs can repair themselves after sublethal mechanical injury (19) and that regenerative capacities are present (20,21). However, in the adult mammalian cochlea, HC loss is currently considered irreversible.

Although mammals have a very limited capacity for replacing lost HCs, continuous HC turnover and ability to regenerate HCs are established features of the mechanosensory organs of many lower vertebrates. The processes of HC development and regeneration may share common molecular pathways, and many of the genes involved in both inner ear and HC development are likely to be responsible for inherited deafness (22). Genes implicated in ear morphogenesis and HC differentiation include various transcription factors, secreted factors, receptor/tyrosine kinases, cyclin-dependent kinase inhibitors, and membrane-bound signaling proteins. We review here (a) the current knowledge of the mechanisms of HC production or regeneration and of the identity of HC progenitors and (b) the various genes implied in HC development and regeneration.

II. MECHANISMS OF HAIR CELL PRODUCTION OR REGENERATION AND CHARACTERIZATION OF HC PROGENITORS

A. Nonmammalian Vertebrates

Studies on birds, amphibians, and fishes led to the suggestion that newly produced HCs result from SC proliferation (for review, see Ref. 23–25). In fishes and amphibians, this perpetual production of HCs leads to a continual increase in the number of HCs, which at least in fishes results in an increase of the size of the sensory epithelium (1,2). Birds appear to be the only warm-blooded animals that demonstrate a robust HC regenerative response beyond the embryonic stages. Jorgensen and Mathiesen (6) first demonstrated that ongoing production of HCs occurs in the vestibular epithelium of adult birds. This regenerative process does not result in an increase in the total number of BrdU-labeled cells over time because there is also a spontaneous and continuous apoptosis of vestibular HCs (7). This ongoing vestibular HC death is postulated to drive the production of new HCs (26). In the basilar papilla (i.e., the auditory portion of the inner ear of birds), new HCs are produced only in response to experimental injury (27). The appearance of new HCs and SCs is preceded by mitosis in the sensory epithelium; the mitotic pool of cells gives rise to new HCs and SCs

(10,11,28–30). It has recently been shown in birds by lineage studies that HCs and SCs are generated from a common pool of precursors and that two morphological types of SCs may exist: a differentiated one and an immature one that could be a precursor cell for both HCs and differentiated SCs (31). There is also evidence that HCs can arise by transdifferentiation of SCs i.e., without an intermediate mitosis, in the lateral line of axolotl and in the basilar papilla of birds (32–34).

B. Mammalian Inner Ear

In the vestibular portion of the mammalian inner ear, different mechanisms for HC recovery following injury, such as ototoxicity induced by aminoglycosides, have been postulated: (a) proliferation of HC progenitors through mitotic division, (b) transdifferentiation of SCs into HCs, and (c) repair of partly damaged HCs. It has been shown that the vestibular epithelium of the mature mammalian inner ear has the ability to produce new HCs by renewed mitotic activity in response to aminoglycosides injury in vitro and in vivo (14–17). However, there is an apparent discrepancy between the number of proliferating cells and the number of immature HCs, characterized by immature stereocilia bundles, which may indicate that other mechanisms are involved in mammalian adult vestibular HC regeneration. HCs were also shown to arise from SCs or from another unidentified cell type of the sensory epithelium by direct transdifferentiation, i.e., without going through a mitotic cycle (35,36). A third possibility is that immature bundles represent a repair process whereby nonlethally damaged HCs replace stereocilia bundles that have been lost due to some traumatic event (37). In addition, experiments with cultured organs of Corti also suggest the possibility of self-repair of the stereociliary bundles after partial damage to HCs (38,39).

In the adult mammalian cochlea, loss of HCs does not induce regeneration or repair but rather results in an epithelial scar whereby SCs contact each other at sites where HCs are missing (40). However, in the developing organ of Corti several data suggest that undifferentiated cells can function as progenitors for new HCs. Laser ablation experiments have demonstrated that regenerated HCs can arise in vitro in the embryonic mouse organ of Corti possibly through direct transdifferentiation of preexisting cells that change from their normal developmental fate (18). HC production has also been suggested to occur in immortalized cell lines derived from organs of Corti of the H2k^btsA58 transgenic mouse (Immortomouse), which carries a conditionally expressed, temperature-sensitive immortalizing gene that perpetuates cell division (41). Isolated organ of Corti cells growing at 33 °C proliferated rapidly and when moved to 39 °C, the cells reduced their rate of proliferation while expressing some specific HC markers such as brn-3c, OCP2, and myosin VIIa (42,43). However, despite the acquisition of HC markers, no demonstration was provided that these cells had functional or ultrastructural features of sensory cells. Production of supernumerary HCs has also been shown in cultured P0 rat organ of Corti explants (44,45). However, in these in vitro experiments, new HCs were never demonstrated to arise after a proliferative phase (46,47).

Several cell types are HC progenitor candidates. Some observations suggest that Deiters' cells of the organ of Corti might have kept a potential to differentiate into HCs, as treatment of young rats with ototoxic concentrations of amikacin leads to the replacement of lost HCs by Deiters' cells with early differentiating stereocilia bundles (48–51). An overproduction of HCs was also observed in vitro at the level of the greater epithelial ridge of cultured organ of Corti when an overexpression of Math1 transcription factor was induced (52). Very recently, we have shown that cultured immature nestin positive cells present in the newborn rat organ of Corti can proliferate and subsequently differentiate into HCs and SCs (53). Interestingly, in these newborn rat organs of Corti, nestin-positive cells are located in the region of the greater epithelial ridge.

III. PRINCIPAL GENES IMPLICATED IN DEVELOPMENT AND REGENERATION OF HC

During both spontaneous and damage-induced HC regeneration, the cellular organization of the sensory epithelium remains precisely maintained. Very little is known about the molecules that control the formation of the correct number, types, and pattern of cells during HC regeneration and which mechanisms are lacking in non- or poorly regenerating systems. The identification of the genes involved in HC development could provide some leads to understand regeneration. Actually, several genes are known to be implicated in inner ear morphogenesis and HC development and differentiation, including genes coding for membrane-bound signaling proteins, various transcription factors, cyclin-dependent inhibitors, and secreted factors, and these genes may also be involved in HC regeneration. Here, we summarize these findings in the prospect of HC regeneration (Table 1).

A. Notch Signaling Pathway

It has been proposed that the formation of the precise array of HCs and SCs is regulated by lateral inhibition that is mediated in several biological systems by the *lin-12/Notch* family of transmembranous receptors and their ligands, *Delta* and *Serrate* or *Delta* and *Jagged*, respectively, in birds and mammals. In that paradigm, nascent HCs express a Notch ligand or ligands and thereby inhibit their immediate neighbors in the developing sensory patch, which express *Notch*, from differentiating in the same way (54,55). Delta-Notch signaling was first implicated in lateral inhibition in sensory cell differentiation based on studies in zebrafish. Misregulation of delta genes and a Serrate homolog have been observed in the zebrafish mind bomb mutant where the ear sensory patches consist solely of HCs (56). There is also a deltaA zebrafish mutant, which has increased numbers of HCs (57). Mouse mutations have made it possible to determine the roles of the various players in this pathway. Mice homozygous for a targeted null mutation of *Jagged2 (Jag2)* develop supernumerary HCs (58), two mice mutant for *Jagged1 (Jag1)* gene, i.e., *slalom* and headturner (Htu) mice, show reduced number of outer HCs (59,60), whereas a mutation in *lunatic fringe (Lfng)*, which encodes an extracellular modulator of the Notch signaling pathway, partly suppresses the effect of the *Jag2* mutation (61). Moreover, the expression patterns of *Notch* and ligands are consistent with their presumed role in lateral inhibition resulting in an ordered array of HCs and SCs (Table 2). In addition, Delta-Notch signaling has been involved during avian HC regeneration. Early after gentamicin-induced HC injury, *Delta1* and *Notch* are highly upregulated in areas of cell proliferation in the basilar papilla, which correspond to HCs progenitors (62).

B. Transcription Factors and HC Differentiation

A number of transcription factors are known to be expressed during inner ear development. In addition, several genetic disorders of inner ear development have recently been identified in human and mouse as being caused by mutations of genes controlling transcription factors. Furthermore, the targeted mutation of several transcription factor genes influences the development of specific inner ear cell types, and suggests a critical role for these factors in controlling inner ear cell lineages.

1. POU-Domain Transcription Factors

The POU proteins are a large family of transcriptional regulators that contains a bipartite DNA recognition domain consisting of a variant homeodomain and a POU-specific domain. Among the POU factors, those of the POU-IV or Brn-3 subclass appear to be especially involved in inner ear development. In mammals, this subclass includes three genes, *Brn-3a*, *Brn-3b*, and *Brn-3c* (also referred to as *Brn-3.0*, *Brn-3.2*, and *Brn-3.1*, respectively), all of which are homologs of the *C. elegans* developmental

Table 1 Principal Genes Implied in Hair Cell Development and Regeneration

Molecule	Cellular expression in the organ of Corti	Cellular defects in mice or humans knockouts	Putative role in HC differentiation and regeneration	Ref.
Notch signaling pathway				
Notch	SCs	n.d.	HC and SC differentiation	56,58,152,153,155,157
Jagged1	SCs	Decrease number of OHCs (slalom and headturner mice)	Upregulation after gentamicin injury in chick	59,60,154,156,157
Jagged2	HCs	Supernumerary HCs	HC differentiation	61,156,158
Transcription factors				
Brn-3c	HCs	Loss of HCs	HC differentiation	70,71
Math1	HCs	Loss of HCs	Overexpression leads to supernumerary HCs	52,78,158
Hes1	GER-LER	Supernumerary HCs	Negative regulator of HC differentiation by antagonizing *Math1*	79,80
Hes5	LER, narrow band of LER	Supernumerary HCs	Negative regulator of HC differentiation by antagonizing *Math1*	80,158
RARα	HCs	Loss of HCs	HC differentiation induced by RA	20,90–92,101
RXRα,γ	HCs	Loss of HCs	HC differentiation induced by RA	
TRβ	GER	Defect in potassium current in IHCs	Accelerated onset of auditory function with TH	108,110
GATA3	All cells before E14, SCs between E14–P5	n.d.	n.d.	111,114,115

SOX10	SCs	Deafness (Waardenburg-Shah syndrome)	n.d.	119,120
Myosin superfamily				
Myo6	HCs	Splayed stereocilia	HC differentiation	126,128,159
Myo7	HCs	Short stereocilia	HC differentiation	122,123,127
Myo15	HCs	Fused stereocilia	n.d.	124,125,129
Cell cycle protein				
p27^{KIP1}	SCs	Supernumerary HCs and SCs	Cell proliferation inhibition	133–135
Growth factors				
FGFR3	SCs	Absence of pillar cells	FGF stimulates mitosis in vestibular sensory epithelium	136,142,143
IGF-I	n.d.	Immature tectorial membrane, abnormal HC's innervation	IGF-I + TGFα + RA enhance regeneration of injured vestibular HCs; Stimulates mitosis in vestibular sensory epithelium	17,141,160
TGFα	EGFR is expressed in HCs and SCs	n.d.	IGF-I + TGFα + RA enhance regeneration of injured vestibular HCs; Stimulates mitosis in vestibular sensory epithelium; Enhances HC regeneration on neonatal	17,145,146,148

n.d. = not determined; SCs = supporting cells; HCs = hair cells; GER = greater epithelial ridge; IER = Lower epithelial ridge.

Table 2 Distinct Expression Patterns of Notch Family Receptors and Ligands: Parallels Between Different Species

	Notch	Serrate/jagged1	Serrate/jagged2	Delta	Ref.
Zebrafish	Highly expressed in the ear rudiment	n.d.	Nascent HC (serrate B)	Nascent HC (delta A, B, and C)	56
Chick, normal	Confined to support cell layer	Marks all cells and downregulated as HCs differentiate, remains high in all SCs	Nascent HC only, ceasing as HC fully differentiated	Nascent HC only, ceasing as HC fully differentiated	152,153
Chick, regeneration	Temporarily upregulated in HCs expressed in SCs	Does not change during the course of drug-induced HC regeneration	n.d.	Upregulated in mitotic progenitors and in early differentiated HC, 3 days postgentamicin	62
Mouse	Expressed throughout the cochlear sensory epithelium	Marks nascent and differentiated SCs	Nascent HCs	HCs (E16.5)	58,154,155
Rat					
E16	Presumptive sensory epithelium	Presumptive sensory epithelium	Absent	n.d.	156
E18–E20	Differentiated SCs	Differentiated SCs	Differentiating HCs	n.d.	
P0-P3	SCs	SCs	HCs	n.d.	

regulator Unc-86 (63,64). *Brn-3a* and *Brn-3b* have been shown to play a role in spiral ganglion neuron development (65,66). In developing and adult mice, *Brn-3c*/*Brn-3.1*/*POU4F3* displays strong expression in the sensory HCs of both the cochlear and vestibular systems. Targeted null mutations of this gene lead to loss of all the cochlear and vestibular HCs, resulting in complete deafness and profound deficit in the vestibular system in the *Brn-3c$^{-/-}$* mice (65,67–70). Therefore, *Brn-3c* seems to play a pivotal role in the development of inner ear sensory HCs. The examination of the development of the cochlea in *Brn-3c$^{-/-}$* mice during embryogenesis indicates that prior to degeneration, HCs become committed and pass through the early stages of development (71). These data indicate that *Brn-3c* is required for maturation, survival, and proper position of HCs, whereas it plays little role in commitment and initial differentiation of HCs.

2. bHLH Transcription Factors

Regulatory cascades of positive and negative basic helix-loop-helix (bHLH) transcription factors play essential roles in mammalian neurogenesis (72–74). The bHLH genes, such as *Math1*, *Mash-1*, and *NeuroD*, are thought to positively regulate neuronal development, i.e., proneural genes, at the level of commitment and postmitotic differentiation (75,76). Other bHLH genes, like *Hes1* and *Hes5*, negatively regulate the transcription of the positive-bHLH genes (77).

Math1, a mouse homolog of the *Drosophila* proneural gene *atonal*, is essential for HC development. Embryonic *Math1*-null mice fail to generate cochlear and vestibular HCs (78). In addition, temporal expression patterns of *Math1* correlate well with the time period for HC differentiation. *Math1* is expressed in differentiating HCs at early embryonic stages, but is down-regulated in SCs and absent in cells outside the sensory epithelium at late embryonic stages (78). In addition, overexpression of *Math1* in postnatal rat organs of Corti induces a production of supernumerary HCs in the greater epithelial ridge (52). These findings demonstrate that *Math1* is necessary and sufficient for the development of cells as HCs, and strongly suggest that *Math1* acts as a "prosensory" gene within the organ of Corti and that the enhancement of *Math1* expression level in the inner ear might be used to stimulate HC regeneration.

The negative bHLH transcription factors *Hes1* and *Hes5* are homologs to the products of *Drosophila hairy* and *Enhancer-of-split* [E(spl)] and have been demonstrated to affect cell fate determination by inhibiting the action of bHLH-positive regulators, such as *Math1*, during neuronal development (74,77). Cochleae from *Hes1-* and *Hes5*-null mice show a significant increase, respectively, in the number of inner and outer HCs (79,80). Cotransfection experiments in cultured postnatal rat organ of Corti explants show that overexpression of *Hes1* prevents HC differentiation induced by *Math1* (79). Therefore, *Hes1* can negatively regulate HC differentiation by antagonizing *Math1*, as has been shown during neurogenesis. These results suggest that a balance between *Math1* and negative regulators such as *Hes1* is crucial for the production of an appropriate number of inner ear HCs.

3.   Steroid/Thyroid Receptor Family

Steroid/thyroid receptor superfamily genes act as nuclear transcription factors and are characterized by a stereotype molecular structure that includes a zinc-finger DNA-binding domain and a conserved ligand-binding/ dimerization region (81). This growing family currently includes more than 50 different genes, including retinoic acid receptors (RAR) and retinoid X receptors (RXR) and thyroid hormone receptors (TR).

Retinoid Signaling and HC Differentiation. Retinoids are a family of molecules derived from vitamin A and include the biologically active metabolite retinoic acid (RA). The cellular effects of RA are mediated through the action of two classes of receptors, the RARs, which are activated by both all-*trans*-RA (tRA) and 9-*cis*-RA, and the RXRs, which are activated only by 9-*cis*-RA (82,83). Three major subtypes, α, β, and, γ, of these receptors have been identified with multiple isoforms due to alternative splicing and differential promoter usage (84). The RARs mediate gene expression by forming heterodimers with the RXRs, while the RXRs can mediate gene expression as homodimers or by forming heterodimers with a variety of orphan receptors (85). Both excess and deficiency of retinoids lead to teratogenic effects including at the inner ear level (86,87). Some of the RAR and RXR receptors are expressed within the developing cochlear duct (88–90). As development continues, the expression of each receptor becomes more intense in cells that will develop as HCs (91). RAR-null mutant studies have shown that these nuclear receptors are critical for normal inner ear development (92). These results clearly suggest that signaling by RAR plays a direct role in the development of the cochlea. Indeed, several lines of evidence have implicated the intracellular receptors for RA in controlling critical steps in cochlear differentiation. RA has been shown by an in vitro reporter assay to be produced endogenously in the inner ear (93). In vitro assays using cultured chick otocysts indicate that RA can inhibit mitogen-induced cellular proliferation and alter normal otocyst morphogenesis as well as induce premature histological differentiation of the cultured cochlear epithelium (94,95). In organotypic cultures of the developing mouse cochlea, exposure to RA results in the formation of supernumerary HCs and SCs (93). In addition, blocking the activation of retinoid receptors in cultures of the embryonic cochlea, with receptor-specific antagonists or inhibitors of retinoic acid synthesis, results in a significant decrease in the number of cells that develop as HCs and a disruption in the development of the organ of Corti (91).

The potential role of RA in HC regeneration has also been studied. As previously described, HC regeneration occurs following ototoxin treatment in the vestibular epithelia of adult mammals but not in the cochleas (96,97). Interestingly, RA and cellular RA-binding protein (CRABP), which controls the level of free intracellular RA and is involved in the transfert of RA from the cytoplasm to the nucleus, are expressed in the adult vestibular epithelia but not in the adult organ of Corti (98,99). In addition, it has been shown that an upregulation in the expression of the RARβ gene appears after noise-induced damage to the chick basilar papilla (100). We have also reported that RA can induce cellular proliferation and HC regeneration in the postnatal rat organ of Corti in culture (20,101).

Thyroid Hormone and Inner Ear Development. Thyroid hormone (triiodothyronine, T3) and its receptors are essential for the development of hearing. Congenital thyroid disorders impair hearing, and profound deafness is common when there is a prevalence of iodine deficiency (102,103). Also, hypothyroidism in rodents causes a pronounced disruption of the organ of Corti especially at the level of the HCs (104,105). T3 receptors (TRs) are ligand-dependent transcription factors encoded by two genes,α and β *c-erbA*, that give rise to three functional TRs, α1, β1, and β2, and to nonthyroid-hormone-binding isotype α2 (106,107). Both TRα1 and TRβ are expressed during embryonic and postnatal development of the cochlea indicating that cochlea is the direct site of T3 action (108,109). TRβ-null mice are severely deaf as assessed by defective auditory-evoked brainstem responses (ABR) whereas TRα1-null mice have normal ABR (110). These results clearly suggest that T3 plays a role in the development of the cochlea.

4. Other Transcription Factors Implicated in HC Differentiation

GATA3. The GATA family of zinc finger transcription factors includes six related proteins and are involved in the development of many different systems including the hematopoietic and the respiratory systems. Among these factors, GATA3 has been shown to be expressed in both the brain and the inner ear (111–114). GATA3 is expressed in all cells of the developing sensory epithelium before HC differentiation, i.e., at E14 in mice. Expression decreases selectively in the HCs as they differentiate progressively from base to apex in the developing organ of Corti. GATA3 subsequently decreases in the SCs and cannot be detected in the adult sensory epithelium. GATA3 has also been shown to be involved in the human hypoparathyroidism, sensorineural deafness, and renal abnormalities (HRD) syndrome (115). Taken together, these results suggest that GATA3 is important for cochlear development and its expression pattern may reflect an inhibitory effect on cell differentiation.

Sox10. More than 20 members of the *Sox* gene family of transcription factors, characterized by a high-mobility group (HMG) domain as DNA-binding motif, play important roles in diverse developmental processes such as chondrogenic differentiation or hematopoiesis (116). Among these factors, the *Sox10* gene is selectively expressed in neural crest cells during early stages of development, in glia cells of the peripheral and central nervous systems, and in the otic vesicle (117,118). *Sox10* mRNA is expressed in the entire epithelia of the developing cochlea at E13.5. At P0 and later, *Sox10* expression is restricted to the SCs of the organ of Corti (119). *Sox10* is also defective in Waardenburg-Shah syndrome characterized by an aganglionic colon as well as sensorineural deafness and pigmentation abnormalities (120). These data suggest that *Sox10* is also important for development of the cochlea.

C. Myosin Superfamily and HC Differentiation

Myosins form a superfamily of proteins that includes the conventional class II myosins and 14 classes of unconventional myosins that are distinguished based on the homology of the motor domains (121). Multiple myosin isozymes are present in the cochlea specifically in the HCs, and they appear to have important nonredundant functions, as evidenced by the different deaf mutants described in both humans and mice. Mutations in the *Myo7a* gene have been found in *shaker1* mouse mutants, Usher type 1B in humans, and both dominant (DNFA11) and recessive (DFNB2) forms of nonsyndromic deafness in humans (122,123). *Myo15* has been reported to underlie both the *shaker2* mouse mutant and another form of human recessively inherited deafness (DNFB3) (124,125). Murine myosin VI (*Myo6*) mutations are responsible for the inner ear abnormalities in the deaf mouse mutant known as *Snell's waltzer* mouse (126). The different myosin gene mutations that result in deafness in both mice and humans underline the crucial role that myosins exert in the actin-rich environment of the cilia of the HCs in the inner ear. The specific functions of the different myosins within the HCs, however, have not yet been determined. Ultrastructural studies of the HCs of all mutant mice, i.e., *shaker 1, shaker 2,* and *Snell's waltzer,* have revealed that the stereocilia bundles are disorganized (127–129). This observation suggests that *Myo6, Myo7a,* and *Myo15* are necessary for normal development of the stereocilia; however, the precise molecular events perturbed by defective specific myosins remain undefined.

D. Cyclin-Dependent Kinase Inhibitors and Cell Differentiation

Inhibitors of cell cycle progression include the cyclin-dependent kinase (CDK) inhibitors, which function in both cell-cycle arrest and differentiation in many cell types. They exert these functions by binding to and inactivating CDK complexes. Two classes of CDK inhibitors have been identified: the INK4 family, which are specific inhibitors of cyclin D–CDK (i.e., CDK4 and CDK6), and the Cip/Kip family including p21, p27, and p57, which inhibit all types of cyclin-CDK complexes (130,131). Cip/Kip proteins have been implicated as critical terminal effectors of the signal transduction pathway that controls cell differentiation. $p27^{KIP1}$ has been shown to be an essential mediator of oligodendrocyte terminal differentiation (132). $p27^{KIP1}$ expression is induced in the primordial organ of Corti between E12 and E14, correlating with the cessation of cell division of the progenitors of the HCs and SCs (133). In wild-type animals, $p27^{KIP1}$ expression is downregulated during subsequent HC differentiation, but persists at high levels in differentiated SCs of the mature organ of Corti. In mice with a targeted deletion of the *p27^{KIP1}* gene, ongoing cell proliferation occurs in the postnatal organ of Corti at time points well after the normal cessation of mitosis, leading to the appearance of supernumerary HCs and SCs (133,134). In the absence of $p27^{KIP1}$, mitotically active cells are still observed in the organ of Corti of P6 animals, suggesting that the persistence of $p27^{KIP1}$ expression in mature SCs may contribute to the maintenance of quiescence in this tissue and, possibly, to its inability to regenerate. In addition, it has recently been shown that $p27^{KIP1}$ antisense oligonucleotides trigger supporting cell proliferation in the mature organ of Corti after aminoglycoside insult (135). Therefore, $p27^{KIP1}$ may become a major target for HC regeneration.

E. Growth Factors and Their Receptors: Implication in HC Regeneration

Several investigators have attempted to stimulate HC regeneration in the chick and mammalian inner ear epithelia by addition of peptidic growth factors or through the manipulation of various second-messenger pathways.

1. Fibroblast Growth Factors

Several fibroblast growth factors (FGFs) and their corresponding receptors have been detected in inner ear sensory epithelium (136–140). FGF-2 has been shown to stimulate mitosis in rat utricular macula in culture (141). Among FGF receptors, recent studies point to a specific receptor tyrosine kinase, FGFR3, as playing a key role in the development and maintenance of the auditory epithelium. FGFR3 is specifically expressed in SCs, and not in HCs, in the basilar papilla and in the organ of Corti of mammals (136). Following HC trauma to the chick or mammalian cochlea, FGFR3 is rapidly modulated in the SCs, suggesting that this receptor plays a role in the response to HC loss (136,142). In addition, deletion of this gene through homologous recombination in mice results in abnormal cochlear development; a particular type of support cell, the pillar cell, fails to develop in these knockout mice (143). These results suggest a possible role for FGFs in HC and SC regeneration.

2. Other Growth Factors

Insulin growth factor-I (IGF-I) and insulin have been shown to induce cell proliferation in the mature avian vestibular sensory epithelium (144). In mammals, studies using organotypic culture indicate that IGF-I (141), transforming growth factor α (TGFα), and epidermal growth factor (EGF) supplemented with insulin (145,146) are mitogenic for SCs in the postnatal and the mature mammalian vestibular sensory epithelium. Perilymphatic infusion of TGFα with insulin induced cell proliferation in the utricular sensory epithelium of adult rats (147). These effects on cell proliferation may be the first step towards HC regeneration. Very recently, it has been shown that growth factor treatment can enhance vestibular HC regeneration in vivo. Infusion of a combination of TGFα, IGF-I, and RA into the perilymphatic space of adult guinea pig vestibule after gentamicin administration results in a significant enhancement of the regeneration of the vestibular HCs (17). Factors able to stimulate cell proliferation in the mammalian cochlea have not been yet identified. In addition, TGFα has been implicated as a factor driving HC regeneration in neonatal organ of Corti cultures (21,148).

3. Second-Messenger Pathways

Binding of growth factors to receptor tyrosine kinases leads to the activation of intracellular cascades composed of enzymes and signaling intermediates that could also be potential targets for therapeutic induction of HC regeneration. High concentrations of forskolin stimulate SC proliferation in chicken cochleae and in mammalian vestibular sensory epithelium in vitro, and inhibitors of protein kinase A reduce that effect (149,150). Phosphatidylinositol 3-kinase (P13-K), the target of rapamycin (TOR), the mitogen-activated protein kinase pathway (MAPK), and some protein kinase C

(PKCs) participate in the induction of S-phase entry in cultured vestibular epithelia from chickens and rats (151). Future studies will be needed to identify the specific isoforms of the kinases that function in the proliferation cascades possibly making it possible to define specific drug targets suitable for the modulation of progenitor cell proliferation and the capacity for regenerative replacement of sensory HCs in mammalian inner ears.

IV. CONCLUSIONS

This brief overview illustrates that significant progress has been achieved to molecularly dissect vertebrate inner ear development and regeneration. However, the patterning process of the ear is not sufficiently known at the moment to provide clues for human HC regeneration. Avian and mammalian auditory epithelia share many anatomical and functional features: they have similar sorts of specialized cell types and mechanisms of sensory signal transduction. Despite these similarities, these two classes of vertebrates clearly possess differences with respect to the ability to form new cells after birth. Studies on nonmammalian vertebrates have shown that HCs can be formed postembryologically, enabling the return of normal structure and function in mature auditory and vestibular organs after damage. In mammals, all cells in the organ of Corti become terminally mitotic by E16 and experimentally induced HC loss does not cause renewed mitotic activity. The failure of renewed proliferation in the mammalian auditory epithelium may be caused by persistent inhibition of mitotic activity among progenitor cells or by the absence of postmitotic stimuli in response to HC loss. However, the recent demonstration that cultured immature nestin-positive cells present in the newborn rat organ of Corti can proliferate in vitro and subsequently differentiate into HCs and SCs, together with the detection of nestin cells in vivo at the spiral limbus in the P15 mature organ of Corti (53), opens new prospects with regard to regeneration of the injured organ of Corti.

Our ability to regenerate or repair damaged HCs therapeutically will certainly be dependent on a better understanding of the many signaling pathways involved in fate specification. Many genes implied in HC development or regeneration have been recently identified, including the Notch signaling pathway, various transcription factors, especially Math1, Brn-3c, RA, and thyroid hormone, cell cycle protein such as $p27^{KIP1}$, and growth factors and their receptors. Activating these systems in the mammalian inner ear will provide real potential for stimulating HC replacement. However, many questions remain unanswered including the ways in which the factors themselves are regulated and interact, the identify of their target genes, and the manner in which the transcription of these genes is influenced. The answer to these questions should lead to identification of the specific molecular and genetic interactions that are required for the development and the regeneration of the inner ear sensory epithelium.

REFERENCES

1. Corwin JT. Postembryonic production and aging in inner ear hair cells in sharks. J Comp Neurol 1981; 201(4):541–553.
2. Corwin JT. Postembryonic growth of the macula neglecta auditory detector in the ray, *Raja clavata*: continual increases in hair cell number, neural convergence, and physiological sensitivity. J Comp Neurol 1983; 217(3):345–356.
3. Popper AN, Hoxter B. Growth of a fish ear. 1. Quantitative analysis of hair cell and ganglion cell proliferation. Hearing Res 1984; 15(2):133–142.
4. Popper AN, Hoxter B. Growth of a fish ear. II Locations of newly proliferated sensory hair cells in the saccular epithelium of *Astronotus ocellatus*. Hearing Res 1990; 45(1–2):33–40.
5. Corwin JT. Perpetual production of hair cells and maturational changes in hair cell ultrastructure accompany postembryonic growth in an amphibian ear. Proc Natl Acad Sci USA 1985; 82(11):3911–3915.
6. Jorgensen JM, Mathiesen C. The avian inner ear. Continuous production of hair cells in vestibular sensory organs, but not in the auditory papilla. Naturwissenschaften 1988; 75(6):319–320.
7. Jorgensen JM. Regeneration of lateral line and inner ear vestibular cells. Ciba Found Symp 1991; 160:151–163.
8. Roberson DF, Weisleder P, Bohrer PS, Rubel EW. Ongoing production of sensory cells in the vestibular epithelium of the chick. Hearing Res 1992; 57(2):166–174.
9. Ruben RJ. Development of the inner ear of the mouse: a radioautographic study of terminal mitoses. Acta Otolaryngol (Stockh) 1967; 220(suppl):1–44.
10. Corwin JT, Cotanche DA. Regeneration of sensory hair cells after acoustic trauma. Science 1988; 240(4860):1772–1774.
11. Ryals BM, Rubel EW. Hair cell regeneration after acoustic trauma in adult coturnix quail. Science 1988; 240:1774–1776.
12. Katayama A, Corwin JT. Cell production in the chicken cochlea. J Comp Neurol 1989; 281(1):129–135.
13. Cotanche DA. Structural recovery from sound and aminoglycoside damage in the avian cochlea. Audiol Neurootol 1999; 4(6):271–285.
14. Forge A, Li L, Corwin JT, Nevill G. Ultrastructural evidence for hair cell regeneration in the mammalian inner ear. Science 1993; 259(5101):1616–1619.
15. Warchol ME, Lambert PR, Goldstein BJ, Forge A, Corwin JT. Regenerative proliferation in inner ear sensory epithelia from adult guinea pigs and humans. Science 1993; 259(5101):1619–1622.
16. Zheng JL, Gao WQ. Analysis of rat vestibular hair cell development and

regeneration using calretinin as an early marker. J Neurosci 1997; 17(21):8270–8282.

17. Kopke RD, Jackson RL, Li G, Rasmussen MD, Hoffer ME, Frenz DA, et al. Growth factor treatment enhances vestibular hair cell renewal and results in improved vestibular function. Proc Natl Acad Sci USA 2001; 98(10):5886–5891.

18. Kelley MW, Talreja DR, Corwin JT. Replacement of hair cells after laser microbeam irradiation in cultured organs of Corti from embryonic and neonatal mice. J Neurosci 1995; 4:3013–3026.

19. Sobkowicz HM, August BK, Slapnick SM. Cellular interactions as a response to injury in the organ of Corti in culture. Int J Dev Neurosci 1997; 15(4–5):463–485.

20. Lefebvre PP, Malgrange B, Staecker H, Moonen G, Van De Water TR. Retinoic acid stimulates regeneration of mammalian auditory hair cells after ototoxic damage in vitro. Science 1993; 260/5108:692–694.

21. Zine A, de Ribaupierre F. Replacement of mammalian auditory hair cells. NeuroReport 1998; 9(2):263–268.

22. Steel KP, Kros CJ. A genetic approach to understanding auditory function. Nat Genet 2001; 27(2):143–149.

23. Cotanche DA, Lee KH, Stone JS, Picard DA. Hair cell regeneration in the bird cochlea following noise damage or ototoxic drug damage. Anat Embryol (Berl) 1994; 189:1–18.

24. Corwin JT, Oberholtzer JC. Fish n' chicks: model recipes for hair-cell regeneration? Neuron 1997; 19(5):951–954.

25. Stone JS, Oesterle EC, Rubel EW. Recent insights into regeneration of auditory and vestibular hair cells. Curr Opin Neurol 1998; 11(1):17–24.

26. Kil J, Warchol ME, Corwin JT. Cell death, cell proliferation, and estimates of hair cell life spans in the vestibular organs of chicks. Hearing Res 1997; 114(1–2):117–126.

27. Cotanche DA, Lee KH. Regeneration of hair cells in the vestibulocochlear system of birds and mammals. Curr Opin Neurobiol 1994; 4(4):509–514.

28. Girod DA, Duckert LG, Rubel EW. Possible precursors of regenerated hair cells in the avian cochlea following acoustic trauma. Hearing Res 1989; 42(2–3):175–194.

29. Duckert LG, Rubel EW. Morphological correlates of functional recovery in the chicken inner ear after gentamycin treatment. J Comp Neurol 1993; 331:75–96.

30. Stone JS, Rubel EW. Cellular studies of auditory hair cell regeneration in birds. Proc Natl Acad Sci USA 2000; 97(22):11714–11721.

31. Fekete DM, Muthukumar S, Karagogeos D. Hair cells and supporting cells share a common progenitor in the avian inner ear. J Neurosci 1998; 18(19):7811–7821.

32. Adler HJ, Raphael Y. New hair cells arise from supporting cell conversion in the acoustically damaged chick inner ear. Neurosci Lett 1996; 205(1):17–20.

33. Jones JE, Corwin JT. Regeneration of sensory cells after laser ablation in the

lateral line system: hair cell lineage and macrophage behavior revealed by time-lapse video microscopy. J Neurosci 1996; 16(2):649–662.

34. Adler HJ, Komeda M, Raphael Y. Further evidence for supporting cell conversion in the damaged avian basilar papilla. Int J Dev Neurosci 1997; 15(4–5): 375–385.

35. Rubel EW, Dew LA, Roberson DW. Mammalian vestibular hair cell regeneration. Science 1995; 267(5198):701–707.

36. Li L, Forge A. Morphological evidence for supporting cell to hair cell conversion in the mammalian utricular macula. Int J Dev Neurosci 1997; 15(4–5):433–446.

37. Zheng JL, Keller G, Gao WQ. Immunocytochemical and morphological evidence for intracellular self-repair as an important contributor to mammalian hair cell recovery. J Neurosci 1999; 19(6):2161–2170.

38. Sobkowicz HM, August BK, Slapnick SM. Epithelial repair following mechanical injury of the developing organ of Corti in culture: an electron microscopic and autoradiographic study. Exp Neurol 1992; 115(1):44–49.

39. Sobkowicz HM, Slapnick SM, August BK. The kinocilium of auditory hair cells and evidence for its morphogenetic role during the regeneration of stereocilia and cuticular plates. J Neurocytol 1995; 24(9):633–653.

40. Raphael Y, Altschuler RA. Reorganization of cytoskeletal and junctional proteins during cochlear hair cell degeneration. Cell Motil Cytoskel 1991; 18: 215–227.

41. Jat PS, Noble MD, Ataliotis P, Tanaka Y, Yannoutsos N, Larsen L, et al. Direct derivation of conditionally immortal cell lines from an H-2Kb-tsA58 transgenic mouse. Proc Natl Acad Sci USA 1991; 88(12):5096–5100.

42. Kalinec F, Kalinec G, Boukhvalova M, Kachar B. Establishment and characterization of conditionally immortalized organ of corti cell lines. Cell Biol Int 1999; 23(3):175–184.

43. Rivolta MN, Grix N, Lawlor P, Ashmore JF, Jagger DJ, Holley MC. Auditory hair cell precursors immortalized from the mammalian inner ear. Proc R Soc Lond B Biol Sci 1998; 265(1406):1595–1603.

44. Abdouh A, Despres G, Romand R. Hair cell overproduction in the developing mammalian cochlea in culture. NeuroReport 1993; 5(1):33–36.

45. Lefebvre PP, Malgrange B, Thiry M, Breuskin I, Van De Water TR, Moonen G. Supernumerary outer hair cells arise external to the last row of sensory cells in the organ of corti. Acta Otolaryngol 2001; 121(2):164–168.

46. Chardin S, Romand R. Factors modulating supernumerary hair cell production in the postnatal rat cochlea in vitro. Int J Dev Neurosci 1997; 15(4–5): 497–507.

47. Lefebvre PP, Malgrange B, Thiry M, Van De Water TR, Moonen G. Epidermal growth factor upregulates production of supernumerary hair cells in neonatal rat organ of Corti explants. Acta Otolaryngol (Stockh) 2000; 120: 142–145.

48. Daudet N, Vago P, Ripoll C, Humbert G, Pujol R, Lenoir M. Characterization of atypical cells in the juvenile rat organ of corti after aminoglycoside ototoxicity. J Comp Neurol 1998; 401(2):145–162.

49. Daudet N, Ripoll C, Lenoir M. Transforming growth factor-α-induced cellular changes in organotypic culture of juvenile, amikacin-treated rat organ of Corti. J Comp Neurol 2002; 442:6–22.

50. Lenoir M, Vago P. Does the organ of Corti attempt to differentiate new hair cells after antibiotic intoxication in rat pups? Int J Dev Neurosci 1997; 15(4–5): 487–495.

51. Parietti C, Vago P, Humbert G, Lenoir M. Attempt at hair cell neodifferentiation in developing and adult amikacin intoxicated rat cochleae. Brain Res 1998; 813(1):57–66.

52. Zheng JL, Gao WQ. Overexpression of Math1 induces robust production of extra hair cells in postnatal rat inner ears. Nat Neurosci 2000; 3(6):580–586.

53. Malgrange B, Belachew S, Thiry M, Nguyen L, Rogister B, Alvarez M-L, et al. Proliferative generation of mammalian auditory hair cells in culture. Mech Dev 2002; 112:79–88.

54. Lewis J. Rules for the production of sensory cells. Ciba Found Symp 1991; 160:25–39.

55. Goodyear R, Holley M, Richardson G. Hair and supporting-cell differentiation during the development of the avian inner ear. J Comp Neurol 1995; 351(1):81–93.

56. Haddon C, Jiang YJ, Smithers L, Lewis J. Delta-Notch signalling and the patterning of sensory cell differentiation in the zebrafish ear: evidence from the mind bomb mutant. Development 1998; 125(23):4637–4644.

57. Riley BB, Chiang M, Farmer L, Heck R. The deltaA gene of zebrafish mediates lateral inhibition of hair cells in the inner ear and is regulated by pax2.1. Development 1999; 126(24):5669–5678.

58. Lanford PJ, Lan Y, Jiang RL, Lindsell C, Weinmaster G, Gridley T, et al. Notch signalling pathway mediates hair cell development in mammalian cochlea. Nat Genet 1999; 21(3):289–292.

59. Tsai H, Hardisty RE, Rhodes C, Kiernan AE, Roby P, Tymowska-Lalanne Z, et al. The mouse slalom mutant demonstrates a role for *Jagged1* in neuroepithelial patterning in the organ of Corti. Hum Mol Genet 2001; 10(5):507–512.

60. Kiernan AE, Ahituv N, Fuchs H, Balling R, Avraham KB, Steel KP, et al. The *Notch* ligand *Jagged1* is required for inner ear sensory development. Proc Natl Acad Sci USA 2001; 98(7):3873–3878.

61. Zhang N, Martin GV, Kelley MW, Gridley T. A mutation in the *lunatic fringe* gene suppresses the effects of a *Jagged2* mutation on inner hair cell development in the cochlea. Curr Biol 2000; 10(11):659–662.

62. Stone JS, Rubel EW. *Delta1* expression during avian hair cell regeneration. Development 1999; 126(5):961–973.

63. Xiang M, Zhou L, Peng YW, Eddy RL, Shows TB, Nathans J. *Brn-3b*: a POU domain gene expressed in a subset of retinal ganglion cells. Neuron 1993; 11(4):689–701.

64. Ryan AF. Transcription factors and the control of inner ear development. Semin Cell Dev Biol 1997; 8(3):249–256.

65. Xiang M, Zhou L, Macke JP, Yoshioka T, Hendry SH, Eddy RL, et al. The *Brn-3* family of POU-domain factors: primary structure, binding specificity, and expression in subsets of retinal ganglion cells and somatosensory neurons. J Neurosci 1995; 15(7 Pt 1):4762–4785.

66. Artinger KB, Fedtsova N, Rhee JM, Bronner-Fraser M, Turner E. Placodal origin of *Brn-3*-expressing cranial sensory neurons. J Neurobiol 1998; 36(4): 572–585.

67. Gerrero MR, McEvilly RJ, Turner E, Lin CR, O'Connell S, Jenne KJ, et al. *Brn-3.0*: a POU-domain protein expressed in the sensory, immune, and endocrine systems that functions on elements distinct from known octamer motifs. Proc Natl Acad Sci USA 1993; 90(22):10841–10845.

68. Erkman L, McEvilly RJ, Luo L, Ryan AK, Hooshmand F, O'Connell SM, et al. Role of transcription factors *Brn-3.1* and *Brn-3.2* in auditory and visual system development. Nature 1996; 381(6583):603–606.

69. Xiang M, Gan L, Li D, Chen ZY, Zhou L, O'Malley BW, et al. Essential role of POU-domain factor *Brn-3c* in auditory and vestibular hair cell development. Proc Natl Acad Sci USA 1997; 94(17):9445–9450.

70. Xiang M, Gan L, Li D, Zhou L, Chen ZY, Wagner D, et al. Role of the *Brn-3* family of POU-domain genes in the development of the auditory/vestibular, somatosensory, and visual systems. Cold Spring Harbor Symp Quant Biol 1997; 62:325–336.

71. Xiang M, Gao WQ, Hasson T, Shin JJ. Requirement for *Brn-3c* in maturation and survival, but not in fate determination of inner ear hair cells. Development 1998; 125:3935–3946.

72. Kageyama R, Sasai Y, Akazawa C, Ishibashi M, Takebayashi K, Shimizu C, et al. Regulation of mammalian neural development by helix-loop-helix transcription factors. Crit Rev Neurobiol 1995; 9(2–3):177–188.

73. Kageyama R, Ishibashi M, Takebayashi K, Tomita K. bHLH transcription factors and mammalian neuronal differentiation. Int J Biochem Cell Biol 1997; 29(12):1389–1399.

74. Lee JE. Basic helix-loop-helix genes in neural development. Curr Opin Neurobiol 1997; 7(1):13–20.

75. Akazawa C, Ishibashi M, Shimizu C, Nakanishi S, Kageyama R. A mammalian helix-loop-helix factor structurally related to the product of *Drosophila* proneural gene atonal is a positive transcriptional regulator expressed in the developing nervous system. J Biol Chem 1995; 270(15):8730–8738.

76. Cau E, Gradwohl G, Fode C, Guillemot F. *Math1* activates a cascade of bHLH regulators in olfactory neuron progenitors. Development 1997; 124(8): 1611–1621.

77. Kageyama R, Nakanishi S. Helix-loop-helix factors in growth and differentiation of the vertebrate nervous system. Curr Opin Genet Dev 1997; 7(5):659–665.

78. Bermingham NA, Hassan BA, Price SD, Vollrath MA, Ben Arie N, Eatock RA, et al. *Math1*: an essential gene for the generation of inner ear hair cells. Science 1999; 284(5421):1837–1841.

79. Zheng JL, Shou J, Guillemot F, Kageyama R, Gao W. *Hes1* is a negative

regulator of inner ear hair cell differentiation. Development 2000; 127(21): 4551–4560.

80. Zine A, Aubert A, Qiu J, Therianos S, Guillemot F, Kageyama R, et al. *Hes1* and *Hes5* activities are required for the normal development of the hair cells in the mammalian inner ear. J Neurosci 2001; 21(13):4712–4720.

81. Mangelsdorf DJ, Thummel C, Beato M, Herrlich P, Schutz G, Umesono K, et al. The nuclear receptor superfamily: the second decade. Cell 1995; 83(6): 835–839.

82. Kastner P, Grondona JM, Mark M, Gansmuller A, LeMeur M, Decimo D, et al. Genetic analysis of RXR alpha developmental function: convergence of RXR and RAR signaling pathways in heart and eye morphogenesis. Cell 1994; 78(6):987–1003.

83. Lohnes D, Dierich A, Ghyselinck N, Kastner P, Lampron C, LeMeur M, et al. Retinoid receptors and binding proteins. J Cell Sci Suppl 1992; 16:69–76.

84. Leid M, Kastner P, Chambon P. Multiplicity generates diversity in the retinoic acid signalling pathways. Trends Biochem Sci 1992; 17:427–433.

85. Mangelsdorf DJ, Evans RM. The RXR heterodimers and orphan receptors. Cell 1995; 83(6):841–850.

86. Bavik C, Ward SJ, Chambon P. Developmental abnormalities in cultured mouse embryos deprived of retinoic by inhibition of yolk-sac retinol binding protein synthesis. Proc Natl Acad Sci USA 1996; 93(7):3110–3114.

87. Morriss-Kay G. Retinoic acid and craniofacial development: molecules and morphogenesis. Bioessays 1993; 15(1):9–15.

88. Dollé P, Ruberte E, Leroy P, Morriss-Kay G, Chambon P. Retinoic acid receptors and cellular retinoid binding proteins. I. A systematic study of their differential pattern of transcription during mouse organogenesis. Development 1990; 110:1133–1151.

89. Dolle P, Fraulob V, Kastner P, Chambon P. Developmental expression of murine retinoid X receptor (RXR) genes. Mech Dev 1994; 45(2):91–104.

90. Romand R, Sapin V, Dolle P. Spatial distributions of retinoic acid receptor gene transcripts in the prenatal mouse inner ear. J Comp Neurol 1998; 393(3): 298–308.

91. Raz Y, Kelley MW. Retinoic acid signaling is necessary for the development of the organ of Corti. Dev Biol 1999; 213:180–193.

92. Lohnes D, Mark M, Mendelsohn C, Dolle P, Dierich A, Gorry P, et al. Function of the retinoic acid receptors (RARs) during development. I. Craniofacial and skeletal abnormalities in RAR double mutants. Development 1994; 120(10):2723–2748.

93. Kelley MW, Xu XM, Wagner MA, Warchol ME, Corwin JT. The developing organ of Corti contains retinoic acid and forms supernumerary hair cells in response to exogenous retinoic acid in culture. Development 1993; 119(4): 1041–1053.

94. Represa J, Sanchez A, Miner C, Lewis J, Giraldez F. Retinoic acid modulation of the early development of the inner ear is associated with the control of c-fos expression. Development 1990; 110(4):1081–1090.

95. Leon Y, Sanchez JA, Miner C, Ariza-McNaughton L, Represa JJ, Giraldez F. Developmental regulation of Fos-protein during proliferative growth of the otic vesicle and its relation to differentiation induced by retinoic acid. Dev Biol 1995; 167(1):75–86.

96. Forge A, Li L, Corwin JT, Nevill G. Ultrastructural evidence for hair cell regeneration in the mammalian inner ear. Science 1993; 259:1616–1619.

97. Warchol ME, Lambert PR, Goldstein BJ, Forge A, Corwin JT. Regenerative proliferation in inner ear sensory epithelia from adult guinea pigs and humans. Science 1993; 259:1619–1622.

98. Ylikoski J, Pirvola U, Eriksson U. Cellular retinol-binding protein type I is prominently and differentially expressed in the sensory epithelium of the rat cochlea and vestibular organs. J Comp Neurol 1994; 349(4):596–602.

99. Romand R, Sapin V, Ghyselinck NB, Avan P, Le Calvez S, Dolle P, et al. Spatio-temporal distribution of cellular retinoid binding protein gene transcripts in the developing and the adult cochlea: morphological and functional consequences in C. Eur J Neurosci 2000; 12(8):2793–2804.

100. Lee KH, Cotanche DA. Potential role of bFGF and retinoic acid in the regeneration of chicken cochlear hair cells. Hear Res 1996; 94(1–2):1–13.

101. Lefebvre PP, Frenz DA, Staecker H, Represa J, Malgrange B, Ruben RJ, et al. Retinoic acid: a primary morphogen that affects both the differentiation and regeneration of mammalian auditory hair cells. In: Salvi R, Henderson D, eds. Auditory System Plasticity and Regeneration. New York: Thieme Medical, 1996:1–12.

102. DeLong GR. Effects of nutrition on brain development in humans. Am J Clin Nutr 1993; 57(2 suppl):286S–290S.

103. Forrest D. Deafness and goiter: molecular genetic considerations. J Clin Endocrinol Metab 1996; 81(8):2764–2767.

104. Uziel A. Periods of sensitivity to thyroid hormone during the development of the organ of Corti. Acta Otolaryngol Suppl 1986; 429:23–27.

105. O'Malley BW, Li D, Turner DS. Hearing loss and cochlear abnormalities in the congenital hypothyroid (hyt/hyt) mouse. Hear Res 1995; 88(1–2):181–189.

106. Brent GA, Moore DD, Larsen PR. Thyroid hormone regulation of gene expression. Annu Rev Physiol 1991; 53:17–35.

107. Lazar MA. Thyroid hormone receptors: multiple forms, multiple possibilities. Endocr Rev 1993; 14(2):184–193.

108. Bradley DJ, Towle HC, Young WS, III. Alpha and beta thyroid hormone receptor (TR) gene expression during auditory neurogenesis: evidence for TR isoform-specific transcriptional regulation in vivo. Proc Natl Acad Sci USA 1994; 91(2):439–443.

109. Lautermann J, Ten Cate WJ. Postnatal expression of the alpha-thyroid hormone receptor in the rat cochlea. Hearing Res 1997; 107(1–2):23–28.

110. Rusch A, Erway LC, Oliver D, Vennstrom B, Forrest D. Thyroid hormone receptor beta-dependent expression of a potassium conductance in inner hair cells at the onset of hearing. Proc Natl Acad Sci USA 1998; 95(26):15758–15762.

111. Rivolta MN, Holley MC. GATA3 is downregulated during hair cell differentiation in the mouse cochlea. J Neurocytol 1998; 27(9):637–647.

112. Pata I, Studer M, van Doorninck JH, Briscoe J, Kuuse S, Engel JD, et al. The transcription factor GATA3 is a downstream effector of Hoxbl specification in rhombomere 4. Development 1999; 126(23):5523–5531.

113. van Doorninck JH, van Der WJ, Karis A, Goedknegt E, Engel JD, Coesmans M, et al. GATA-3 is involved in the development of serotonergic neurons in the caudal raphe nuclei. J Neurosci 1999; 19(12):RC12.

114. Lawoko-kerali G, Rivolta MN, Holley M. Expression of the transcription factors GATA3 and Pax2 during development of the mammalian inner ear. J Comp Neurol 2002; 442:378–391.

115. Van Esch H, Devriendt K. Transcription factor GATA3 and the human HDR syndrome. Cell Mol Life Sci 2001; 58(9):1296–1300.

116. Wegner M. From head to toes: the multiple facets of Sox proteins. Nucleic Acids Res 1999; 27(6):1409–1420.

117. Kuhlbrodt K, Herbarth B, Sock E, Hermans-Borgmeyer I, Wegner M. *Sox10*, a novel transcriptional modulator in glial cells. J Neurosci 1998; 18(1):237–250.

118. Pusch C, Hustert E, Pfeifer D, Sudbeck P, Kist R, Roe B, et al. The *SOX10/Sox10* gene from human and mouse: sequence, expression, and transactivation by the encoded HMG domain transcription factor. Hum Genet 1998; 103(2): 115–123.

119. Watanabe K, Takeda K, Katori Y, Ikeda K, Oshima T, Yasumoto K, et al. Expression of the *Sox10* gene during mouse inner ear development. Brain Res Mol Brain Res 2000; 84(1–2):141–145.

120. Sham MH, Lui VC, Chen BL, Fu M, Tam PK. Novel mutations of *SOX10* suggest a dominant negative role in Waardenburg-Shah syndrome. J Med Genet 2001; 38(9):E30.

121. Hasson T, Mooseker MS. The growing family of myosin motors and their role in neurons and sensory cells. Curr Opin Neurobiol 1997; 7(5):615–623.

122. Mburu P, Liu XZ, Walsh J, Saw D, Cope MJ, Gibson F, et al. Mutation analysis of the mouse myosin VIIA deafness gene. Genes Funct 1997; 1(3): 191–203.

123. Weil D, Kussel P, Blanchard S, Levy G, Levi-Acobas F, Drira M, et al. The autosomal recessive isolated deafness, DFNB2, and the Usher 1B syndrome are allelic defects of the myosin-VIIA gene. Nat Genet 1997; 16(2):191–193.

124. Wang A, Liang Y, Fridell RA, Probst FJ, Wilcox ER, Touchman JW, et al. Association of unconventional myosin *MYO15* mutations with human non-syndromic deafness DFNB3. Science 1998; 280(5368):1447–1451.

125. Probst FJ, Fridell RA, Raphael Y, Saunders TL, Wang A, Liang Y, et al. Correction of deafness in *shaker-2* mice by an unconventional myosin in a BAC transgene. Science 1998; 280(5368):1444–1447.

126. Avraham KB, Hasson T, Steel KP, Kingsley DM, Russell LB, Mooseker MS, et al. The mouse *Snell's waltzer* deafness gene encodes an unconventional myosin required for structural integrity of inner ear hair cells. Nat Genet 1995; 11(4):369–375.

127. Self T, Mahony M, Fleming J, Walsh J, Brown SD, Steel KP. *Shaker-1* mutations reveal roles for myosin VIIA in both development and function of cochlear hair cells. Development 1998; 125(4):557–566.

128. Self T, Sobe T, Copeland NG, Jenkins NA, Avraham KB, Steel KP. Role of myosin VI in the differentiation of cochlear hair cells. Dev Biol 1999; 214(2):331–341.

129. Anderson DW, Probst FJ, Belyantseva IA, Fridell RA, Beyer L, Martin DM, et al. The motor and tail regions of myosin XV are critical for normal structure and function of auditory and vestibular hair cells. Hum Mol Genet 2000; 9(12):1729–1738.

130. Sherr CJ, Roberts JM. Inhibitors of mammalian G1 cyclin-dependent kinases. Genes Dev 1995; 9(10):1149–1163.

131. Sherr CJ, Roberts JM. CDK inhibitors: positive and negative regulators of G1-phase progression. Genes Dev 1999; 13(12):1501–1512.

132. Durand B, Gao FB, Raff M. Accumulation of the cyclin-dependent kinase inhibitor p27/Kip1 and the timing of oligodendrocyte differentiation. EMBO J 1997; 16(2):306–317.

133. Chen P, Segil N. p27^{Kip1} links cell proliferation to morphogenesis in the developing organ of Corti. Development 1999; 126(8):1581–1590.

134. Lowenheim H, Furness DN, Kil J, Zinn C, Gultig K, Fero ML, et al. Gene disruption of p27^{Kip1} allows cell proliferation in the postnatal and adult organ of Corti. Proc Natl Acad Sci USA 1999; 96(7):4084–4088.

135. Gu R, Griguer CE, Lynch ED, Kil J. p27 antisense oligonucleotides triggers supporting cell proliferation in the organ of Corti in vivo. Abstracts of XXXth ARO, St Petersburg 2001; 21490.

136. Pirvola U, Cao Y, Oellig C, Suoqiang Z, Pettersson RF, Ylikoski J. The site of action of neuronal acidic fibroblast growth factor is the organ of Corti of the rat cochlea. Proc Natl Acad Sci USA 1995; 92(20):9269–9273.

137. Malgrange B, Rogister B, Lefebvre PP, Mazy-Servais C, Welcher AA, Bonnet C, et al. Expression of growth factors and their receptors in the postnatal rat cochlea. Neurochem Res 1998; 23(8):1135–1140.

138. Pickles JO, Harter C, Rebillard G. Fibroblast growth factor receptor expression in outer hair cells of rat cochlea. NeuroReport 1998; 9(18):4093–4095.

139. Pirvola U, Spencer-Dene B, Xing-Qun L, Kettunen P, Thesleff I, Fritzsch B, et al. FGF/FGFR-2(IIIb) signaling is essential for inner ear morphogenesis. J Neurosci 2000; 20(16):6125–6134.

140. Pickles JO. The expression of fibroblast growth factors and their receptors in the embryonic and neonatal mouse inner ear. Hearing Res 2001; 155(1–2):54–62.

141. Zheng JL, Helbig C, Gao WQ. Induction of cell proliferation by fibroblast and insulin-like growth factors in pure rat inner ear epithelial cell cultures. J Neurosci 1997; 17(1):216–226.

142. Bermingham-McDonogh O, Stone JS, Reh TA, Rubel EW. FGFR3 Expression during development and regeneration of the chick inner ear sensory epithelia. Dev Biol 2001; 238(2):247–259.

143. Colvin JS, Bohne BA, Harding GW, McEwen DG, Ornitz DM. Skeletal overgrowth and deafness in mice lacking fibroblast growth factor receptor 3. Nat Genet 1996; 12(4):390–397.

144. Oesterle EC, Tsue TT, Rubel EW. Induction of cell proliferation in avian inner ear sensory epithelia by insulin-like growth factor-I and insulin. J Comp Neurol 1997; 380(2):262–274.

145. Lambert PR. Inner ear hair cell regeneration in a mammal: identification of a triggering factor. Laryngoscope 1994; 104(6 Pt 1):701–718.

146. Yamashita H, Oesterle EC. Induction of cell proliferation in mammalian inner-ear sensory epithelia by transforming growth factor alpha and epidermal growth factor. Proc Natl Acad Sci USA 1995; 92(8):3152–3155.

147. Kuntz AL, Oesterle EC. Transforming growth factor α with insulin stimulates cell proliferation in vivo in adult rat vestibular sensory epithelium. J Comp Neurol 1998; 399(3):413–423.

148. Staecker H, Lefebvre PP, Malgrange B, Moonen G, Van De Water TR. Regeneration of mammalian auditory hair cells. Science 1995; 267:707–711.

149. Navaratnam DS, Su HS, Scott SP, Oberholtzer JC. Proliferation in the auditory receptor epithelium mediated by a cyclic AMP-dependent signaling pathway. Nat Med 1996; 2(10):1136–1139.

150. Montcouquiol M, Corwin JT. Brief treatments with forskolin enhance S-phase entry in balance epithelia from the ears of rats. J Neurosci 2001; 21(3):974–982.

151. Montcouquiol M, Corwin JT. Intracellular signals that control cell proliferation in mammalian balance epithelia: key roles for phosphatidylinositol-3 kinase, mammalian target of rapamycin, and S6 kinases in preference to calcium, protein kinase C, and mitogen-activated protein kinase. J Neurosci 2001; 21(2):570–580.

152. Eddison M, Le R, I, Lewis J. Notch signaling in the development of the inner ear: lessons from *Drosophila*. Proc Natl Acad Sci USA 2000; 97(22):11692–11699.

153. Adam J, Myat A, Le R, I, Eddison M, Henrique D, Ish-Horowicz D, et al. Cell fate choices and the expression of *Notch, Delta* and *Serrate* homologues in the chick inner ear: parallels with *Drosophila* sense- organ development. Development 1998; 125(23):4645–4654.

154. Morrison A, Hodgetts C, Gossler A, Hrabe d, Lewis J. Expression of *Delta1* and *Serrate1* (*Jagged1*) in the mouse inner ear. Mech Dev 1999; 84(1–2):169–172.

155. Lewis AK, Frantz GD, Carpenter DA, de Sauvage FJ, Gao WQ. Distinct expression patterns of Notch family receptors and ligands during development of the mammalian inner ear. Mech Dev 1998; 78(1–2):159–163.

156. Zine A, Van De Water TR, de Ribaupierre F. Notch signaling regulates the pattern of auditory hair cell differentiation in mammals. Development 2000; 127(15):3373–3383.

157. Weir J, Rivolta MN, Holley MC. Notch signaling and the emergence of auditory hair cells. Arch Otolaryngol Head Neck Surg 2000; 126(10):1244–1248.

158. Lanford PJ, Shailam R, Norton CR, Gridley T, Kelley MW. Expression of *Math1* and *HES5* in the cochlea of wildtype and *Jag2* mutant mice. JARO 2000; 1(2):161–171.
159. Muller U, Littlewood E. Mechanisms that regulate mechanosensory hair cell differentiation. Trends Cell Biol 2001; 11(8):334–342
160. Leon Y, Vazquez E, Sanz C, Vega JA, Mato JM, Giraldez E, et al. Insulin-like growth factor-I regulates cell proliferation in the developing inner ear, activating glycosylphosphatidylinositol hydrolysis and Fos expression. Endocrinology 1995; 136(8):3494–3503.

29

Genetic Testing: Possibilities and Attitudes

Tim Hutchin
Children's Hospital, Birmingham, England

Karen Thompson and Robert Mueller
St. James's University Hospital, Leeds, England

I. INTRODUCTION

Hearing impairment is a common disorder in humans affecting individuals of all ages. For the 1 in 1000 children born with moderate to profound hearing impairment, particularly in families in which there is no previous history of deafness, the diagnosis has a major impact on that family. Concerns arise about communication with and the education of the child, as well as their development in a hearing world. Although hearing impairment later in life may not have such dramatic consequences it will nevertheless still have a major impact on that individual's life. Technologies such as cochlear implants and hearing aids are constantly improving, as are methods for communication, making it easier for deaf people to integrate into a hearing society. The last few years have also seen rapid advances in our understanding of the genetic causes of deafness in children. With these advances come prospects of improved genetic testing and counseling and ultimately the potential of therapies to prevent or cure deafness.

However, these advances also raise several issues that need consideration, not least so that this information can best benefit the public and, most notably, the ethical implications raised. Indeed many deaf persons view their deafness as a distinguishing characteristic and not as a handicap, impairment, or medical condition requiring treatment or a "cure," with many opposing cochlear implants or genetic testing (1,2). On the other hand, some 90–95% of deaf children are born to hearing parents who are likely to ask many questions such as "Why is my child deaf?" "Will his or her hearing get worse?" or "Will my other children be similarly affected?" (Table 1). Not surprisingly, then, most of these parents are in favor of genetic testing (3).

Only upon establishing the precise cause of a child's deafness can we begin to answer questions such as those above with any degree of certainty. At least half of all prelingual cases of deafness have a genetic etiology, with at least 80% being inherited in an autosomal recessive manner (4–7). Thus upon presentation of a case of isolated deafness within a family wanting recurrence risks for deafness, only genetic testing can confirm a genetic etiology. Without a confirmed cause one can only provide the family with an empirical or average recurrence risk, which is usually given as somewhere between 1 in 5 to 1 in 18 in such cases (8,9). With our rapidly increasing understanding of the genetic causes comes the prospect of providing many families with a precise genetic cause and hence accurate recurrence risks and perhaps more information on issues such as the severity or progression of deafness, carrier status, and perhaps even prenatal diagnosis.

Many genetic disorders are caused by mutations in a single gene, e.g., cystic fibrosis, Huntington's disease, and as such genetic counseling is largely straightforward. With perhaps as many as a hundred genes involved in deafness, however, genetic screening and counseling is a big challenge. Yet already research findings are having a positive impact, most notably the finding that mutations in a single gene, connexin 26 (*GJB2*), can account for up to 60% of prelingual nonsyndromic hearing impairment in some populations (10,11). Consequently the precise cause of a significant proportion of such cases can be determined with a relatively quick and simple diagnostic test. Unfortunately, the genetic heterogeneity of hearing impairment means that a single, simple genetic test for all affected individuals is not yet available. Despite the rapid pace of genetic studies caution needs to be taken to ensure expectations of the general public are not raised too high and that the ethical implications of this work are fully realized, not least those of the

Table 1   Reasons for Genetic Testing

Define diagnosis/cause
Provide recurrence risks
Alter medical management
Determine carrier status
Prenatal diagnosis
   Prepare for future, e.g., language and schooling needs
   Terminate pregnancy

Deaf community themselves many of whom are fearful of the impact of this work. Note that "Deaf" refers to individuals who are culturally deaf, viewing deafness from the cultural or sociological perspective where deafness is a condition to be understood and preserved.

II. TESTING FOR DEAFNESS

Prelingual hearing impairment has a dramatic effect on speech acquisition and consequently cognitive social development and education. The birth of a hearing-impaired child to hearing parents can often cause great concerns. With early identification and appropriate intervention before a child reaches 6 months language development can often be normal, while late diagnosis can have a devastating effect on language acquisition, communications development, confidence, and social skills (12–14).

Depending upon where a child is born his or her chances of being detected at such an early age can vary. In England it is estimated than around 50% of the 840 children born each year with a permanent hearing impairment will not be identified until they are 18 months old, with 25% still left undiagnosed at 3 years old (15). Steps to introduce universal neonatal hearing screening, a noninvasive test measuring otoacoustic emissions, will hopefully lead to early detection in a much higher proportion of newborns (16).

In addition to the 1 in 1000 children with a prelingual hearing impairment a similar number will develop a hearing impairment before their teens (17). Although language will have been acquired by this age a prompt diagnosis is still essential to ensure the child's continued educational and social development.

The most common form of hearing impairment is that affecting adults. Approximately half of all adults over the age of 65 have a significant hearing impairment, which we tend to accept as part of getting old (18). The causes of this age-related hearing loss are less well understood and are likely to be much more complicated than childhood hearing loss. Nevertheless age-related hearing impairment has a significant social impact and it seems likely that much of what we learn from studying childhood-onset deafness will help us to develop therapies to slow down or prevent age-related hearing loss. Since certain genetic backgrounds may make persons more sensitive to environmental factors such as noise, the issue of predictive testing for adult-onset deafness also exists. In fact it is already known that individuals with a particular mutation of the mitochondrial DNA (A1555G) will suffer a permanent hearing loss shortly after taking aminoglycoside antibiotics (19).

Although genetic testing has the potential to detect children or adults who will become or are at risk of becoming deaf it seems highly unlikely, particularly given the costs, that genetic testing will be used to screen all newborns for deafness genes. At present, genetic testing will be of most value in establishing the precise cause of deafness in an individual who is deaf, which will help him and his family answer many questions they might have.

III. DEAFNESS GENES

Just a cursory glance of the contents of this book shows the remarkable progress that has been made in the last 5 years in establishing the genetic causes of hearing impairment. More than 90 loci for nonsyndromic hearing impairment have been identified; 51 autosomal dominant, 39 autosomal recessive, and six X-linked. To date more than 20 of these genes have been identified. In addition, more than 30 genes causing syndromic forms of deafness have also been characterized (7,20). As we isolate more genes and study their effects more closely the complex nature of these deafness genes becomes apparent. Mutations in the same gene can cause both syndromic and nonsyndromic deafness (e.g., *MYO7A* can cause Usher syndrome type 1b or NSSHI), others can cause both dominant and recessive forms (e.g., both *DFNA8/12* and *DFNB21* are caused by mutations in the *TECTA* gene), while the effects of others may be modified by other genes (e.g., *DFNM1* protects against *DFNB26*). Such findings are fascinating for the scientist researching these genes, posing many more questions, but also highlight the difficulties sometimes facing the genetic counselor when dealing with a family with deafness.

IV. ESTABLISHING THE GENETIC CAUSE

With perhaps as many as 100 different genes involved in hearing impairment where does one start? Clearly screening all of these genes is not practical so steps must be taken to narrow down the number of potential genes as much as possible. Three key steps in this process are: clinical diagnosis, pattern of inheritance, and appropriate genetic testing. These are not mutually exclusive as the identification of the genetic cause may help establish the precise nature of a syndromic form of deafness for example.

An accurate clinical diagnosis is important not only for the individual's health but also in directing the appropriate genetic testing. Approximately 70% of genetic hearing impairment is nonsyndromic whilst the remaining 30% is syndromic of which many hundreds of syndromes have been described (9). Identifying a syndromic deafness significantly reduces the number of genes to screen, to perhaps half a dozen or fewer.

In the absence of any family history establishing the precise clinical phenotype can be difficult, particularly where some features may not manifest themselves until later in life. For example in Usher syndrome type 1, retinitis pigmentosa does not normally develop until the end of the first decade or shortly thereafter. Appropriate genetic testing, however, could lead to an early diagnosis of a syndromic form before many clinical features manifest themselves, allowing extremely early treatment of such conditions. Conversely, genetic testing may be able to exclude the possibility of such conditions developing in a deaf child, thus allaying any fears the parents may have.

The presence of other affected family members will of course help establish a diagnosis and can help determine the pattern of inheritance of the genetic defect, directing genetic testing. In large enough families linkage analysis can be used, at the very least to exclude certain loci. Deafness in more than one generation may imply an autosomal dominant gene while the absence of any family history suggests the trait is most likely autosomal recessive, especially if consanguinity is present, but one cannot rule out the possibility of a new, spontaneous mutation.

In determining the pattern of inheritance one needs to beware of possible confounding factors such as reduced penetrance or the presence of modifier genes. Quite often other family members may not be available for examination and thus a verbal account of a distant relative being deaf needs to be taken with caution, especially in cases of late, adult-onset hearing impairment. Likewise environmental causes, such as meningitis, ototoxic drugs, or infection mother had in pregnancy, must also be excluded as the presence of a phenocopy may give the impression of an incorrect pattern of inheritance.

Having established whether the deafness is syndromic or nonsyndromic, its pattern of inheritance, and any other information, one now has a much better idea of which gene(s) is likely the cause. For example *Cx26* is likely in a child with prelingual, severe, recessive deafness whereas a child with postlingual, low-frequency hearing loss inherited in a dominant manner is much more likely to have a mutation in the *WFS1* gene. In fact, autosomal dominant deafness appears to be more varied than autosomal recessive deafness; i.e., some forms are prelingual though most are postlingual, some affect high frequencies while others affect low frequencies. Consequently in dominant families it is possible to narrow down, somewhat, the number of candidate genes based on the clinical phenotype. Unfortunately this does not appear to be the case for the recessive genes, and as such, determining a genetic cause is probably most challenging for nonsyndromic deafness.

At present screening of only a handful of deafness genes is carried out by DNA diagnostic laboratories on a routine service basis. Most mutation detection is only done on a research basis but it is likely that as more genes are identified and mutations within these genes are characterized more of this work will be moved to a service-based setting. Which genes are screened and which are not will depend primarily on how common a cause each is of deafness. Thus routine screening for the *Cx26* gene is now common and is offered by DNA laboratories all over the world.

Strategies for screening genes will also need to be developed with the primary aim being to identify the genetic mutation in as many cases as possible. Thus routine screening of *Cx26* usually takes account of the fact that a deletion of a single guanine in a stretch of six G's (35delG) accounts for 70–80% of *DFNB1* cases in many Caucasian populations (10,11,21). However, the *35delG* mutation appears to be almost absent in some parts of the world, e.g., Asia and Africa (22,23). In Japan the *235delC* mutation is much more common, being present in 1–2% of cases (22,23), while the *167delT* is present in 4% of Ashkenazi Jews (24). Specific screening strategies will therefore have to be developed for each country or population.

Cx26 has a single coding exon and as such is simple to screen. However, many of the other genes causing deafness are considerably larger, several having 50 or more exons. In these cases the best way of screening is to follow the example of the cystic fibrosis (CF) gene. The CF gene has 27 exons but from numerous studies it has become apparent that certain mutations are much more common than others. Consequently screening the CF gene now involves using a kit to detect the 10 or so most common mutations within that population. Such a strategy will be most appropriate for many of the deafness genes, though at present such data are available on very few of these gene to allow us to build up such a mutation profile of each gene. One example is the PDS gene where, from several surveys, it appears that mutations in certain exons are more common than in others; e.g., in Caucasians about 60% of PDS mutations lie in exons 6, 8, and 10 (25). Thus a strategy for screening the PDS gene would begin with these exons, though again, population differences are likely to exist.

Ultimately any diagnostic service offered will of course be largely limited by costs. Screening a very large gene that perhaps accounts for less than 1% of cases is unlikely to be offered on a routine basis. As technology advances so will the capability to screen for increasing numbers of mutations. The costs of such a service will also have to be balanced against the benefits to the individual. At present, apart from providing accurate genetic counseling, the identification of the defective gene in nonsyndromic deafness offers little direct health benefits to that individual. However, this may change as therapies are developed and genetic testing is already beneficial in determining whether or not the deafness is syndromic.

V.   POTENTIAL PITFALLS AND PROBLEMS

Given that we have not yet identified all of the genes involved in deafness, it is clear that the genetic cause in many cases cannot yet be established. Even where the gene has been identified there are still some instances in which it may be difficult to interpret with any certainty the effect of a particular mutation that is found (Table 2). In some cases these may even raise more problems than they solve, making genetic counseling difficult.

The first question asked upon finding a new mutation within a gene is what effect does that mutation have on the gene product? In the case of nonsense or frameshift mutations it is apparent that a truncated gene product is unlikely to function normally. Further studies to assess the mutation frequency in the general population and deaf persons will help determine whether a mutation is indeed pathogenic or merely a polymorphism. Missense mutations or those that might perturb a splice site are more difficult to interpret. Proving that a particular mutation causes deafness can sometimes be very difficult.

Learning more about the gene product helps us understand which nucleotides and amino acids are most important and likely to be pathogenic if altered. Animal models provide an excellent way of studying the role of specific genes in hearing, though species differences can prove problematic. The most notable example is that of *Cx26* where the knockout is embryonic lethal in mice owing to differences between the human and mouse placenta (26). Similarly, functional and mRNA splicing studies, which are usually beyond the scope of diagnostic laboratories, do not always extrapolate to humans. One excellent example of this is also provided by mutations in the *Cx26* gene. Using in vitro expression systems such as *Xenopus* oocytes, the *M34T* mutation has been shown to cause impaired intercellular coupling and abnormalities of trafficking and targeting of *Cx26* (27,28). Although this work suggests the *M34T* mutation is dominant, clinical data in humans suggest it is recessive or even just a benign polymorphism (29–31). Thus the status of this mutation remains uncertain and providing counseling for families with such mutations is difficult as the genetic cause has not been determined for certain.

Although screening *Cx26* can establish the genetic cause of perhaps 50% of autosomal recessive cases, the high carrier frequency of *Cx26* muta-

Table 2 Potential Difficulties in Establishing a Genetic Cause

No family history
Genetic heterogeneity—which gene to look at?
Is the mutation pathogenic? (e.g., missense)
Only 1 recessive mutation found
Animal/functional studies may not extrapolate to humans
Does the mutation cause syndromic or nonsyndromic deafness?
Reduced penetrance of some mutations
Mutation does not predict severity/age of onset
Ethical considerations

tions [1 in 31 in Spain and Italy (20)] can also cause problems. Many deaf persons will be incidental carriers of *Cx26* mutations, a separate gene being the cause of their deafness. Yet it would be unwise to dismiss the presence of a single recessive mutation in the *Cx26* gene in a deaf child. A recent study has shown that a large deletion just upstream of the *Cx26* gene, acting in trans with a mutation in the other copy of the *Cx26* gene, or in the homozygous state, leads to deafness, possibly through disrupting the regulatory region of the *Cx26* gene (32).

Such a scenario highlights how the absence of a mutation in a gene must be treated with caution and not taken as absolute and demonstrates how genetic testing needs to be continually updated as further findings come to light. In fact, the vast majority of deafness-causing mutations reported to date have been in the gene transcript. Yet the possibility remains that mutations in regulatory regions of these genes also exist that contribute to deafness. For instance, mutations in the PDS gene are thought to account for as much as 10% of childhood deafness (9) and as such the carrier frequency of mutations within the PDS gene may be relatively high. There are several reports of deaf individuals with inner ear defects and mapping to *DFNB4* in whom only a single mutation in the coding region of the PDS gene has been found (25). As the regulatory regions of the PDS gene have not been characterized it is not possible to determine for certain whether the PDS gene is the cause of these individuals' deafness.

Although identification of a genetic mutation can confirm a genetic cause there is often no clear genotype-phenotype correlation. For example, even siblings homozygous for *Cx26 35delG* may display variation in age of onset and severity of hearing impairment. This is even more extreme where mutations in a single gene can lead to both syndromic and nonsyndromic forms of deafness, e.g., *COL11A2*-Stickler syndrome or *DFNA13*; *MYO7A*-Ush1b or *DFNB2*; PDS- Pendred syndrome or *DFNB4*; WFS1- Wolfram syndrome or *DFNA6/14* (7). In some instances the identification of a mutation in the relevant gene can confirm a diagnosis of a syndromic form. On the other hand, the identification of a mutation in, for example, the *MYO7A* or *CDH23* genes in a child with prelingual hearing loss raises the possibility that that child may develop ocular problems later in life as part of Usher syndrome. Since we do not yet understand how mutations in these genes lead to Usher syndrome as opposed to nonsyndromic deafness, advising the family can be extremely difficult. While one does not unnecessarily wish to cause parents concern they are likely to want know as early as possible if their child has Usher syndrome so that they can prepare for the future of that child. Of course, the identification of mutations in another gene, such as *Cx26*, can exclude the possibility of syndromic deafness and help reassure the parents.

Many more genes remain to be identified and mutations within these genes detected and characterized. It will be important to determine the prevalence and penetrance of the various mutations and also to gather phenotypic information such as the degree of hearing loss, its age of onset, and rate of progression. Only then can we determine what effect a mutation in a particular gene will have on an individual's hearing.

VI. GENETIC TESTING AND THE PUBLIC

Despite the above difficulties it seems likely that diagnostic, carrier, and perhaps prenatal diagnosis (PND) for deafness will become part of clinical practice. With increasing public awareness of genetics there is likely to be more call for genetic testing but with this are likely to come misconceptions, false expectations, and perhaps fears about what can be achieved. Thus it is important that any genetic testing is backed up with appropriate genetic counseling for all who want it and that the issues are fully explained, particularly in the case of PND. However, even if a simple gene test for deafness became available, one cannot assume that this would be viewed as good news by everyone as attitudes toward genetic testing differ between individuals and groups of individuals.

When hearing parents have a deaf child they may find this more difficult to cope with than would deaf parents, perhaps perceiving deafness as a handicap. Parents may feel shock, guilt, or grief and be concerned about how they will communicate with their child and how that child will cope in a predominantly hearing world. Knowing little or nothing of deafness and its causes, the parents are likely to arrive at incorrect conclusions. Identifying the precise cause can help alleviate such misconceptions.

The majority of people who want such a test for themselves or their child do so for similar reasons: to try and understand why a certain disease is affecting them, what the risk might be to their family or any future children, and to help with future medical management (Table 1). Genetic testing for a monogenic disorder such as cystic fibrosis (CF) can be more easily explained than for a disorder such as deafness, for which the cause may not be so clear-cut. Genetic testing for CF is well established and as there is some correlation between the genotype and phenotype, genetic testing can be used to predict the progression and type of CF in the individual. With this information parents can make an informed, albeit difficult, choice about having further children.

As discussed above, genetic testing for deafness is complex given the many genetic and environmental factors involved and as yet no simple gene test is available. Genetic testing for deafness can be described as specific but not sensitive (33) as a negative test result may rule out mutations in a specific gene but since the cause could be a mutation in a different gene it does not rule out genetic factors completely. Prior to genetic testing parents therefore need to be made fully aware of the possible consequences and that, at present, in many cases the genetic cause will not be found.

To provide effective genetic testing and counseling for deafness the needs and views of individuals need to be considered. Although a number of surveys have shown that many people would welcome genetic testing for deafness they have also shown that people often have misconceptions, with many, mostly those who are deaf themselves, opposing genetic testing (2,3,34,35).

Brunger et al. (3) found that 96% of hearing parents, with one or more deaf children, had a positive attitude toward genetic testing for deafness. The most common reason given for having a genetic test was to identify the cause of deafness. Other reasons were to help the affected child's medical management in the future and to determine a recurrence risk. Most people surveyed said they would be interested in having such testing themselves. Some parents said their decision to have other children might be affected by genetic test results but none said they would choose to terminate pregnancy.

However, a significant proportion of parents wanting testing for their children felt there was no need for testing themselves or their other children as they were not deaf (3). Some parents even disapproved of testing, one being "opposed to eugenics." Such apprehension and fears are consistent with other studies of public attitude toward testing for other diseases (36,37) and illustrate the variance in attitude toward genetic testing.

Such views are much more common among culturally Deaf people who have predominantly negative attitudes toward genetic testing, 55% of Deaf individuals feeling it would do more harm than good, 46% feeling it devalues deaf people, and 21% being "horrified" at the prospects of genetic testing (2). Such fears of the Deaf are deep rooted as, all too often throughout history, eugenics programs have included deafness as a condition to be removed from society (9,38). Whereas many hearing parents may view their deaf child as being disabled, people in the Deaf community do not view themselves as being disabled and often would prefer to have deaf children. They want to protect their Deaf culture and many see genetics as another way for the medical community to eradicate deafness (3).

Some deaf persons refuse genetic counseling for fear of being told not to have children (39). That results of genetic testing may deter some hearing parents from having further children is also a major concern to the Deaf community who feel this could lead to a reduction in the number of deaf children (2). Many deaf couples' preference for deaf children and opposition to genetic testing is perhaps warranted as such testing is likely to confirm that most with recessive deafness will have hearing children, unless they have mutations in the same gene. Thus while the majority of people welcome genetic testing for deafness, the views of the Deaf community need to be respected and taken into account.

With genetic testing also comes the possibility of PND. Most hearing parents feel that prenatal testing for deafness should be offered (3), primarily to allow parents to prepare, e.g., learn sign language themselves and look for schooling needs. Only 21% of deaf persons approved of PND, with 8% of these preferring deaf children and 2% saying they would consider aborting a hearing fetus (35). Conversely, 6% of deaf and 16% of hearing persons with a deaf child or parent would consider a termination of pregnancy if the fetus were deaf. However, the majority of deaf individuals do not mind if their child is deaf or not (2,35). The decision to perform prenatal diagnosis for a nonlethal condition such as deafness relies largely upon the discretion of the clinician involved. In an international study looking at attitudes toward PND it was found that 35% of British and 9% of American genetic professionals would perform PND for a deaf couple wanting to have deaf children (40). That there is no obvious consensus of opinion on this matter highlights the need for discussion on such issues.

With the results of genetic testing known, whether positive or negative, comes the need to convey their meaning to the family. Somewhat worryingly, it has been found that parents who have received genetic counseling still have no better understanding of the genetics of deafness than those who have not had counseling (3,34). Parents frequently had little idea of the relative risk they had been given and almost none knew the chance for their deaf child of having deaf children. One third of those who received negative *Cx26* testing, i.e., normal, felt their child "does not have the deafness gene," while many of those where *Cx26* was the cause became more fearful after the result and so may be less likely to have further children (3). Such misunderstandings are not surprising given the complexities of the genetics of deafness and with the parents already concerned about their child they are likely to be overwhelmed with the information given to them. Establishing a program of both pre- and posttest counseling will be important to enable parents and patients to fully understand the meaning and implications of any test result and thus make informed decisions about what is best for them and/or their child.

The role of the genetic counselor and clinical geneticists involved with a family is of course central to this process. Robin et al. (41) also found that although most pediatric otolaryngologists have a good understanding of genetics, many gave incorrect recurrence risks in some examples. Given the heterogeneity of deafness and the rapid advances being made, it is not surprising that otolaryngologists and genetic counselors will need to keep abreast of the genetic studies of deafness.

VII. FUTURE PROSPECTS

The potential for identification of the genetic defect in inherited deafness is now becoming a reality. It will enable families and individuals to be advised appropriately about the chance for other individuals in that family to be affected and what the future will hold for them. In the longer term, there is the possibility of potential preventive and/or therapeutic interventions for individuals and families with or at risk for hearing impairment due to genetic and acquired causes, with the prospect of maintaining the status of their hearing.

There have already been significant health gains arising from research in clinical and molecular studies in inherited hearing impairment, most notably the development of routine diagnostic genetic testing for mutations in connexin 26 in children presenting with congenital/early-childhood nonsyndromal sensorineural hearing impairment. This means that a significant proportion of families presenting with a child sporadically affected with nonsyndromic deafness can be provided with definitive recurrence risks.

As our understanding of genetics advances, issues such as PND, designer babies, and cloning may become more of a reality. Society therefore has to address complicated and emotional issues sensitive to both hearing and deaf people. Surveys have shown that the overwhelming majority of parents with deaf children want genetic counseling and appropriate genetic testing but have a poor understanding of the issues. Prior to clinical implementation of genetic testing, several issues must be addressed to assess the utility of such tests. Many unresolved issues remain regarding the prevalence and penetrance of mutations in various populations, the clinical significance of these mutations, and the short- and long-term impact of such testing and counseling on individuals and their families. With these in mind the continued advances in genetics will begin to yield significant benefits to deaf individuals and their families. Finally, it is recognized that there are unique challenges pertaining to genetic testing for deafness and hearing impairment because these conditions are not universally considered to be disabling or undesirable.

REFERENCES

1. Gibson WPR. Opposition from deaf groups to the cochlear implant. Med J Aust 1991; 155:212–214.
2. Middleton A, Hewison J, Mueller RF. Attitudes of deaf adults toward genetic testing for hereditary deafness. Am J Hum Genet 1998; 63:1175–1180.

3. Brunger JW, Murray GS, O'Riordan M, Matthews AL, Smith RJH, Robin N. Parental attitudes toward genetic testing for pediatric deafness. Am J Hum Genet 2000; 67:1621–1625.

4. Fraser GRThe Causes of Profound Deafness in Childhood. Baltimore: Johns Hopkins University Press, 1976.

5. Parving A. Epidemiology of hearing loss and aetiological diagnosis of hearing impairment in childhood. Int J Ped Otorhinolaryngol 1983; 5:151–165.

6. Newton V. Aetiology of bilateral sensorineural hearing loss in young children. J Laryngol Otol 1985; 10(suppl):1–57.

7. van Camp G, Smith RJH. Hereditary hearing loss home page. World Wide Web URL: http://dnalab-www.uia.ac.be/dnalab/hhh/.

8. Koehn D, Morgan K, Fraser FC. Recurrence risks for near relatives of children with sensorineural deafness. Genet Couns 1990; 1:127–132.

9. Gorlin RJ, Toriello JV, Cohen MM. Hereditary Hearing Loss and Its Syndromes. New York: Oxford University Press, 1995.

10. Denoyelle F, Weil D, Maw MA, Wilcox SA, Lench NJ, Allen-Powell DR, Osborn AH, Dahl H-HM, Middleton A, Houseman MJ, Dode C, Marlin S, Boulila-ElGaied A, Grati M, Ayadi H, BenArab S, Bitoun P, Lina-Granade G, Godet J, Mustapha M, Loiselet J, El-Zir E, Aubois A, Joannard A, Petit C. Prelingual deafness: high prevalence of a *30delG* mutation in the connexin 26 gene. Hum Mol Genet 1997; 6:2173–2177.

11. Zelante L, Gasparini P, Estivill X, Melchionda S, D'Agruma L, Govea N, Mila M, Della Monica M, Lutfi J, Shohat M, Mansfield E, Delgrosso K, Rappaport E, Surrey S, Fortina P. Connexin26 mutations associated with the most common form of non-syndromic neurosensory autosomal recessive deafness (*DFNB1*) in Mediterraneans. Hum Mol Genet 1997; 6:1605–1609.

12. Downs PM, Yoshinaga-Itano C. The efficacy of early identification and intervention for children with hearing impairment. Pediatr Clin North Am 1999; 46:79–87.

13. Moeller MP. Early intervention and language development in children who are deaf and hard of hearing. Pediatrics 2000; 106:E43.

14. Yoshinaga-Itano C, Coulter D, Thomson V. The Colorado newborn hearing screening project: effects on speech and language development for children with hearing loss. J Perinatol 2000; 20:S132–137.

15. http://www.rnid.org.uk/index.htm.

16. Department of Health. Piloting the introduction of universal neonatal hearing screening in England. www.doh.gov.uk/uhnspilots/index.htm.

17. Fortnum HM, Summerfield AQ, Marshall DH, Davis AC, Bamford JM. Prevalance of permanent childhood hearing impairment in the United Kingdom and implications for universal neonatal hearing screening: questionnaire based ascertainment study. Br Med J 2001; 323:1–6.

18. Morton NE. Genetic epidemiology of hearing impairment. In: Genetics of Hearing Impairment. NY Acad Sci 1991; 630:16–31.

19. Hutchin TP. Sensorineural hearing loss and the 1555G mitochondrial DNA mutation. Acta Otolaryngol (Stockh) 1999; 118:48–52.

20. Resendes BL, Williamson RE, Morton CC. At the speed of sound: gene discovery in the auditory system. Am J Hum Genet 2001; 69:923–935.

21. Estivill X, Fortina P, Surrey S, Rabionet R, Melchionda S, D'Agruma L, Mansfield E, Rappaport E, Govea N, Mila M, Zelante L, Gasparini P. Connexin-26 mutations in sporadic and inherited sensorineural deafness. Lancet 1998; 351:394–398.

22. Abe S, Usami S, Shinkawa H, Kelley PM, Kimberling WJ. Prevalent connexin 26 gene (GJB2) mutations in Japanese. J Med Genet 2000; 37:41–43.

23. Kudo T, Ikeda K, Kure S, Matsubara Y, Oshima T, Watanabe K, Kawase T, Narisawa K, Takasaka T. Novel mutations in the connexin 26 gene (*GJB2*) responsible for childhood deafness in Japanese. Am J Med Genet 2000; 90:141–145.

24. Morell RJ, Kim HJ, Hood LJ, Goforth L, Friderici K, Fisher R, Van Camp G, Berlin CI, Oddoux C, Ostrer H, Keats B, Friedman TB. Mutations in the connexin 26 gene (*GJB2*) among Ashkenazi Jews with nonsyndromic recessive deafness. N Engl J Med 1998; 339:1500–1505.

25. Campbell C, Cucci RA, Prasad S, Green GE, Edeal JB, Galer CE, Karniski LP, Sheffield VC, Smith RJ. Pendred syndrome, *DFNB4*, and PDS/SLC26A4 identification of eight novel mutations and possible genotype-phenotype correlations. Hum Mutat 2001; 17:403–411.

26. Gabriel HD, Jung D, Butzler C, Temme A, Traub O, Winterhager E, Willecke K. Transplacental uptake of glucose is decreased in embryonic lethal connexin26-deficient mice. J Cell Biol 1998; 140:1453–1461.

27. White TW, Deans MR, Kelsell DP, Paul DL. Connexin mutations in deafness. Nature 1998; 394:630–631.

28. Martin PE, Coleman S, Casalotti SO, Forge A, Evans WH. Properties of connexin 26 gap junctional proteins derived from mutations associated with non-syndromal hereditary deafness. Hum Mol Genet 1999; 13:2369–2376.

29. Griffith AJ, Chowdhry AA, Kurima K, Hood LJ, Keats B, Berlin CI, Morell RJ, Friedman TB. Autosomal recessive nonsyndromic neurosensory deafness at *DFNB1* not associated with the compound-heterozygous *GJB2* (connexin 26) genotype *M34T/167delT*. Am J Hum Genet 2000; 67:745–749.

30. Houseman MJ, Ellis LA, Pagnamenta A, Di WL, Rickard S, Osborn AH, Dahl HH, Taylor GR, Bitner-Glindzicz M, Reardon W, Mueller RF, Kelsell DP. Genetic analysis of the connexin-26 *M34T* variant: identification of genotype *M34T/M34T* segregating with mild-moderate non-syndromic sensorineural hearing loss. J Med Genet 2001; 38:20–25.

31. Marlin S, Garabedian E-N, Roger G, Moatti L, Matha N, Lewin P, Petit C, Denoyelle F. Connexin 26 gene mutations in congenitally deaf children: pitfalls for genetic counselling. Arch Otolaryngol Head Neck Surg 2001; 127:927–933.

32. Lerer I, Sagi M, Ben-Neriah Z, Wang T, Levi H, Abeliovich D. A deletion mutation in *GJB6* cooperating with a *GJB2* mutation in trans in non-syndromic deafness: a novel founder mutation in Ashkenazi Jews. Hum Mutat 2001; 18:460.

33. Brunger JW, Matthew AL, Smith RH, Robin NH. Genetic testing and genetic counselling for deafness: the future is here. Laryngoscope 2001; 111:715–718.
34. Parker MJ, Fortnum HM, Young ID, Davis AC. Genetics and deafness: what do families want? J Med Genet 2000; 37:e26.
35. Middleton A, Hewison J, Mueller RF. Prenatal diagnosis for inherited deafness—what is the potential demand? J Genet Couns 2001; 10:121–131.
36. Chapple A, May C, Campion P. Lay understanding of genetic disease: a British study of families attending a genetic counseling service. J Genet Couns 1995; 4:281–300.
37. Hietala M, Hakonen A, Aro AR, Niemela P, Peltonen L, Aula P. Attitudes toward genetic testing among the general population and relatives of patients with a severe genetic disease: a survey from Finland. Am J Hum Genet 56: 1493–1500.
38. Bahan B. What if . . . Alexander Graham Bell had gotten his way? In: Wilcox S, ed. American Deaf Culture. Silver Spring, MD: Linstock Press, 1989; 83–87.
39. Israel J. An Introduction to Deafness: A Manual for Genetic Counselors. Washington, DC: Gallaudet University and National Society of Genetic Counselors Special Projects Fund, 1995.
40. Wertz D. Ethics and genetics: in global perspective. Unpublished document. 1999.
41. Robin N, Dietz C, Arnold J, Smith RJH. Pediatric otolaryngologists' knowledge and understanding of genetic testing for deafness. Arch Otolaryngol Head Neck Surg 2001; 127:937–940.

Index